W0043622

NEUROPOISONS
THEIR PATHOPHYSIOLOGICAL ACTIONS

Volume 1 – Poisons of Animal Origin

CONTRIBUTORS

Edward Barry Adams — *Department of Medicine, University of Natal, Congella, Durban, South Africa.*

Eleanor Condrea — *Department of Biochemistry, Tel-Aviv University Medical School, and Rogoff-Wellcome Medical Research Institute, Beilinson Hospital, Petah Tikva, Israel.*

D. R. Curtis — *Department of Physiology, Australian National University, Canberra, Australia.*

Wolf-Dietrich Dettbarn — *Department of Pharmacology, Vanderbilt University School of Medicine, Nashville, Tennessee, U.S.A.*

André de Vries — *Department of Medicine, Tel-Aviv University Medical School, and Rogoff-Wellcome Medical Research Institute, Beilinson Hospital, Petah Tikva, Israel.*

Daniel B. Drachman — *Department of Neurology, The Johns Hopkins University School of Medicine and Hospital, Baltimore, Maryland, U.S.A.*

Peter W. Gage — *School of Physiology, University of New South Wales, Kensington, New South Wales, Australia.*

M. Glenn Koenig — *Department of Medicine, Vanderbilt University School of Medicine, Nashville, Tennessee, U.S.A.*

C. Y. Lee — *Pharmacological Institute, College of Medicine, National Taiwan University, Taipei, Taiwan, China.*

Yasumi Ogura — *Department of Pharmacology, Faculty of Dentistry, Tohoku University, Sendai, Japan.*

Philip Rosenberg — *Division of Pharmacology, School of Pharmacy and Pharmacy Research Institute, The University of Connecticut, Storrs, Connecticut, U.S.A.*

Edward J. Schantz — *Biological Science Laboratories, Fort Detrick, Frederick, Maryland, U.S.A.*

Michael F. Sheff — *Ayer Laboratory, Pennsylvania Hospital, Philadelphia, Pennsylvania, U.S.A.*

Lance L. Simpson — *Laboratory of Chemical Biodynamics, University of California, Berkeley, California, and Division of Neuroscience, New York State Psychiatric Institute, New York, New York, U.S.A.*

Anthony T. Tu — *Department of Biochemistry, Colorado State University, Fort Collins, Colorado, U.S.A.*

James A. Vick — *Department of Pharmacology, Walter Reed Army Institute of Research, Walter Reed Army Medical Center, Washington, D.C., U.S.A.*

Sumner I. Zacks — *Department of Pathology, University of Pennsylvania School of Medicine, and Ayer Laboratory, Pennsylvania Hospital, Philadelphia, Pennsylvania, U.S.A.*

NEUROPOISONS
THEIR PATHOPHYSIOLOGICAL ACTIONS

Volume 1– Poisons of Animal Origin

Edited by Lance L. Simpson

Laboratory of Chemical Biodynamics
University of California
Berkeley, California
and
Division of Neuroscience
New York State Psychiatric Institute
New York, New York

℗ PLENUM PRESS · NEW YORK-LONDON · 1971

Library of Congress Catalog Card Number 76-128511

ISBN-13: 978-1-4684-2942-8   e-ISBN-13: 978-1-4684-2940-4
DOI: 10.1007/978-1-4684-2940-4

© 1971 Plenum Press, New York
Softcover reprint of the hardcover 1st edition 1971
A Division of Plenum Publishing Corporation
227 West 17th Street, New York, N.Y. 10011

United Kingdom edition published by Plenum Press, London
A Division of Plenum Publishing Company, Ltd.
Donington House, 30 Norfolk Street, London W.C. 2, England

All rights reserved

No part of this publication may be reproduced in any form
without written permission from the publisher

Preface

Poisons are topics of multidisciplinary concern. The clinician and the pathologist are sensitive to instances of human poisoning. The laboratory researcher, whether pharmacologist, physiologist, or biochemist, is oriented toward molecular modes of poison action. Both clinician and researcher are eager to learn of poisons that can be used as therapeutic agents or methodological tools.

This volume is an attempt to underscore the multidisciplinary character of neuropoisons. Six poisons of animal origin which are receiving considerable clinical and research attention are discussed. Each poison is presented first as a clinical entity, then as a topic of investigative research, and finally as an agent useful to the study of nerve function.

Because no single volume on neuropoisons can be exhaustive, an attempt at balance is offered as compensation. Two snake venoms, two marine poisons, and two bacterial toxins are presented in detail. In the sequel to this volume, attention will be focused on representative neuropoisons of plant origin.

Lance L. Simpson

New York City
September, 1970

v

Contents

Chapter 3
Symptomatology of Experimental and Clinical Crotalid Envenomation ... 71
by James A. Vick

Chapter 4
The Mechanism of Snake Venom Actions—Rattlesnakes and Other Crotalids 87
by Anthony T. Tu

Chapter 5
The Use of Snake Venoms as Pharmacological Tools in Studying Nerve Activity 111
by Philip Rosenberg

Chapter 11
Biochemical and Physiological Aspects of Tetanus Intoxication..............225
by Sumner I. Zacks and Michael F. Sheff

Chapter 12
Tetanus Toxin as a Neuropharmacological Tool...............................263
by D. R. Curtis

Chapter 13
The Clinical Aspects of Botulism...283
by M. Glenn Koenig

Chapter 14
The Neuroparalytic and Hemagglutinating Activities of Botulinum Toxin...303
by Lance L. Simpson

Chapter 15
Botulinum Toxin as a Tool for Research on the Nervous System...............325
by Daniel B. Drachman

Chapter 1

Clinical Aspects of Elapid Bite

André de Vries and Eleanor Condrea

Departments of Medicine and Biochemistry
Tel-Aviv University Medical School; and
Rogoff-Wellcome Medical Research Institute
Beilinson Hospital, Petah Tikva, Israel

I. INTRODUCTION

Although the elapid family comprises numerous species, the rationale of dealing with the clinical aspects of their bites jointly is their having in common neurotoxic symptomatology as the preponderant feature. In this characteristic they differ from the Viperidae and the Crotalidae whose bites mainly produce blood clotting disturbances, hemorrhage, and necrosis. Indeed, the clinical picture following snake bite often may serve indirectly to identify the responsible snake and determine treatment accordingly. On the other hand, these clinical disturbances are not absolute since necrosis may be produced by elapid bite, as for instance in the case of the Malayan cobra (Reid, 1964). Therefore, knowledge of both the species locally prevalent and the characteristic symptoms produced by their bite is imperative.

II. ELAPIDAE

A. Classification

The Elapidae are a family belonging to the group of Proteroglypha, of which all are poisonous although not all are dangerous to man. Their two fangs, placed in the front part of the upper jaw, have an inner tubular duct which evolved by the closing of a groove still visible on the anterior face of

1

the fang. The venom, stored in the reservoir of the venom gland, is pressed during the bite by the jaw muscles through a duct into the basal lumen of the fang. Thus, the venom is injected into the victim's tissue under pressure. Continuous replacement keeps the fangs sharp. The Elapidae are characterized by fixed fangs, except for the snakes belonging to the genus *Dendroaspis* (mambas) whose fangs, similar to those of the Viperidae, move forward when biting (Phisalix, 1940).

B.   Geographic Distribution

The 41 genera and numerous species of the elapid family are found all over the world with the exception of Europe (Klemmer, 1963; Rosenfeld, 1963). As listed by Rosenfeld (1963) there are two genera in south Africa, one in Central America, two in North America, seven in Asia, ten in Africa, sixteen in the East Indies, and sixteen in Australia. The genus *Micrurus* (coral snake) is found only on the American continent; *Dendroaspis* (mamba) and *Hemachatus* (ringhals) are specific for the African continent; *Bungarus* (krait) and *Ophiophagus* (king cobra) for Asia and the East Indies; *Notechis* (tiger snake), *Denisonia* (copperhead), *Acanthophis* (death adder), *Demansia* (brown snake), and *Oxyuranus* (taipan) for Australia. The genus *Naja* (cobra) is found in Africa, Asia, and the East Indies, while *Pseudechis* (black snake) is shared by Australia and the East Indies. The distribution of elapid genera for the various regions of central and south Africa is given by Broadley (1968), for India and southeast Asia by Reid (1968), for north Africa and north and west Asia by Klemmer (1968), for North America by Boys and Smith (1959), and for South America by Bücherl (1963).

C.   Venom Toxicity

All elapid venoms are neurotoxic, producing paralytic symptoms, and death from respiratory depression and cardiac arrest.

Reports on venom toxicity of various elapid species are numerous, but a comparison of the data is rendered difficult by variations in type of experimental animal, route of administration, and definition and pharmacological expression of lethal dose. Furthermore, venom toxicity has been found to vary within one species (Minton, 1957, 1967b). The values tabulated by Christensen (1955) from converted data of various investigators illustrate important variations in toxicity extimates. On the other hand, relative toxicity estimations on different snake venoms, tested under identical conditions, give a more reliable picture, viz., the data of Devi (1968) and Morgan (1956) on elapids from India and Australia, of Vick *et al.* (1967) from India and America, and of Christensen (1968) from Africa. Outstanding is the extreme toxicity of the Australian tiger snake and Indian krait, which are lethal to the mouse in doses of 2–5 μg (Minton, 1957).

D. Venom Yield

The danger of a snake to man depends not only on the toxicity of its venom but also on its aggressiveness, the amount of venom it delivers, and the depth of its bite. Snakes usually inject much less venom than the yield obtained by milking. However, knowledge of the venom yield, together with observation of the clinical symptoms, may serve in estimating the amount of antivenin to be used. Amounts of venom delivered by milking vary greatly with the snake species. Even within the same species, variations according to sex, season, and habitat have been reported (Deoras, 1966). Venom yields of some elapids are given in Table I.

Although extrapolation of venom toxicity from animal to man can be misleading (Minton, 1957), it may, in conjunction with knowledge of the venom yield, furnish an estimate of potential danger. Such an approximation shows that a coral snake might deliver 1–2 human LD_{100}, a blue krait 7, an Indian cobra 12–15, a mamba 5–15, and a tiger snake 20 (Minton, 1957; Boys and Smith, 1959).

E. Epidemiology

1. General Incidence and Mortality

Tropical countries with predominantly manual labor show the highest incidence of snake bite. As pointed out by Swaroop and Grab (1956) in their study on snake bite mortality in the world, statistics of snake bite in tropical regions are underestimates, since they are based solely on the accidents occurring within reach of a medical institution. Bites from remote villages may not be registered. Statistics of bites related to particular snake species are scarce. From Swaroop and Grab's book of world statistics (1956), data that comes from Australia, Papua, and New Guinea can be dependably attributed to elapid bite, since all poisonous snakes in these regions belong to the elapid family. In Australia, the annual snake bite death rate reported by these authors is 0.07 per 100,000 population. In Papua during the years 1949–1952, of 118 persons admitted to hospitals, 9 died. In New Guinea there was no fatality among 123 persons hospitalized.

In a statistic of snake bite in India over the years 1940–1953 reported by Ahuja and Singh (1956), the fatality rate on a total of 280 hospitalized elapid bite cases was 27.5% (77 deaths). In this patient material there were 131 cases of cobra (*Naja naja*) bite with a fatality rate of 8.4%, 35 cases of krait (*Bungarus caeruleus*) bite with a fatality rate of 77.1%, and 114 cases of bite by unidentified elapids with a fatality rate of 33.2%. The extremely high fatality rate of the krait bite in contrast to that of cobra bite was attributed to the inefficacy of the antivenom used, which at that time had no neutralizing action against krait venom. The relatively low fatality rate of

Table I.
Venom Yield of Some Elapid Snakes

Species	Number	Size, cm	Average yield ml	Average yield Wet weight, g	Average yield Dry weight, g	Percentage solid w/v	Reference
Sepedon hemachatus	10	90–120	0.35			23.9	Christensen (1955)
Naja flava	150		0.42			24.0	Grasset *et al.* (1935)
Naja flava	1	140	0.11			27.1	Christensen (1955)
	45		0.26			42.7	Christensen (1955)
	10		0.41			43.4	Christensen (1955)
Naja haje	1	150	0.12			33.5	Christensen (1955)
Naja naja (Male)	5		0.6			34.1	Deoras (1966)
Naja naja (Female)	5		0.4			35.3	Deoras (1966)
Naja naja Kept in room	801				0.157		Deoras (1966)
Naja naja Kept at farm	253				0.181		Deoras (1966)
Micrurus corallinus	116		0.082			18.4	Bücherl (1963)
Micrurus frontallis	78		0.069			37.0	Bücherl (1963)
Notechis scutatus	67	medium		0.1		26.3	Tidswell (1906)
Pseudechis porphyriacus	32			0.04		29.1	Tidswell (1906)
Bungarus caeruleus Kept in room	1.059				0.009		Deoras (1966)
Bungarus caeruleus Kept at farm	381				0.012		Deoras (1966)
Dendroaspis angusticeps	?				0.1		Grasset *et al.* (1935)

Naja naja bite, 4.2 %, is evident also in a report by Reid (1964) on 47 cases from Malaya.

Reports from the south African area reveal a relatively low incidence of elapid bite. The data of Christensen (1955) show that the cape cobra, the mamba, and the ringhals caused about 20 bites each out of a total of 359 registered in south Africa during a five-year period. Out of 40 cases of elapid bite hospitalized in Natal (Chapman, 1968a) 10 were lethal. *Dendroaspis* (mamba) was responsible for the high death toll, with 7 deaths in 7 cases. Chapman (1968a) stresses the low incidence of *Naja* bite (in spite of the prevalence of this genus), as well as its low mortality. In the United States, an average of 14 snake bite deaths a year, constituting an annual death rate 0.09 per 1,000,000 population, is reported by Parrish (1957). From all bites by venomous reptiles less than 2 % were inflicted by coral snakes (Russell, 1961).

2. *Seasonal Incidence and Time of Bite*

Large variations in incidence of snake bite according to season have been reported, the peak occurring in the hot, humid summer months in southern Africa (Christensen, 1955; Chapman, 1968a) and India (Ahuja and Singh, 1956). Although venom output is known to be larger after hibernation, the data of Ahuja and Singh (1956) do not show a seasonal variation of mortality. The above data are not specific for elapids and refer to snake bite in general.

Although cobras are generally reported to bite more frequently at night, the data of Reid (1964) as well as of Ahuja and Singh (1956) do not confirm this. Daylight bite was also found to be less effective by the latter authors, but more effective by the former. Chapman (1968a) observed that elapid bite, particularly by *Dendroaspis*, occurred more often in daylight. While cobras are active in the field, kraits infest occupied dwellings. They frequently bite sleeping humans, as shown by 29 nocturnal bites among 35 cases analyzed by Ahuja and Singh (1956).

3. *Age, Sex, and Occupation*

Reid's (1964) Malayan statistics show that the highest frequency of cobra bite is in males of the age group 20 to 49, reflecting the occupational nature of snake bite. The preponderance of Malayan cobra bite in male versus females corresponds to the general distribution of snake bite in India, with a male:female ratio of 4:1 (Ahuja and Singh, 1956).

4. *Site of Bite*

Most snake bite occurs on the lower extremities during barefoot work in the fields. Some southern African elapids like cobra and ringhals rear to strike, and their bites often occur on the thigh or higher (Chapman, 1968a). Others, like the mambas, are arboreal and also strike on the upper parts of the body. In the 47 Malayan cobra bite cases reported by Reid (1964), more than half of the victims were bitten on foot or toe. Eight were bitten on the upper part of the leg by rearing snakes.

Some importance has been attached to the site of a bite in determining its severity, based on the assumption that thin extremities offer a better hold for the snake's jaw than flat body surfaces; therefore, the bite would be more efficient. The data of Ahuja and Singh (1956), relating mainly to krait bites, do not confirm this; the mortality of bites on fingers and toes was slightly lower than that on other parts of the body. Chapman (1968a) considers the bites on head and trunk as particularly dangerous, because the abundant blood supply allows rapid absorption of the venom; moreover, it is impossible to apply ligature.

III. SYMPTOMATOLOGY OF ELAPID BITE

A. General Characteristics

Because of the wide distribution of Elapidae and the low frequency of elapid bite, exhaustive clinical descriptions are few. Authoritative clinical information can be found in the articles by Reid (1968) on land-snake bite in India and southeast Asia, on cobra bite specifically (Reid, 1964), on African snakes by Chapman (1968a), on snakes in the Pacific area by Campbell (1964, 1969) and on North American coral snakes by Russell (1967), and Ramsey and Klickstein (1962).

As for snake bite in general, elapid bite is not synonymous with envenomation. Indeed, out of Reid's 47 cobra-bitten patients, 25, or 53%, had no or negligible symptoms.

A common feature of elapid bite is muscle paralysis ensuing from peripheral neuromuscular block (Campbell, 1969). The description by Calmette in 1907 in his classic book "Les Venins, les Animaux Venimeux et la Sérothérapie Antivenimeuse," clearly illustrates the neurotoxic basis of the clinical symptoms and death:

> La morsure de cobra, même de grande taille, n'est pas très douloureuse. Elle est surtout caractérisée par de l'engourdissement qui survient dans la partie mordue, se propage rapidement dans tout le corps et produit des syncopes, des défaillances. Bientôt le blessé éprouve une sorte de lassitude et de sommeil invincible; ses jambes le portent à peine; il respire difficilement et sa respiration prend le type diaphragmatique. L'assoupissement et l'anxiété respiratoire augmentent peu à peu; le pouls, d'abord plus rapide, se ralentit et s'affaiblit graduellement; la bouche se contracte, devient baveuse; la langue semble

gonflée; les paupières restent tombantes, après quelques hoquets qu'accompagnent souvent des vomissements alimentaires et des émissions involontaires d'urine ou de matières fécales, la malheureuse victime tombe dans le coma le plus profond et meurt.

Still, neurotoxicity is not the only feature of elapid bite. Indeed, other symptomatology may be present or even be preponderant, such as local necrosis in bites by Malayan cobras (*Naja naja leucodira* and *Naja naja kaouthia*) (Reid, 1964), or hemorrhage and hemolysis in bites by elapids from the Pacific area (*Pseudechis papuanus, Oxyuranus scutellanus canni*) (Campbell, 1964, 1969). These symptoms are due to separate toxins which, however, are less important, because they do not appear to be lethal in themselves (*see* Chap. 2; Sec. III). Bites by certain elapids produce severe abdominal pain, for example, the Indian cobra (Chatterjee, 1965) and the Indian krait (*Bungarus caeruleus*) (Ahuja and Singh, 1956). Eye symptoms (ophthalmia), result from spitting by *Naja nigricollis* and *Hemachatus haemachatus* (Corkill, 1956; Gilkes, 1959; Chapman, 1968a).

Generally one may distinguish, as Reid has done (1964), symptoms due to local poisoning (pain, swelling, blistering, hemorrhage, necrosis) and those due to systemic poisoning (neurotoxicity, cardiovascular manifestations, hemolysis, hemorrhage). Although neurotoxic signs are prominent in elapid envenomation and though the mode of death is generally considered to be neurotoxic, mainly through respiratory paralysis, venom cardiotoxicity has been implicated. Autopsies in elapid bite are not revealing, except for necrosis, edema, and findings secondary to respiratory paralysis consistent with the clinical picture (Chapman, 1968a).

B. Local Poisoning

Early literature on necrosis following cobra bite was reviewed by Reid (1964). Local pain often starts immediately after Malayan cobra bite (Reid, 1964), and lasts, on the average, 10 days, depending on the development and severity of necrosis. Swelling usually starts a few hours after the bite and reaches a maximum in 1 or 2 days. It is mostly localized, but, rarely, involves the whole limb, often with a dusky discoloration around the bite mark; eventually sanguineous blisters and necrosis appear, the latter sometimes involving large areas of sloughing. Extensive necrosis may require excision and skin grafting, and healing may be delayed for months. Even extensive necrosis may occur without neurotoxic signs.

According to Chapman (1968a), swelling and pain are not clinically prominent in southern African elapid bite. American coral snake bite (*Micrurus corallinus, fulvius, lemniscatus*) is reported to cause intense local pain but no swelling (Amaral, 1951). The bite by the strongly neurotoxic common krait (*Bungarus caeruleus*) does not produce any local reaction

(Amaral, 1951). Christensen (1955) in discussing elapid bite (*Naja, Sepedon, Dendroaspis*) mentions pain and local swelling but no necrosis. Bleeding from the bite wound or first aid incision may occur in Australian elapid bite (*Pseudechis papuanus, Oxyuranus scutellanus canni*) (Campbell, 1969).

Conjunctivitis with pain and photophobia are caused by a local action of the venom spat by *Hemachatus haemachatus* or *Naja nigricollis* (Chapman, 1968a). Symptoms last a few days and are reversible, although, rarely, blindness may occur (FitzSimons, 1962).

C. Systemic Poisoning

1. Neurotoxic Effects

The preponderance of neurotoxic symptomatology in the clinical picture varies greatly with the elapid species. It constitutes the main or only manifestation of the bite by some species, for instance, the krait (Ahuja and Singh, 1956), the mamba (Le Gac and Lepesme, 1940; Lefrou, 1951; Chapman, 1968a), and the coral snake (Russell, 1967), it is less prevalent in others, as for instance, the Malayan cobra (Reid, 1964).

The neurotoxic symptomatology following bites by different elapid species varies in rapidity of appearance and in fatality rate, but varies little in type of neurological disturbance (mainly a flaccid paralysis). Ptosis, external ophthalmoplegia, facial paresis, difficulty in swallowing and speaking, difficulty in lifting the head (broken neck syndrome), and loss of tendon reflexes, are described by Reid (1964) for Malayan cobra envenomation. Twitching but no convulsions occurred.

Campbell (1964; 1969) in his observations on Australian elapids (*Pseudechis papuanus, Oxyuranus scutellatus canni, Acanthophis antarcticus*) describes similar neurotoxic symtoms. Death is due to respiratory obstruction from accumulation of secretion, to mechanical obstruction caused by paralysis of tongue and jaw muscles, or to respiratory insufficiency resulting from paralysis of chest muscle and diaphragm.

There are only slight differences in description of the neurotoxic signs of envenomation by a wide variety of elapid species. We might mention *Naja tripudians* from Thailand (Puranananda, 1968), *Micruroides euryxanthus* from North America (Ramsey and Klickstein, 1962; Russell, 1967), and the Pacific area elapids (*Pseudechis papuanus, Oxyuranus scutellatus, Acanthophis antarcticus*) (Campbell, 1964, 1969). Convulsions have been observed from American coral snake bite (*Micrurus corallinus, fulvius, lemniscatus*) (Amaral, 1951). Acute ascending spinal paralysis with death from respiratory causes has been described for cobra bite in Nigeria (Onuaguluchi, 1960).

Whereas flaccid muscular paralysis accounts for much of the above described symptomatology, central nervous system action of elapid venom (demonstrated experimentally by Krupnick *et al.*, 1968), may be clinically manifest. *Hemachatus haemachatus* bite may rapidly produce unconsciousness as the initial symptom (Gray, 1962); the drowsiness in Malayan cobra bite (Reid, 1964) seems to be unrelated to the peripheral symptomatology, as is the early sudden loss of consciousness in snake bite in the Pacific area (Campbell, 1969).

2. Cardiovascular Effects

Reid (1964) describes in Malayan cobra bite an initially slow pulse, later rising when necrosis accompanied by fever occurs. According to him, the mode of death in cobra bite remains obscure, but cardiotoxicity may be an important cause. Sudden collapse in *Naja nivea* bite has been ascribed to a cardiotoxic effect of the venom (FitzSimons, 1962). On the other hand, in Australian elapid bite no primary circulatory changes were detected; even in severely paralyzed patients without obvious respiratory movements, the blood pressure was well maintained and the electrocardiogram remained normal (Campbell, 1964). Neither is there clear evidence for cardiotoxic symptomatology in southern African elapid bite, circulatory effects possibly being secondary to anoxia induced by respiratory paralysis (Chapman, 1968a).

3. Hematological Effects

Bites by elapids of the Australian region may cause two types of hematological disturbance (Campbell, 1969): bleeding tendency and intravascular hemolysis. Continued bleeding from the bite wound or first-aid incision, spitting, vomiting, or coughing of blood may occur in bites by *Pseudechis papuanus* and *Oxyuranus scutellanus canni*, due to coagulant factors and/or hemorrhagin. Hemolysis ensues in hemoglobinuria in the bite of *Pseudechis papuanus*. In systemic poisoning following Malayan cobra bite, Reid (1964) reports laboratory findings indicating mild hemolysis. The king cobra or hamadryad (*Naja hannah*) is mentioned to have a slight hemolytic effect (Amaral, 1951). Southern African elapid bite is not characterized by hemorrhage or hemolysis, although the venoms of these snakes may possess anticoagulant and hemolytic properties (Chapman, 1968a).

4. Allergy

Reid (1964) describes urticaria of face and limbs in a patient bitten by a Malayan cobra, and not treated with antivenin. Itching, allergic rhinitis, and conjunctivitis were described by Mendes *et al.* (1960) in personnel handling snake venom from elapids and others.

IV. TREATMENT

A. Indigenous and Chemical Treatment

Corkill (1956) describes indigenous practices in prevention and treatment of snake bite in the Sudan. Written charms worn in leather cases are thought to prevent poisoning of the wearer as well as of nine of his best friends. Treatment consists of scarification, suction, and cauterization followed by ingestion of milk, eggs, and decoctions of plants and of rhinoceros horn fragments. Wounds are dressed with roots and plants. On the skin around the bite the sign of Solomon, Lord of the Jinn, is drawn to drive away the evil spirits. Since the person bitten by a cobra shows increasing torpor, dancing, beating of drums, and playing music is thought to prevent the victim from falling into a sleep with no wakening. Ahuja and Singh (1956) describe the use of herbs, charms, and snake-stones in India, adding a remark on the confusion concerning the value of these practices in the minds not only of laymen but also of physicians. Christensen (1955) tested African native remedies consisting of dry vegetable matter, whose actual composition is a closely guarded secret. They were found harmless to mice and rabbits, but of no protective value whatsoever.

British medical officers in India in the late eighties initiated the use of potassium permanganate in the treatment of snake bite. Led by the observations of Lacerda and of Blyth on the neutralizing action of potassium permanganate on viper and cobra venom, Rogers (1904a, 1904b, 1905), stationed in Calcutta, advised rubbing permanganate crystals into an incision made at the site of the bite. He devised an instrument consisting of a lancet and a container for the crystals "to be sold at very low figure and bring it within the reach of even the poorest classes in India and elsewhere" (Rogers, 1904b). The use of potassium permanganate became general in cobra bite, whether rubbed in the wound, injected around it, or even given orally in combination with antivenins or other drugs (Condon, 1899; Rogers, 1904a, 1905; Haw, 1907; Bose, 1910; Fox, 1915). Although it has been stressed recently that permanganate treatment not only is useless but indeed harmful since it promotes necrosis and sloughing (Ahuja and Singh, 1956; Corkill, 1959), it was applied in India (Basu, 1939; Pern, 1941) as well as in Africa (Le Gac and Lepesme, 1940), in addition to or in the absence of available antivenin.

Other remedies that have been used but with less claim for success are "chloride of gold" (Calmette, 1892; Kanthack, 1892), "liquor potassae" (Shortt, 1882), various dyes, and colloidal solutions of silver, sulfur, and iodine (Ahuja and Singh, 1956). Local injection of carbolic soap in elapid bite is opposed by Reid (1957), but advocated by Ahuja and Singh (1956) on the basis of their own experimental data as well as the work of Christensen and De Waal (1947). The procedure is thought to be of value as a first aid measure in delaying absorption of venom until the patient can receive antivenin. Corkill (1959) recommends injection of plain soap solution around elapid bite wounds. Although antivenins are increasingly available, the search for a cheap miracle drug has not been abandoned, as illustrated by a recent report on the virtues of Higgins India Ink (Grab *et al.*, 1955).

B. First Aid

According to Reid (1968) first-aid treatment means "measures taken by the victim or associates before receiving medical treatment." Immobilization, ligature, incision, and suction are the common first-aid measures in snake bite.

1. Immobilization and Reassurance

Complete immobilization of the victim, or at least of the bitten limb, will help check the spread of venom (Barnes and Trueta, 1941; Corkill, 1959; Ad Hoc Committee, 1963). The limb should be kept in a horizontal position during hospitalization (Chapman, 1968a; Reid, 1968). Prompt reassurance of the snake bite victim is considered of major importance; emotional shock is held to be deleterious. A placebo injection (Reid, 1968), a small dose of tranquilizer (Chapman, 1968a), or simple encouragement by a physician (Corkill, 1959) are advocated.

2. Ligature

Ligature can be applied with anything at hand—cloth, handkerchief, even grass (Reid, 1968). It may, however, be dangerous, as discussed in detail by Chapman (1968a). Obviously, ligature in elapid bite is of no use if not applied immediately (Ahuja and Singh, 1956). In view of the experimental evidence for the spreading of venom from tissue to blood stream by the lymphatic system (Barnes and Trueta, 1941), ligature, as proposed by many clinicians, should aim at arrest of superficial venous and lymphatic return but not of arterial flow (Ad Hoc Committee, 1963; Reid, 1968; Shannon, 1956). However, while in experimental animals lymphatic obstruction checks the spreading of tiger snake venom, it does not prevent that of cobra venom (Barnes and Trueta, 1941). Chapman (1968a) prefers an arterial tourniquet, periodically released, and discarded following antivenin administration. The arterial tourniquet should be placed high on the upper arm or thigh, as opposed to the conventional lymphatic–venous tourniquet, which is applied proximal to the bite. Gradually moving the tourniquet in advance of the swelling has been recommended (Shannon, 1956; Lefrou, 1951).

3. Incision and Suction

As true for the tourniquet, the efficacy of incision and suction in elapid bite is a function of time. Elapid venoms contain highly dialyzable, low-molecular-weight toxins (Mebs, 1969) and, in addition, some of them, such as *Bungarus caeruleus* venom, have high hyaluronidase activity (Jaques, 1955; 1956). In view of the fast spreading of such venoms, the use of incision and suction is often questioned (Ahuja and Singh, 1956; Chapman, 1968a; Reid, 1968) and even altogether dismissed, as for instance by the staff of the Miami Serpentarium, who rely on the treatment of accidental bites by antivenins alone (Christy, 1967).

C. Antivenins

1. History

At the turn of the century, British medical officers stationed in India suggested that local snake charmers gained immunity by letting themselves be bitten repeatedly by young or freshly-milked specimens, which deliver small amounts of venom (Bawa, 1898). The pioneer work of Phisalix, Bertrand, and Calmette, followed by Fraser, demonstrated that animals injected with small doses of venom became immune and that their sera acquired antivenin properties. Large-scale production of antivenomous sera was started by Calmette at the Pasteur Institute of Lille, by immunizing horses with the venom of the Indian cobra, *Naja tripudians*. This antivenin was used in India, Algeria, Egypt, west Africa, America, the West Indies, the Antilles, etc., both for human and domestic animals, regardless of the species of the snake that inflicted the bite. The numerous reports of success following the use of Calmette's antivenin (Rennie, 1896; Keatinge and Ruffer, 1897; Hazard, 1897; De Lavigne, 1897; Hanna and Lamb, 1901) reflect as much the real virtues of the preparation as the prestige and the authority that Calmette enjoyed. In 1896 Calmette presented his results before a commission of the Royal College of Physicians and Surgeons in London and claimed universal preventive and curative properties for his antivenin (Calmette, 1897, 1898). An official statement was issued recommending the use of his antivenin in all cases of snake bite (Calmette, 1897).

However, the universal use of Calmette antivenin was challenged by Martin (1898) who showed its low efficacy against Australian snake venoms. The work of Rogers (1904b) in London and of Arthus' group in Lausanne soon demonstrated that the neutralizing action of Calmette's anti-cobra serum was weak against the venoms of other elapids, such as *Bungarus caeruleus* (krait) (Galperine, 1912), or *Ophiophagus elaps* (king cobra) (Ittine, 1911; Rapoport, 1913), thus supporting the views of Martin (1898) and Tidswell (1906) that antivenins are specific to the venom used for immunization.

2. Commercial Preparations

A first list of antivenins available for the treatment of snake bite, including elapid bite, appeared in 1952 (Oliver and Goss, 1952), soon to be followed by more comprehensive lists, which included potency, mode of production, and degree of purification (Taub, 1964; Keegan, 1956; Russell and Lauritzen, 1966). Prompted by the lack of international standards of antivenin potency and by the inadequate knowledge of their paraspecific neutralizing activity, Minton (1967a) tested 17 elapid antivenins. His results, suggesting that a few well-chosen antivenins might achieve protection against a wide range of venoms, are of considerable practical importance.

An antivenin specific for the South American coral snakes, *Micrurus corallinus* and *Micrurus frontalis*, is "Soro Elapidico" manufactured by the Butantan Institute. As indicated by the manufacturers, by Keegan *et al.* (1961), and by Flowers (1966), it also offers protection against the North American coral species, and indeed has been used in bites by *Micrurus fulvius* (Ramsey and Klickstein, 1962) and *Micrurus euryxanthus* (Russell, 1967). Antivenins specific for *Micrurus fulvius* venom that provide protection against *Micrurus euryxanthus* have been prepared recently by Gennaro (mentioned by Russell, 1967), and by Kocholaty *et al.* (1967).

3. Time and Route of Administration

Although it is the only unquestioned antidote to snake venom, antivenin therapy is not without danger. Therefore, since snake bite is not equal to envenomation, antivenin therapy should be started when there are signs of systemic poisoning (Reid, 1968). This attitude seems justified in cases of bite by Malayan elapids (mainly *Naja naja*) where systemic poisoning develops in the minority of the cases, and specific antivenin administration can be effective even if given hours or days after the bite (Reid, 1968). Ahuja and Singh report that moribund patients have recovered completely following antivenin treatment: "While the victim of an Indian cobra is still alive, it is never too late to begin serum treatment. . . ." (Ahuja and Singh, 1956.) It has been pointed out, however, that some elapid venoms, such as of that of the African mambas, are so strongly neurotoxic that, unless antivenin is given immediately, there is little chance of survival (Christy, 1967). Chapman (1968a), dealing with African elapid bite, recommends immediate use of the antivenin without even taking time to estimate sensitivity.

Soon after Calmette anti-cobra serum became available in the early nineties, experimental studies established that a maximal neutralizing effect is obtained by intravenous administration (Loubo, 1912). In 1904, Rogers (1904a, 1904b) advised that the serum be injected intravenously, so as to obtain the most rapid action possible. It has been agreed ever since that in elapid bite the intravenous route is the best. Local injections are opposed as useless if not given immediately (Chapman, 1968a); they also increase the tension in an already edematous limb, which, moreover, has a diminished capacity to take up subcutaneously injected antivenin (Stahnke *et al.*, 1957).

4. Dosage

According to the severity of the symptoms, amounts of 100–200 ml are given by Reid (1968) by intravenous drip as a first dose, with 100 ml to follow if no improvement occurs. Chapman stresses the importance of giving at least the amount recommended by the manufacturer in one large dose, and adding subsequent doses, up to a total of 200 ml in serious bites (Chapman, 1968a). Campbell (1964) calculates the dose of antivenin to neutralize double the average venom yield of each of the three elapid snakes responsible for the bites in one area; this represents 180–190 ml of serum. Estimating that a large cobra may introduce an amount of venom equivalent to about 150 mg dry weight, Christensen (1955) indicates that about 60 ml of the locally produced antivenin would neutralize it *in vitro*, and that the doses used in southern Africa were usually below this amount. There is no agreement as to whether children should receive the same dose as adults (Chapman, 1968a; Christensen, 1955), smaller doses (Reid, 1968), or larger ones (Amaral, 1951).

5. Efficacy

Statistics on 52 cases of elapid (*Oxyuranus scutellatus, Acanthophis antarcticus, Pseudechis papuanus*) bite in Papua, treated with specific antivenin, tracheotomy, and artificial respiration, show a mortality of 4%. Although the author (Campbell, 1964) stresses the importance of respiratory support, antivenin is considered to have prevented serious paralysis in 17% of the cases. The success of polyspecific antivenin therapy in African elapid bite is illustrated by the course in 25 severe envenomations listed by Chapman (1968a), in 14 of which obvious improvement was noticed within a few hours after serum administration. Reid (1964), reviewing 47 cases of *Naja naja* bite in Malaysia when monospecific and polyspecific antivenins were used, judges the treatment effective though not as dramatic as in cases of viper or sea-snake bites. Improvement was observed in the systemic symptoms only; neither specific *Naja naja* antivenin nor polyvalent antivenin prevented or ameliorated local necrosis. Reporting on the treatment of snake bite, including cobra bite, in Thailand, Puranananda (1968) claims that if the dose of antivenin is large enough, it always saves the victim's life.

D. Cryotherapy

Cryotherapy is controversial in snake bite. Stahnke (Stahnke *et al.*,

1957; Stahnke and McBride, 1966) claims that cryotherapy prevents tissue destruction by arresting the action of venom enymes and bacteria, and slows the absorption of neurotoxins. He successfully applied cryotherapy to bites by crotalid snakes, whose venoms contain mainly large-molecular-weight proteins with strong proteolytic activity and relatively slow absorption. In contrast, use of cryotherapy in cobra bite seems less rational in view of the fast spreading of the low-molecular-weight cobra venom neurotoxins (see Chap. 2, Sec. II). A report on successful use of cryotherapy in a case of cobra bite (Mullins and Naylor, 1960) raised severe criticism by Shannon (1956; 1961), who considers this form of treatment dangerous to an already anoxic tissue, increasing the hazard of gangrene and amputation, and useless in checking the spread of the cobra toxins.

E. Tracheostomy and Artificial Respiration

Artificial respiration has been used in early studies on experimental envenomation by various elapids (Semenoff, 1912; Calame, 1913; Lvova, 1913), since it was established that heart action continues after arrest of respiration. The importance of respiratory aid in elapid bite is now unanimously stressed. Campbell (1964; 1969), summarizing the therapeutic problems in Australian elapid snake bite, considers relief of respiratory obstruction and insufficiency to be as important as antivenin treatment. Respiratory obstruction, resulting from accumulation of oral secretions in the paralyzed larynx, was relieved by tracheostomy and aspiration in 32 of the 73 cases reported. Respiratory insufficiency by paralysis of respiratory muscles prompted the use of some form of artificial respiration in 17 patients. Use of these measures is believed to have saved at least 25 % of the patients who would have otherwise died. Similar treatment is advised by Chapman (1968a) in the management of envenomation by African elapids, by Reid (1968) for Indian and southeast Asian elapid poisoning, and by Corkill (1959) for snake bite in the tropics in general. Oxygen and positive-pressure breathing are advocated by Russell (1967) when respiratory deficit develops following Sonoran coral snake (*Micruroides euryxanthus*) bite.

F. Antibiotics and Tetanus Antitoxin

Bacterial contamination in snake bite is frequent, especially when incision is performed with no regard to asepsis, and even more so when indigenous medication has been used. Furthermore, it has been shown that bacteria are prevalent in the mouth and venom glands of the snake (Parrish *et al.*, 1956). Indeed, commercial preparations of venoms are sometimes contaminated with bacteria, including clostridia (Kellaway and Williams, 1933; Prévot, 1951; Boys *et al.*, 1960). It was therefore suggested that wide-spectrum antibiotics should be used in routine treatment of snake bite

(Parrish *et al.*, 1956; Chapman, 1968a; Ramsey and Klickstein, 1962), as well as in experimental envenomation (Boys *et al.*, 1960).

In a report of the Ad Hoc Committee of the National Academy of Sciences (1963) on the treatment of snake bite, use of antibiotics as first aid is not recommended but is advised when symptoms develop. Reid (1964) holds the same view, specifically for the treatment of cobra bite. The more severe the local necrosis, the stronger the indication for antibiotics, even though necrosis is not always due to bacterial infection (Reid, 1964).

Tetanus antitoxin was used in every case of snake bite in central and southern Africa by Chapman (1968a) and is also recommended by Russell (1967) and by the Ad Hoc Committee (1963).

G.   Corticosteroids, Antihistaminics, and Other Drugs

A decrease in lethality of *Naja naja* venom in dogs by large doses of hydrocortisone has been reported by Morales *et al.* (1961); the effect is related to the ability of the drug to decrease the pooling of blood in the envenomated animal (Bangananda and Perry, 1962). It should be pointed out that the steroid dose used in these studies was massive.

Use of corticosteroids and ACTH in snake bite in the human has been both advocated (Gupta *et al.*, 1960; Benyajati *et al.*, 1960; Wig and Vaish, 1960) and opposed (Schöttler, 1954). Shannon (1961), commenting specifically on the treatment of cobra bite, strongly opposes early use of corticosteroids, since they act synergistically with the venom in predisposing to bacterial invasion. In spite of the still inconclusive clinical evidence, hydrocortisone is still given in elapid bite (Campbell, 1964; Mullins and Naylor, 1960). Use of corticosteroids together with antihistaminics in the treatment of anaphylactic shock following administration of antivenin is common practice (Puranananda, 1968; Ad Hoc Committee, 1963; Reid, 1964; Chapman, 1968b).

The use of antihistaminics in cobra bite is based on experimental evidence for the liberation of histamine from lung and diaphragm by cobra venom (Feldberg and Kellaway, 1937; Dutta and Narayanan, 1952), and on the resemblance between some circulatory effects of the venom and those of histamine (Chopra and Chowan, 1939). However, it was shown that administration of antihistaminics does not alter the time of survival of rats receiving Indian cobra venom intravenously (Dutta and Narayanan, 1952). Lefrou and Michard (1956) demonstrated in animals receiving *Dendroaspis* venom that death was accelerated by antihistaminic treatment, presumably due to its hypotensive action. Schöttler (1954), relating this harmful effect of antihistaminic drugs to high dosage, maintains that low doses might be beneficial. Antihistaminics are generally advised when the patient develops an anaphylactic reaction to antivenin (Puranananda, 1956).

An early treatment of cardiac failure in elapid envenomation was administration of strychnine. In 1892, Banerjee reported two cases of krait bite in India treated with repeated strychnine injections "until twitching of the face appeared." Drinking of "liquor strychninae" was used in treatment of cobra bite (Haw, 1907) sometimes together with digitalis (Bose, 1910). Even recently, Burette (1947) reported the successful treatment of five cases of mamba (*Dendroaspis*) bite with intravenous strychnine only. Strychnine together with coffeine and camphor is still used in association with antivenin in mamba bite (Le Gac and Lepesme, 1940; Lefrou, 1951).

Christensen (1955) tested the value of a series of drugs on mice injected intravenously with *Naja flava* venom. Prostigmine, British Anti-Lewisite ergotamine, dihydroergotamine, and calcium gluconate all failed to modify the survival rates of the experimental animals.

Trethewie and Day (1948b) found that heparin had no effect on the mortality of mice given *Pseudechis porphyriacus* venom, but, if combined with Neoantergan, it markedly reduced mortality. Heparin alone delayed the death time of guinea pigs and mice injected with *Pseudechis porphyriacus* and *Notechis scutatus* venoms (Trethewie and Day, 1948a). Macht (1943) found that heparinization of cats prior to intravenous administration of cobra venom diminished the toxicity. The effect of heparin was related to the clotting activity of these venoms. Clinical evidence for a beneficial action of heparin is as yet lacking.

H. Treatment of Ophthalmia

Fox (1915) recommended washing the eyes with canned milk. In the case of ophthalmia caused by *Naja nigricollis* venom reported by Ridley (1944), treatment by irrigations and atropine was satisfactory; no antivenin was given. Simple lavage with water or some other bland fluid is considered adequate by Chapman (1968a). Christensen (1955) recommends additional instillation with diluted antivenin. Gilkes (1959) treated a patient with conjunctivitis due to *Naja nigricollis* venom by irrigations and penicillin–streptomycin ointment.

V. REFERENCES

Ad Hoc Committee, National Academy of Sciences. National Research Council on Snakebite Therapy, 1963, *Toxicon*, 1:81.

Ahuja, M. L. and G. Singh (1956), Snakebite in India, in "Venoms" (E. Buckley and N. Porges, eds.), American Association for the Advancement of Science, Washington, D.C., p. 341.

Amaral, A. (1951), Snake Venenation (Ophidism), *in* "Clinical Tropical Medicine" (R. B. H. Gradwohl, L. B. Soto, and O. Felsenfeld, eds.), C. V. Mosby Co., St. Louis, p. 1238.

Banerjee, R. P. (1892), *Lancet*, 1:1183.

Banganada, K. and J. F. Perry, Jr. (1962), *Proc. Soc. Exp. Biol.*, **110**:229.

Barnes, J. M. and J. Trueta (1941), *Lancet*, **1**:623.

Basu, U. P. (1939), *Amer. J. Trop. Med.*, **19**:385.

Bawa, H. (1895), *Brit. Med. J.*, **2**:1199.

Benyajati, C., N. Kooplung, and R. Sribhibhadh (1960), *J. Trop. Med. Hyg.*, **63**:254.

Bose, N. (1910), *Lancet*, **1**:643.

Boys, F. and H. M. Smith (1959), "Poisonous Amphibians and Reptiles," Charles C. Thomas, Springfield, Illinois, p. 72.

Boys, F., D. Beamer, and H. M. Smith (1960), *J. Amer. Med. Assoc.*, **174**:306.

Broadley, D. G. (1968), The venomous snakes of Central and South Africa, *in* "Venomous Animals and Their Venoms," vol. 1 (W. Bucherl, E. Buckley, and U. Deulofeu, eds.), Academic Press, New York, p. 403.

Bucherl, W. (1963), Über die Ermittlung von Durchschnitts- und Höchst-Giftmengen bei den häufigsten Giftschlangen Südamerikas, *in* "Die Giftschlangen der Erde," Behringwerk-Mitteilungen, N. G. Elwert Universitäts- und Verlags-Buchhandlung, Marburg/Lahn, p. 67.

Burette, J. (1947), *Ann. Soc. Belge Méd. Trop.*, **27**:195.

Calame, S. (1913), Nouvelles recherches sur le venin de *Bungarus Caeruleus* où krait de l'Inde, *thèse, Fac. de Méd. Lausanne.*

Calmette, A. (1892), *Ann. Inst. Pasteur*, **6**:160.

Calmette, A. (1897), *Ann. Inst. Pasteur* **11**:214.

Calmette, A. (1898), *Brit. Med. J.*, **1**:1253.

Calmette, A. (1907), "Les Venins, les Animaux Venimeux et la Serothérapie Antivenimeuse," Masson et Cie., Paris.

Campbell, C. H. (1964), *Trans. Roy. Soc. Trop. Med. Hyg.*, **58**:263.

Campbell, C. H. (1969), *Toxicon*, **7**:25.

Chapman, D. S. (1968a), The symtomatology, pathology and treatment of the bites by venomous snakes of Central and Southern Africa, *in* "Venomous Animals and their Venoms," vol. 1 (W. Bücherl, E. Buckley, and V. Deulofeu, eds.), Academic Press, New York, p. 463.

Chapman, D. S. (1968b), Snake bites, *in* "Companion to Surgery in Africa" (W. W. Davey, ed.), Livingston, pp. 127–134; quoted from *Toxicon*, **6**:228.

Chatterjee, S. C. (1965), *J. Indian Med. Assn.*, **45**:654.

Chopra, R. N. and J. S. Chowhan (1939), *Ind. Med. Gaz.*, **74**:422.

Christensen, P. A. (1955), "South African Snake Venoms and Antivenoms," The South African Institute for Medical Research, Johannesburg.

Christensen, P. A. 1968, The venoms of Central and South African snakes, *in* "Venomous Animals and their Venoms, vol. 1" (W. Bucherl, E. Buckley, and U. Deulofeu, eds.), Academic Press, New York, p. 437.

Christensen, P. A. and M. De Waal (1947), *South African Med. J.*, **21**:680.

Christy, N. P. (1967), *Amer. J. Med.*, **42**:107.

Condon, de V. (1899), *Brit. Med. J.*, **1**:271.

Corkill, N. L. (1956), Snake poisoning in the Sudan, *in* "Venoms" (E. Buckley and N. Porges, eds.), American Association for the Advancement of Science, Washington, D.C., p. 331.

Corkill, N. L. (1959), *Practitioner*, **183**:354.

De Lavigne (1897), *Arch. Méd. Nav.*, **67**:449.

Deoras, P. J. (1966), *Mem. Inst. Butantan Simp. Internac.*, **33**:767.

Devi, A. (1968), The protein and nonprotein constituents of snake venoms, *in* "Venomous Animals and Their Venoms," vol. 1 (W. Bücherl, E. Buckley, and V. Deulofeu, eds.), Academic Press, New York, p. 119.

Dutta, N. K. and K. G. A. Narayanan (1952), *Nature*, **169**:1064.

Feldberg, W. and C. H. Kellaway (1937), *Austr. J. Exp. Biol. Med. Sci.*, **15**:81.

FitzSimons, V. F. M. (1962), "Snakes of Southern Africa," Purnell, Cape Town.

Flowers, H. H. (1966), *Amer. J. Trop. Med. Hyg.*, **15**:1003.

Fox, J. C. (1915), *Brit. Med. J.*, **1**:632.

Galperine, A. (1912), Etudes sur le venin de *Bungarus caeruleus* (krait), thèse, fac. de Méd. Lausanne.
Garb, S., A. Schiabine, B. B. Roy, V. Venturi, and M. Penna (1955), *J. Lab. Clin. Med.*, 45:580.
Gilkes, M. J. (1959), *Brit. J. Ophtal.*, 43:638.
Grasset, E., A. Zoutendyk, and A. W. Schaafsma (1935), *Trans. Roy. Soc. Trop. Med. Hyg.*, 28:601.
Gray, H. H. (1962), *Trans. Roy. Soc. Trop. Med. Hyg.*, 56:390.
Gupta, P S., S. P. Bhargava, and M. L Sharma (1960), *J. Indian Med. Assn.*, 35:387.
Hanna, W. and G. Lamb (1901), *Lancet*, 1:25.
Haw, W. H. (1907), *Lancet*, 1:1154.
Hazard, A. (1897), *Arch. Méd. Nav.*, 67:219.
Ittine, C. (1911), Etudes sur le venin de *Naja bungarus* (king cobra), thèse, Fac. de Méd. Lausanne.
Jaques, R., 1955, *Helv. Physiol. Acta*, 13:113.
Jaques, R. (1956), The hyaluronidase content of animal venoms, *in* "Venoms" (E. Buckley and N. Porges, eds.), American Association for the Advancement of Science, Washington, D.C., p. 291.
Kanthack, A. A. (1892), *Lancet*, 1:1296.
Keatinge, H. P. and M. A. Ruffer (1897), *Brit. Med. J.*, 1:9.
Keegan, H. L. (1956), Antivenins available for treatment of envenomation by poisonous snakes, scorpions and spiders, *in* "Venoms" (E. Buckley and N. Porges, eds.), American Association for the Advancement of Science, Washington, D.C., p. 413.
Keegan, H. L., F. W. Whittemore, Jr., and J. F. Flanigan (1961), *Public Health Report, Washington*, 76:540.
Kellaway, C. H. and F. E. Williams (1933), Investigation of toxicity and sterility of commercial preparations containing modified snake venom, *Med. J. Australia*, 19:581.
Klemmer, K. (1963), Liste der rezenten Giftschlangen, *in* "Die Giftschlangen der Erde," Behringwerk-Mitteilungen, N. G. Elwert Universitäts- und Verlags-Buchhandlung, Marburg/Lahn, p. 225.
Klemmer, K. (1968), Classification and distribution of European, North African and North and West Asiatic venomous snakes, *in* "Venomous Animals and Their Venoms," vol. 1 (W. Bucherl, E. Buckley, and V. Deulofeu, eds.), Academic Press, New York, p. 309.
Kocholaty, W. F., B. D. Ashley, and T. A. Billing (1967), *Toxicon*, 5:43.
Krupnick, J., H. I. Bicher, and S. Gitter (1968), *Toxicon*, 6:11.
Le Gac, P. and P. Lepesme (1940), *Bull. Soc. Pathol. Exot.*, 33:256.
Lefrou, G. (1951), *Bull. Soc. Pathol. Exot.*, 44:234.
Lefrou, G. and V. Michard (1956), *Bull. Soc. Pathol. Exot.*, 49:936.
Loubo, V. (1912), Etudes sur le sérum antivenimeux. Des injections intramusculaires de serum antivenimeux, thèse, Fac. de Med. Lausanne.
Lvova, F. (1913), Le venin de *Naja haje*, thèse, Fac. de Méd. Lausanne.
Macht, D. I. (1943), *Ann. Int. Med.*, 18:772.
Martin, C. J. (1898), *Brit. Med. J.*, 2:1805.
Mebs, D. (1969), *Toxicon*, 6:247.
Mendes, E., A. U. Cintra, and A. Corréa (1960), *J. Allergy*, 31:68.
Minton, S. A. (1957), *Sci. Amer.*, 196:114.
Minton, S. A. (1967a), *Toxicon*, 5:47.
Minton, S. A. (1967b), Observations on toxicity and antigenic make up of venoms from juvenile snakes, *in* "Animal Toxins" (F. E. Russell, and P. R. Saunders, eds.), Pergamon Press, London, p. 211.
Morales, F., H. D. Root, and J. F. Perry, Jr. (1961), *Proc. Soc. Exp. Biol. Med.*, 108:522.
Morgan, F. G. (1956), The Australian Taipan Oxyuranus scutellatus scutellatus (Peters), *in* "Venoms" (E. Buckley and N. Porges, eds.), American Association for the Advancement of Science, Washington, D.C., p. 359.

Mullins, J. F. and D. Naylor (1960), *J. Amer. Med. Assn.*, **174**:1677.
Oliver, J. and L. Goss, (1952), *Copeia*, **4**:270.
Onuaguluchi, G. O. (1960), *Trans. Roy. Soc. Trop. Med. Hyg.*, **54**:265.
Parrish, H. M. (1957), *Public Health Rep.*, **72**:1027.
Parrish, H. M., A. W. MacLaurin, and R. L. Tuttle (1956), *Virginia Month.*, **83**:383.
Pern, S. (1941), *Brit. Med. J.*, **1**:338.
Phisalix, M. (1940), *Bull. Soc. Pathol. Exot.*, **33**:258.
Prèvot, A. R. (1951), *Ann. Inst. Pasteur*, **81**:665.
Puranananda, C. (1956), Treatment of snakebite cases in Bangkok, *in* "Venoms" (E. Buckley and N. Porges, eds.), American Association for the Advancement of Science, Washington, p. 353.
Ramsey, G. F. and G. D. Klickstein (1962), *J. Amer. Med. Assn.*, **182**:949.
Rapoport, T. (1913), L'immunisation antivenemeuse est-elle spécifique?, thèse, Fac. de Méd. Lausanne.
Reid, H. A. (1957), *Lancet*, **2**:697.
Reid, H. A. (1964), *Brit. Med. J.*, **2**:540.
Reid, H. A. (1968), Symptomatology, Pathology and Treatment of Land Snake Bite in India and Southeast Asia, *in* "Venomous Animals and Their Venoms," vol. 1 (W. Bücherl, E. Buckley, and V. Deulofeu, eds.), Academic Press, New York, p. 611.
Rennie, S. J. (1896), *Brit. Med. J.*, **2**:1501.
Ridley, H. (1944), *Brit. J. Ophthalm.*, **28**:568.
Rogers, L. (1904a), *Brit. Med. J.*, **2**:670.
Rogers, L. (1904b), *Lancet*, **1**:349.
Rogers, L. (1905), *Brit. Med. J.*, **2**:1290.
Rosenfeld, G. (1963), Unfälle durch Giftschlangen, *in* "Die Giftschlangen der Erde," Behringwerk-Mitteilungen, N. G. Elwert Universitäts- und Verlags-Buchhandlung, Marburg/Lahn, p. 161.
Russell, F. E. (1961), *J. Amer. Med. Assoc.*, **177**:903.
Russell, F. E. (1967), *Toxicon*, **5**:39.
Russell, F. E. and L. Lauritzen (1966), *Trans. Roy. Soc. Trop. Med. Hyg.*, **60**:797.
Schöttler, W. H. A. (1954), *Am. J. Trop. Med. Hyg.*, **3**:1083.
Semenoff, E. (1912), Parallèle des venins de *Naja tripudians* et de *Crotalus adamanteus*, thèse, Fac. de Méd. Lausanne.
Shannon, F. A. (1956), Comments on the treatment of reptile poisoning, *in* "Venoms" (E. Buckley and N. Porges, eds.), American Association for the Advancement of Science, Washington, D.C., p. 405.
Shannon, F. A. (1961), *J. Amer. Med. Assn.*, **176**:387.
Shortt, J. (1882), *Lancet*, **1**:725.
Stahnke, H. L. and A. McBride, 1966, *J. Occup. Med.*, **8**:72.
Stahnke, H. L., F. M. Allen, R. V. Horan, and J. H. Tenery (1957), *Amer. J. Trop. Med. Hyg.*, **6**:323.
Swaroop, S. and B. Grab (1956), The snakebite mortality problem in the world, *in* "Venoms" (E. Buckley and N. Porges eds.), American Association for the Advancement of Science, Washington, D.C., p. 439.
Taub, A. M. (1964), *Toxicon*, **2**:71.
Tidswell, F. (1906), "Researches on Australian Venoms, Snake Bite, Snake Venom and Antivenin," Sydney.
Trethewie, E. R. and A. J. Day (1948a), *Austr. J. Exp. Biol. Med. Sci.*, **26**:37.
Trethewie, E. R. and A. J. Day (1948b), *Austr. J. Exp. Biol. Med. Sci.*, **26**:153.
Vick, J. A., P. Ciuchta, and J. H. Manthei (1967), Pathophysiological studies of ten snake venoms, *in* "Animal Toxins" (F. E. Russell and P. R. Saunders, eds.), Pergamon Press, London, p. 269.
Wig, K. L. and S. K. Vaish (1960), *J. Indian Med. Assn.*, **35**:307.

Chapter 2

Mode of Action of Cobra Venom and Its Purified Toxins

C. Y. Lee

Pharmacological Institute, College of Medicine
National Taiwan University, Taipei
Taiwan, China

I. INTRODUCTION

The cobra is a common snake throughout Asia and Africa. There are at least twelve cobra species in six genera; most of them are found in Africa, and only two species, *Naja naja* and *Ophiophagus hannah*, are present in Asia. However, many subspecies of *Naja naja* have been recognized in different parts of Asia, except Japan, Korea, and northern China (*see* Table I).

The literature reporting experimental work with cobra venom is prodigious. The venoms of *Naja naja*, *Naja naja atra*, *Naja haje*, *Naja nigricollis*, and *Hemachatus haemachatus* have been most extensively studied. Although the toxicity and other pharmacological properties, as well as the chemical constituents of cobra venom may vary quantitatively from one species to another, there appear to be no marked qualitative differences among venoms from different species so far studied. Therefore, the expression "cobra venom" will be retained in this review for description of various properties held in common.

Cobra venom, like the venom of most snakes, is a complex mixture, chiefly of proteins, many of which have enzymatic activities. Although the most toxic fractions have been shown to be neurotoxins, other constituents such as cardiotoxin and some of the enzymes certainly contribute to the overall toxicity of the venom. In addition, the envenomated organism may release several autopharmacologic substances which render study of the

21

Table I.
Classification and Distribution of Cobras[a]

Species	Common name	Distribution
Genus *Naja* Laurenti, 1768		
Naja naja	Indian cobra, Asiatic cobra	Indian subcontinent
Naja naja atra	Chinese cobra, Formosan cobra	South China east to Viet Nam, Thailand, Hainan, Taiwan
Naja naja kaouthia	Monocellate cobra	West Bengal, East Pakistan, Burma, Thailand, Malaya, Southwest China
Naja naja sputatrix	Malay cobra	Malay peninsula, Indonesia
Naja naja miolepis	Borneo cobra	Borneo, Palawan (Philippines)
Naja naja philippinensis	Philippine cobra	Philippines
Naja naja oxiana	Oxus cobra	Near and Middle East
Naja haje	Egyptian cobra	Northern Africa, Near and Middle East
Naja nigricollis	Spitting cobra	Savannah areas of Africa, southern of the Sahara
Naja nivea (*Naja flava*)	Yellow cobra, Cape cobra	Southern Africa, central southwest Africa
Naja melanoleuca	Forest cobra	Western and central Africa
Genus *Ophiophagus* Günther, 1864		
Ophiophagus hannah	King cobra	India, southeast Asia, Philippines
Genus *Hemachatus* Fleming, 1822		
Hemachatus haemachatus	Ringhals	Southern Africa
Genus *Boulengerina* Dollo, 1886		
Boulengerina annulata	Banded water cobra	Central Africa
Boulengerina christyi		″
Genus *Paranaja* Loveridge, 1944		
Paranaja multifasciata	Burrowing cobra	Western central Africa
Genus *Pseudohaje* Günther, 1858		
Pseudohaje goldii	Gold's tree cobra	Central and western Africa
Pseudohaje nigra		″

[a] Cited from "Poisonous Snakes of the World" (NAVMED P-5099).

pathogenesis of syndromes caused by the whole venom even more difficult. Indeed, the complexity of the venom actions is chiefly, if not entirely, due to combined effects of different components contained in the same venom. The success in isolation of cobra neurotoxin, cardiotoxin, phospholipase A, and other enzymes from cobra venom in pure or fairly pure state in recent years has made it possible to elucidate the mode of action of individual components, and thus contributed tremendously to better understanding of the pathogenesis of syndromes caused by the whole venom.

II. CHEMISTRY OF COBRA VENOM

The chemistry of snake venoms has been reviewed by Slotta (1955), Christensen (1955), Kaiser and Michl (1958), and more recently by Boquet (1966). Cobra venom contains about 90% proteins, most of which migrate toward the cathode on electrophoresis. Several biologically active components such as neurotoxin, cardiotoxin, direct lytic factor (DLF), cytotoxin, phospholipase A, and some proteins having other enzymatic activities have been separated from cobra venom.

A. Neurotoxins

In most animal species the main cause of death due to cobra venom is peripheral respiratory paralysis caused by neurotoxin(s) (*see* Sec. III, A,C). Cobra neurotoxin is a basic polypeptide, which is heat stable at acidic pHs. The content of the neurotoxin in Formosan cobra venom was found to be about 10% of the total protein (Lo *et al.*, 1966), but it may vary from one species to another. Moreover, there is ample evidence that more than one neurotoxin is present in the same venom (Porath, 1966; Lee *et al.*, 1968; Larsen and Wolff, 1968a).

1. Isolation and Nomenclature

Various early authors have prepared fractions of cobra venom with high toxicity and low enzymic activity by fractional precipitation, adsorption, electrodialysis, and electrophoresis. These preparations have been called "neurotoxin" without any specific proof of their purity (for references *see* the above-mentioned reviews).

From the venom of the Formosan cobra, Sasaki (1957a,b) prepared, by acetone and ammonium sulfate fractionation, a neurotoxin which is paper-electrophoretically homogeneous. Determination of its amino acid composition indicated a molecular weight of 6000. Its N-terminal and C-terminal amino acids were determined as leucine and glycine, respectively. More recently, Yang (1965) has succeeded in obtaining a neurotoxin in crystalline state from the same venom by ammonium sulfate fractionation followed by repeated chromatography on carboxymethyl (CM)-cellulose column, and named it "cobrotoxin." Its molecular weight was at first reported to be 11,000 but later calculated to be 6949 from amino acid composition (Yang *et al.*, 1969a). The same neurotoxin was also prepared by column chromatography on CM-Sephadex (Lo *et al.*, 1966), and contamination of phospholipase A in this neurotoxin could be eliminated by repeated rechromatography on CM-cellulose column (Hsieh and Lee, unpublished). Chromatographic fractionation of the same venom with sulphoethyl-Sephadex column has also been reported (Brisbois *et al.*, 1968).

A neurotoxin, called "toxin a," has been isolated from the venom of *Naja nigricollis* by ion-exchange chromatography on Amberlite IRC-50 (Karlsson *et al.*, 1966), and another neurotoxin, also called "toxin α" was recently isolated from the venom of *Naja haje haje* by gradient chromatography on Amberlite CG-50, followed by gel filtration on Sephadex G-50 (Botes and Strydom, 1969).

Among the three toxic fractions isolated from *Hemachatus haemachatus* venom, peaks 3 and 5 represent highly toxic neurotoxins (Porath, 1966), whereas peak 12 appears to be identical with the direct lytic factor (DLF) isolated from the same venom by Aloof-Hirsch *et al.* (1968), judging from the amino acid composition (*see* Table III).

2. *Amino Acid Composition and Sequence*

The amino acid compositions of five neurotoxins so far isolated from different cobra venoms are compared with those of neurotoxins isolated from sea-snake venoms in Table II. All of the cobra-neurotoxins are composed of 61–62 residues of 15 common amino acids but devoid of alanine, methionine, and phenylalanine. All of them consist of a single peptide chain cross-linked by four disulfide bonds and terminated by leucine and asparagine at its amino and carboxyl ends, respectively.

It is interesting to note that the neurotoxins isolated from sea-snake venoms (Tamiya and Arai, 1966; Tamiya and Sato, 1967; Sato and Tamiya, 1968) also consist of 61–62 amino acid residues in a single chain cross-linked by four disulfide bonds. The similarity in amino acid composition is also remarkable; they are all basic polypeptides and devoid of alanine and methionine in their molecules.

In Fig. 1, the amino acid sequences of three cobra neurotoxins, cobrotoxin from *Naja naja atra* (Yang *et al.*, 1969b), toxin α from *Naja haje haje* (Botes and Strydom, 1969) and toxin α from *Naja nigricollis* (Eaker and Porath, 1967), are compared with that of erabutoxin b from *Laticauda semifasciata* (Sato and Tamiya, 1968). It is evident that a remarkable degree of similarity exists, especially among the three cobra neurotoxins. The two α toxins are identical from the amino terminus to position 26 and also in their carboxyl terminal sequences from positions 52 to 61. In the region from position 27 to 51, only seven amino acid differences are found between the two neurotoxins. There are also only eight amino acid differences between cobrotoxin and toxin α from *Naja nigricollis* if serine at position 18 in cobrotoxin is disregarded. It is noteworthy that half-cystinyl residues in these neurotoxins which form four disulfide bonds for maintaining the

Table II.
Amino Acid Composition of Neurotoxins Isolated from Cobra and Sea-snake Venoms

Amino acid	Naja nigricollis (toxin α)	Naja haje haje (toxin α)	Naja naja atra (cobrotoxin)	Hemachatus haemachatus (peak 3)	Hemachatus haemachatus (peak 5)	Laticauda semifasciata (erabutoxin) a	Laticauda semifasciata (erabutoxin) b	Laticauda laticaudata (laticotoxin a)
Lysine	6	6	3	4	6	4	4	4
Histidine	2	2	2	2	2	1	2	2
Arginine	3	4	6	5	4	3	3	5
Aspartic acid	7	7	8	9	5	5	4	9
Threonine	8	7	8	7	9	5	5	4
Serine	2	4	4	3	4	8	8	5
Glutamic acid	6	7	7	5	8	8	8	7
Proline	5	4	2	5	4	4	4	5
Glycine	5	5	7	5	5	5	5	5
Alanine	0	0	0	0	0	0	0	0
Half-cystine	8	8	8	8	8	8	8	8
Valine	2	1	1	1	1	2	2	1
Methionine	0	0	0	0	0	0	0	0
Isoleucine	3	3	2	3	1	4	4	2
Leucine	2	1	1	2	2	1	1	1
Tyrosine	1	1	2	0	1	1	1	1
Phenylalanin	0	0	0	1	0	2	2	1
Tryptophane	1	1	1	1	1	1	1	1
Amide NH$_3$	7	9	9	10	8	10	10	
Total	61	61	62	61	61	62	62	61
N-terminal	Leucine	Leucine	Leucine			Arginine	Arginine	Arginine
C-terminal	Asparagine	Asparagine	Asparagine			Asparagine	Asparagine	Asparagine
Molecular weight	6787	6835	6949	6828	6823	6837	6857	6880
Reference	Karlson et al. (1966)	Botes and Strydom (1969)	Yang et al. (1969a)	Porath (1966)		Sato and Tamiya (1968)		Tamiya and Sato (1967)

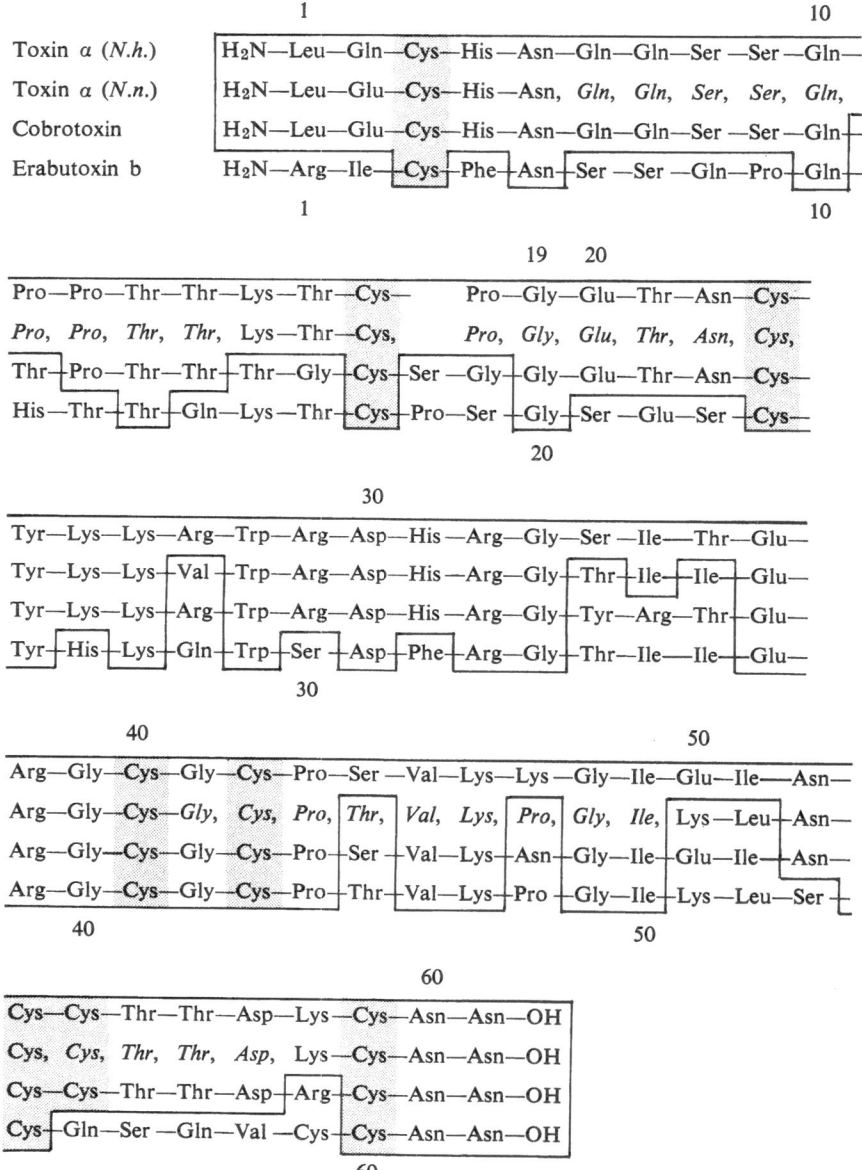

Fig. 1. Comparison of amino acid sequences of toxin α of *Naja haje haje* (*N.h.*) (Botes and Strydom, 1969), toxin α of *Naja nigricollis* (*N.n.*) (Eaker and Porath, 1967), cobrotoxin of *Naja naja atra* (Yang *et al.*, 1969) and erabutoxin b of *Laticauda semifasciata* (Sato and Tamiya, 1968). The parts of the *Naja nigricollis* toxin sequence in *italics* were assigned by similarity to the sequences of other two toxins.

polypeptides in their active conformation are in the same positions. The similarity in amino acid sequence is found not only among cobra neurotoxins but also between erabutoxin b on one hand and cobra neurotoxins on the other. Thus, 28 amino acid residues are found to be common to these neurotoxins, and seven out of eight half-cystinyl residues are in the same positions. Similar amino acids tend to be clustered together in their molecules, and the location of all of the half-cystinyl residues near the ends of the molecules leaves the center sequence from 24–25 to 39–40 free. It has been speculated that this central non-cross-linked sequence containing most of the basic amino acids and all of the aromatic amino acids in close order might be the "active site" of the neurotoxin molecules (Eaker and Porath, 1967).

None of these purified neurotoxins has been shown to be glycoprotein as reported by Braganca and Patel (1965). The low-molecular-weight toxins separated from the venoms of *Naja naja* and other cobras by thin-layer chromatography on silicic acid might be fragments of these larger neurotoxins (Fisher and Kabara, 1967), but so far no evidence has been obtained to support such a possibility.

B. Cardiotoxin, Cobramines, DLF, Toxin γ, and Cytotoxin

Cardiotoxin, cobramines A and B, direct lytic factor (DLF), toxin γ, and cytotoxin are all strongly basic polypeptides isolated from cobra venom. They are very closely related, if not entirely identical, and may be regarded as "isotoxins."

1. Cardiotoxin

A fraction producing systolic arrest of the isolated frog or mammalian heart was separated from Indian cobra venom by fractional precipitation and called "cardiotoxin" (Sarkar, 1947a). Sarkar (1947b) found its molecular weight to be about 46,200 by a diffusion method, but it was subsequently shown to be not a single protein (Raudonat and Holler, 1958; Tseng, 1964). Using gradient chromatography on a CM-Sephadex column, three cardiotoxic fractions were separated from the venom of *Naja naja atra* (Lo *et al.*, 1966), and the major fraction was called "cardiotoxin" (Lee *et al.*, 1968). Together they constitute more than 50% of the venom protein. After repeated rechromatography on a CM-cellulose column, this cardiotoxin was found to be free from phospholipase A activity, and its homogeneity was verified by microzone and disc gel electrophoresis, amino acid analysis, and endgroup analysis. Its molecular weight was about 6400 from equilibrium centrifugation measurements, and 6734 on the basis of amino acid analysis (60 residues) (Narita and Lee, 1970). Cardiotoxin was heat stable at acidic pHs but not at alkaline pHs.

2. *Cobramines A and B*

Two basic proteins that inhibit iodide accumulation by thyroid slices have been purified from *Naja naja* venom by CM-cellulose chromatography, gel filtration, and ammonium sulfate crystallization (Larsen and Wolff, 1968b). They were named cobramines A and B and together constitute about 40% of the venom protein. Their isoelectric points were 11.9 and 12.6, respectively. Cobramine B was found to be homogeneous on paper and disc gel electrophoresis and by ultracentrifugation ($S_{20,w} = 0.98$). Its molecular weight was 6400 by equilibrium centrifugation measurements and 5840 on the basis of amino acid analysis (52 residues).

3. *Direct Lytic Factor (DLF)*

The so-called "direct lytic factor" (DLF) of cobra venom is also one of the strongly basic polypeptides, first separated by paper electrophoresis from the venoms of *Naja naja* and *Hemachatus haemachatus* (Condrea *et al.*, 1964), and recently purified by successive application of trichloroacetic acid and salt precipitation from the venom of *Hemachatus haemachatus* (Aloof-Hirsch *et al.*, 1968). The purified DLF was homogeneous by ultracentrifugal and electrophoretic criteria. It consisted of 57 amino acid residues in a single chain cross-linked by four disulfide bridges and terminated by leucine and serine at its amino and carboxyl ends, respectively. Its molecular weight determined by Yphantis technique was 7000. The hemolytic activity of DLF was rather low, particularly when compared to the corresponding substance, melittin, from bee (*Apis mellifera*) venom (Slotta *et al.*, 1967). Although DLF from cobra venom and melittin are both strong basic polypeptides and share a variety of pharmacological effects, they do not appear to be identical, since the molecular weight of melittin is only 2850 and its amino acid composition is also different from that of DLF (Habermann and Reiz, 1965; Habermann and Jentsch, 1967).

4. *Toxin γ*

From the venom of *Naja nigricollis* another basic polypeptide, in addition to toxin α, called toxin γ, has recently been isolated by Sephadex G-75 gel filtration and gradient chromatography on Biorex 70 (Izard *et al.*, 1969a). Toxin γ was homogeneous on disc gel electrophoresis and by ultracentrifugation ($S_{20,w} = 0.891$). Its molecular weight was about the same as that of toxin α. Toxin γ was found to be cardiotoxic but devoid of any lytic effect on human erythrocytes even in the presence of phospholipase A (Izard *et al.*, 1969b).

5. *Cytotoxin*

A cytotoxic protein, selectively destructive to Yoshida sarcoma cells and relatively nontoxic to animals, has been separated from *Naja naja* venom by gradient chromatography on CM-cellulose column after $HClO_4$ treatment, followed by ammonium sulfate fractionation, Sephadex G-50 gel filtration, and acetone precipitation, successively (Braganca *et al.*, 1967). The cytotoxin migrated as a single band in agarose electrophoresis, and the isoelectric point was above 9.4. The molecular weight was estimated to be 10,500 by gel filtration on Sephadex G-50 and G-75 columns. The cytotoxin was stable to heat and acid or alkali treatment. The purified cytotoxin was found to be devoid of direct lytic effect on human and rat erythrocytes.

Table III.
Amino Acid Composition of Cardiotoxin, Cobramine B, and DLF

Amino acid	Cardiotoxin (*Naja naja atra*)	Cobramine B (*Naja naja*)	DLF (*Hemachatus haemachatus*)	Peak 12 (DLF ?) (*Hemachatus haemachatus*)
Lysine	9	8	10	11
Histidine	0	0	1	1
Arginine	2	2	1	1
Aspartic acid	6	5	6	6
Threonine	3	3	3	3
Serine	2	2	3	3
Glutamic acid	0	0	1	1
Proline	5	4	5	5
Glycine	2	2	2	2
Alanine	2	2	1	1
Half-cystine	8	6	8	8
Valine	7	6	4	4
Methionine	2	2	2	3
Isoleucine	1	1	2	2
Leucine	6	5	6	7
Tyrosine	3	3	1	1
Phenylalanine	2	1	1	1
Tryptophan	0	0	0	0
Amide NH_3	3	3–4	7	4
Total	60	52	57	60
N-terminal	Leucine		Leucine	
C-terminal	Asparagine		Serine	
Molecular weight	6734	5840	6334	6707
Reference	Narita and Lee (1970)	Larsen and Wolff (1968)	Aloof-Hirsch *et al.* (1968)	Porath (1966)

6. Identification of DLF, Cobramines, Toxin γ, and Cytotoxin with Cardiotoxin

The possibility was first suggested by Meldrum (1965a) that DLF is identical with cardiotoxin. Slotta and Vick (1969) have found that the most basic polypeptide isolated from *Naja naja* venom by chromatography on a CM-Sephadex column comprises the total, rather low, direct lytic activity and also the total, very strong, cardiotoxic activity of the cobra venom. They suggested, therefore, that it should be named "cardiotoxin" rather than DLF. Similarly, cobramines A and B isolated from the same venom have been shown to possess a weak hemolytic as well as cardiotoxic activity (Larsen and Wolff, 1967b, 1968a). Lee *et al.*, (1970) also found that the cardiotoxin isolated from *Naja naja atra* venom has a weak direct hemolytic activity on washed erythrocytes of the guinea-pig and cat, but not on those of rabbit, rat, mouse and goat. Both the contracture-inducing and direct-lytic activities of cardiotoxin can be potentiated by phospholipase A and prevented by polyanions (gangliosides, RNA, and heparin), as in the case of the inhibition of iodide accumulation in thyroid slices by cobramine B (Wolff *et al.*, 1968). Moreover, as shown in Table III, the amino acid composition of cardiotoxin was recently found to be very similar to that of cobramine B and DLF (Narita and Lee, 1970). Both cardiotoxin and cobramine B are devoid of histidine, glutamic acid, and tryptophan in their molecules. All these findings indicate that cardiotoxin, cobramine B, and DLF are at least biologically identical, and that cardiotoxin from different venoms may vary in its amino acid composition, just as in the case of cobra neurotoxin.

On the other hand, both toxin γ and cytotoxin have been claimed to be devoid of direct lytic effect on human and rat erythrocytes (Izard *et al.*, 1969b; Braganca *et al.*, 1967). However, since both rat and human erythrocytes are also rather resistant to cardiotoxin (Lee *et al.*, 1970), it remains to be shown that these two basic polypeptides are really different from DLF or cardiotoxin.

C. Enzymes

The enzymes of snake venoms and their biological significance have been reviewed by Zeller (1948, 1951), Meldrum (1965a), and Boquet (1964, 1966). Cobra venom contains a variety of enzymes, such as phospholipase A, acetylcholinesterase, phosphodiesterase, phosphomonoesterase, 5'-nucleotidase, glycerophosphatase, ATPase, L-amino acid oxidase, peptidases, and hyaluronidase (Suzuki and Iwanaga, 1958; Yang *et al.*, 1959; Detrait *et al.*, 1959; Bjork and Boman, 1959; Bjork, 1961; Master and Rao, 1961; Lo *et al.*, 1966). The distribution pattern of enzymes in cobra venom differs from that of crotalid or viperid venoms in at least two aspects: (1) the presence of acetylcholinesterase, and (2) little or no proteinase (Tu *et al.*,

1965; Suzuki, 1966). Among these enzymes, some have been claimed to contribute to "neurotoxicity" and others to circulatory effects of the venom. The toxicity of enzymes is mostly the result of their action on substrates. The destruction of the substrate itself may be responsible for the effects observed, or the effects may be mediated by compounds liberated in the course of the enzymic reaction.

1. Phospholipase A (Phosphatide Acyl-hydrolase, EC 3.1.1.4)

Two excellent reviews on venom phospholipase A have recently appeared (Condrea and De Vries, 1965; Meldrum, 1965a). This enzyme catalyzes the hydrolysis of one ester bond at the β position of phosphatide molecules with formation of lysophosphatides and release of free fatty acids, mostly unsaturated. The unique feature of phospholipase A is that both products of its hydrolytic action are pharmacologically active and potentially toxic (see Sec. III). The enzyme is not uniform, even in one given venom; several isozymes seem to exist in cobra venom which can be separated but which have only small differences in their actions (Wakui and Kawachi, 1961; Bjork, 1961; Neelin, 1963; Braganca and Sambray, 1967). Dawson (1963) found that a phospholipase from Naja naja venom had an isoelectric point at pH 5.2, as compared with values of 8.55 and 8.62 found by De (1944) for crystalline "hemolysin" prepared from the same venom. The molecular weight of the crystalline phospholipase A isolated from the same venom by ammonium sulfate fractionation and chromatography on CM-Sephadex C-25 has been estimated to be approximately 24,000 (Currie et al., 1968). Phospholipase A is remarkably heat stable at pHs below 5.9, but is inactivated by boiling at pHs higher than 7 (Hughes, 1935; Lin and Chang, 1957; Rimon and Schapiro, 1959).

2. Phospholipases B (EC 3.1.1.5) and C (EC 3.1.4.3)

Phospholipase B splits off the fatty acid of α-acyl lysophosphatide, whereas phospholipase C effects hydrolytic rupture of diesteratic phosphorus with formation of a diglyceride. Phospholipase B activity has recently been demonstrated in a wide range of snake venoms including Naja naja venom (Doery and Pearson, 1964), but not in the venom of Hemachatus haemachatus (Klibansky and De Vries, 1964). Nothing is known of its pharmacology.

Phospholipase C activity has recently been demonstrated in the cytotoxic protein of Naja naja venom (Braganca and Khandeparkar, 1966), but other authors were unable to detect it in the venom of Naja naja atra (Hsieh and Lee, unpublished). This enzyme has striking pharmacological effects including hemolysis, increase of serum potassium, increase of capillary permeability, and effects on smooth and skeletal muscle in vitro (Habermann, 1960; Habermann and Krusche, 1962; Albuquerque and Thesleff, 1967).

3. *Acetylcholinesterase (EC 3.1.1.7)*

Hydrolysis of acetylcholine by *Naja naja* venom was first demonstrated by Iyergar *et al.* (1938). They suggested that the neurotoxin of cobra venom is probably identical to the cholinesterase of cobra venom. However, subsequent authors noticed that the neurotoxin of cobra venom does not have any cholinesterase activity (Ghosh *et al.*, 1939; Sarkar *et al.*, 1942). Moreover, cholinesterase is completely inactivated by heating at 60°C for 10 min, whereas the neurotoxin is heat stable (Chang and Lee, 1955). This enzyme is found in all elapid venoms but not in the Viperidae, Crotalidae, or Hydrophiidae (Zeller, 1947, 1948). Studies of the substrate specificity of the enzyme have shown it to be an acetylcholinesterase (Zeller, 1947; Bovet-Nitti, 1947; Chaudhuri, 1949; Mounter, 1951; Augustinsson, 1951; Chang and Lee, 1955).

The instability of acetylcholinesterase of cobra venom was found to be due to coexistence of an inactivating factor (Chang and Lee, 1955). This anticholinesterase factor is heat labile and is reversibly inhibited by various cations, especially magnesium (Lee *et al.*, 1956). This factor is not effective against the cholinesterase activity of mammalian tissue preparations.

4. *Phosphodiesterase (Orthophosphoric Diester Phosphohydrolase, EC 3.1.4.1)*

This enzyme acts as an exonucleotidase, releasing 5'-nucleotides in a sequential fashion from polynucleotides (Bjork, 1961; Bjork and Boman, 1959; Razzell and Khorana 1959a, 1959b; Felix *et al.*, 1960; Williams *et al.*, 1960). It has been suggested that this enzyme is also responsible for the ATP pyrophosphohydrolase and the dinucleotide nucleotidehydrolase (nucleotide pyrophosphatase) activity of venoms (Bjork and Boman, 1959). The optimum activity is around pH 9.0, both for calcium di-*p*-nitrophenyl phosphate and for DNA.

The possibility has been suggested that venom phosphodiesterase may be responsible for the immediate fall in blood pressure following the intravenous injection of many venoms (*see* Meldrum, 1965a). Adenosine 5'-phosphate (formed by the action of venom phosphodiesterase) and adenosine (formed by the further action of 5'-nucleotidase) both produce in cats and dogs a transient fall in blood pressure with a time course closely resembling that produced by venoms or phosphodiesterase preparations (Green and Stoner, 1950; Angelakos and Glassman, 1965).

5. *Phosphomonoesterase (Orthophosphoric Monoester Phosphohydrolase, EC 3.1.3.1)*

This nonspecific alkaline monophosphatase was detected in a variety of snake venoms by Gulland and Jackson (1938a). It hydrolyses 3'-AMP nearly as fast as 5'-AMP and also releases phosphate from ATP, ribose 5-phosphate, dinucleotides, etc. It shows optimum activity at pH 9.5. It is present in much greater amounts in cobra venom than in crotalid venoms (Richards *et al.*, 1965). Nothing is known about its pharmacology.

6. 5'-Nucleotidase (5'-Ribonucleotide Phosphohydrolase, EC 3.1.3.5)

5'-Nucleotidase (or AMPase) is known to occur in various animal tissues, bacteria, potato, and in all snake venoms so far tested (Gulland and Jackson, 1938b; Zeller 1950; Sulkowski *et al.*, 1963). It hydrolyses 5'-mononucleotides to the ribonucleoside and orthophosphate. The purified enzyme from *Naja naja atra* venom has a molecular weight of about 10,000. It shows optimum activity at pH 6.5–7.0, is activated by Mg^{2+} or Mn^{2+} and inhibited by Zn^{2+} or Ni^{2+}. It is completely inactivated by heating at 80°C for 2 min (Chen and Lo, 1968). Purified 5'-nucleotidase from *Hemachatus haemachatus* venom has a pH optimum between 8.0 and 9.0, and is inactivated at 60°C at pH 6.0 or 9.0 (Bjork, 1964). 5'-Nucleotides are produced by the action of venom phosphodiesterase on naturally occurring substrates, and secondary pharmacological effect could follow their conversion to nucleosides.

7. ATP Pyrophosphohydrolase (α-β-"ATPase," EC 3.6.1.8)

Many venoms rapidly convert ATP to AMP and pyrophosphate (Zeller, 1950; Johnson *et al.*, 1953; Yang and Chang, 1954; Kaye, 1960), and this activity has been assigned to an α-β-"ATPase." It displays many features in common with phosphodiesterase, including optimum activity near pH 9.0, marked activation by Mg^{2+} and less by Ca^{2+}, and complete inactivation on heating to 60°C for 15 min at pH 8.3. It has been suggested that this enzyme may play a part in toxic effects, especially if the other phosphatases assist by destroying substances as important for the resynthesis of ATP as glucosephosphate and NAD (Zeller, 1951).

D. Nonproteins

A nonprotein fraction with maximum absorbance at 252 mμ has been separated from Formosan cobra venom (Lo *et al.*, 1966) and subsequently identified as a mixture of guanosine, adenosine, and inosine (Lo and Chen, 1966). Cholesterol, free lecithin, and protein-bound lecithin have been also found in Indian cobra venom (Ganguly and Malkana, 1936).

Of inorganic substances, the zinc content is rather high (5 mg/g) in cobra venom and lower in krait, viper, and other venoms (Delezenne, 1919; Ray, 1940; Kaye, 1955). Zn^{2+} is a powerful inhibitor of 5'-nucleotidase and ATPase. Possibly, by inhibiting the phosphatases and other enzymes, it protects the venom gland from damage by its own secretion (Fleckenstein

Table
The Lethal Doses (mg/kg) of Venoms from

Venom	Mouse		LD$_{50}$ iv	Rat sc	Minimal lethal			
					Guinea pig		Rabbit	
	sc	ip			sc	ip or iv	sc	iv
Naja naja	0.45[h]	0.35[j] 0.7[n]	0.25[a] 0.276[w] 0.32[b] 0.39[f] 0.45[n]	0.66[c]	0.3[d] 0.4[c]	0.2[d] iv	0.3[d] 0.5[c]	0.2[d]
Naja naja atra	0.63[s] 0.67[r]	0.44[s] 0.6[j]	0.395[p]	0.7[u]	0.15[u] 0.2[x]	0.15[x] ip	0.2[x] 0.35[u]	0.1[x]
Ophiophagus hannah		2.0[j]						
Naja nivea	0.65[m] 0.72[h]	0.6[j]	0.2[a] 0.57[h]	0.2[m] 0.75[i]	0.4[m]		0.33[m]	0.15[e] 0.15[m]
Naja haje	1.7[h] 2.5[m]	1.3[j]	0.42[f] 0.6[a] 1.24[h]	1.5[m]	0.8[m]			0.6[l]
Naja nigricollis	2.5[m] 2.8[h]	3.0[j]	0.6[a] 0.62[b] 0.71[f] 1.4[h]	1.5[m]	0.8[m]		1.6[m]	0.35[o] 0.53[m] 0.8[l]
Hemachatus haemachatus	1.8[h] 3.7[m]	1.5[j] 1.5[n]	0.38[a] 0.75[n] 1.7[h]	1.25[m] 1.6[k]	0.6[m]		1.33[m] 1.0[k]	0.5[e] 0.6[m] 0.65[l]

[a] Boquet (unpublished).
[b] Boquet *et al.* (1967a).
[c] Calmette (1907).
[d] Césari and Boquet (1936).
[e] Césari and Boquet (1937).
[f] Cheymol *et al.* (1967).
[g] Chopra and Iswariah (1931).
[h] Christensen (1966) (calculated from dose/animal to dose/kg).
[i] Epstein (1930).
[j] Fischer and Kabara (1967).
[k] Fraser and Gunn (1909).
[l] Grasset and Christensen (1947) (calculated from dose/animal to dose/kg).

IV.
Different Cobras for Various Animals

dose (MLD) (LD$_{50}$–LD$_{100}$)

Cat		Dog		Monkey		Pigeon		Fowl	Frog
sc or im	iv	sc	iv	sc	iv	sc or im	iv	sc	sc
1.5–2^g im	1.0^t 1.04^t	0.8^c	0.15^v	0.35^v	0.2^v	0.5^g im			10^c
25^u sc	1.0^p	0.6^u		0.4^u		0.4^x sc 0.43^q sc 0.5^u sc		0.4^u	40^x 70^u
			1.5^v						
3.5^t sc	1.5^t		0.5^v			1.25^m sc	0.25^m	0.5^m	4^m
			1.75^v			2.5^m sc	0.75^m	1.5^m	
			0.6^v				0.33^m	1.25^m	
15^k sc			1.5^v			1.9^m sc 3.3^k sc	0.63^m	1.25^m	1.2^k

^{m} Grasset *et al.* (1935) (calculated from dose/animal to dose/kg).
^{n} Grotto (unpublished).
^{o} Guyot and Boquet (1960).
^{p} Lee (unpublished).
^{q} Lee and Tseng (1969).
^{r} Lee *et al.* (1962).
^{s} Lee *et al.* (1968).
^{t} Macht (1936).
^{u} Oh (1942).
^{v} Vick (unpublished).
^{w} Vick *et al.* (1967).
^{x} Yamaguti (1923).

and Gerhardt, 1952; Fleckenstein and Jaeger, 1952). Protein-bound copper was found in *Naja naja* venom at a concentration of 1.1–1.6 mg/g (Gitter *et al.*, 1963). Besides, Mg, Ca, K, Na, Cl, SO_4, and P_2O_5 have been detected in the ash of Formosan cobra venom (Ueda *et al.*, 1951).

III. PHARMACOLOGICAL ACTIONS OF COBRA VENOM

A. Toxicity, Symptoms Produced in Animals, and Cause of Death

1. Toxicity

An impression of the toxicity of venoms from different cobras for a number of laboratory animals may be obtained from Table IV, which summarizes the findings of different workers. Although the figures recorded are not strictly comparable, certain conclusions may be drawn from the table: (1) the venoms of *Naja naja*, *Naja naja atra*, and *Naja nivea* appear to be more toxic than those of *Naja haje*, *Naja nigricollis*, and *Hemachatus haemachatus*, although the differences among venoms from different cobras are not great (*see* also Christensen, 1955); (2) the lethal doses by different routes of administration are very close in most animals, except in the cat, indicating fast absorption of the venom component (neurotoxin) which is responsible for the respiratory paralysis; (3) there are no great differences in susceptibility to cobra venom among most laboratory animals except the cat and the frog. The cat is highly resistant to cobra venom if given subcutaneously (Oh, 1942), because its skeletal muscle is highly resistant to the neuromuscular blocking action of cobra neurotoxin (Lee and Tseng, 1969). If given intravenously, cobra venom causes circulatory failure rather than respiratory paralysis in the cat (Epstein, 1930; Lee and Peng, 1961). On the other hand, the frog is quite resistant to cobra venom, most probably because of the unique cutaneous respiratory mechanism of this animal, which precludes skeletal muscle paralysis as a primary cause of death.

Among the components separated from cobra venom, the neurotoxin is most toxic, being about 6–10 times more toxic than the original venom when assayed in mice (Peng, 1951; Yang, 1965; Su *et al.*, 1967; Karlsson *et al.*, 1966). If assayed in frogs, however, the lethality of the neurotoxin is no greater than that of the whole venom (Peng, 1951; Su *et al.*, 1967). The neurotoxin may also lack a high lethal index in cats. In contrast, phospholipase A, which is almost nontoxic to mice, is quite toxic to cats (Lee *et al.*, unpublished). The toxic effects of phospholipase A have been shown to be due to liberation of pharmacologically active substances such as histamine, 5-hydroxytryptamine and slow-reacting substance (SRS) in the animal body, and mice appear to be resistant to such autopharmacological reactions. On the other hand, cardiotoxin is toxic to both mice and cats, although its lethality in mice is much lower than that of crude venom (Lee *et al.*, 1968). The high ratio between subcutaneous LD_{50} and intraperitoneal LD_{50} of cardiotoxin can be accounted for by its slow absorption from the subcutaneous tissue (Tseng *et al.*, 1968).

2. Symptoms Produced in Warm-blooded Animals

Flaccid paralysis is the outstanding feature of poisoning with cobra venom (Brunton and Fayrer, 1873; Fraser and Gunn, 1909; Epstein, 1930; Iwase 1933; Césari and Boquet, 1936; 1937; Peng, 1951). After an initial period of restlessness and excitement, probably due to local irritation, the animal becomes dull and drowsy, with unsteady movements and dropping head. The movements of the head are typical in the rabbit; the head gradually sinks lower and lower, to be raised again in one quick movement when it almost touches the ground. This repeats itself until the head can no longer be supported, at which stage the respirations are markedly labored and froth may be seen around the mouth and nostrils. Death, often heralded by asphyxial convulsions, is due to respiratory paralysis in most animals except the cat; the heart continues to beat for some time after cessation of the respiratory movements.

3. Cause of Death

Although many early workers (Ragotzi, 1890; Arthus, 1910; Cushny and Yagi, 1918; Kellaway and Holden, 1932; Kellaway *et al.*, 1932; Gautrelet *et al.*, 1934) supported the view that peripheral paralysis of the respiratory muscles is the primary cause of death in cobra venom poisoning, other workers have claimed a direct action on the respiratory center to be more important (Elliot, 1905; Rogers, 1905; Fraser and Gunn, 1909; Chopra and Iswariah, 1931; Venkatachalam and Ratnagiriswaran, 1934) or possibly equally important (Brunton and Fayrer, 1874; Vollmer, 1893; Epstein, 1930; Bicher, 1966). The criticisms of the theory include observations that stimulation of the phrenic nerve in the animal dead from cobra venom produces a perceptible contraction of the diaphragm—but the same is true after poisoning with curare (Kellaway *et al.*, 1932)—and that direct application of smaller doses of the venom to the floor of the fourth ventricle produces respiratory arrest. However, subsequent evidence clearly established that the respiratory failure produced by the venom stems from a peripheral action (Kellaway *et al.*, 1932; Lee and Peng, 1961; Vick *et al.*, 1965). Thus, action potentials can be recorded from the phrenic nerve even after complete disappearance of the electromyograms (EMG) of the diaphragm and intercostal muscle. The intensity of the action potentials increases during asphyxia produced by interrupting artificial respiration or during the administration of 5% CO_2, thus demonstrating the persistence of central respiratory control. The continued activity of the central respiratory mechanism is also indicated by the presence of Hering–Breuer reflex in the paralyzed, artificially respired animal (Cushny and Yagi, 1918; Kellaway *et al.*, 1932).

B. Absorption, Distribution, and Fate

1. Absorption

Barnes and Trueta (1941) stated that cobra venom is readily absorbed from the subcutaneous tissue into the blood stream by passing through the capillary wall, whereas black tiger snake and Russell's viper venoms, whose molecular weights exceed 20,000, are absorbed by the lymph stream.

A recent study by Tseng *et al.* (1968), using ^{131}I-labeled cobra venom and its purified toxins, revealed that absorption of cardiotoxin after subcutaneous injection is very slow (about 30% within 4 hr), while absorption of the neurotoxin is much faster (about 60% within 2 hr). Since the molecular weights of both cobra neurotoxin and cardiotoxin have been estimated to be about 7000 the delay of absorption of cardiotoxin appears to be due not to the difference in the route of absorption but rather due to its strong affinity for the tissue.

Literature on the absorption of cobra venom by the oral route is contradictory. While many authors believed that snake venom introduced by the oral route is not toxic (Fraser, 1897a, 1897b; Buglia and Barbieri, 1923; Epstein, 1930; Chopra and Iswariah, 1931), several authors claimed that cobra venom produces a lethal effect in rabbits and guinea pigs when given by mouth or by stomach tube in sufficiently large doses (Brunton and Fayrer, 1874; Macht and Kehoe, 1943; Christensen, 1955). In view of the fact that both the neurotoxin and cardiotoxin of cobra venom are basic polypeptides, absorption of cobra venom from the intact gastrointestinal tract should be extremely slow, if not impossible. Moreover, the venom may be destroyed by the proteolytic enzymes of the gastrointestinal tract.

2. Distribution

The highest concentration of radioactivity is found in kidneys, with marked localization in the cortex, when labeled cobra venom is injected into animals (Sumyk *et al.*, 1963; Tseng *et al.*, 1968). Relatively high levels of radioactivity are also found in spleen, liver, and lungs. After intravenous injection, the plasma level of cardiotoxin declines much faster than that of the neurotoxin, probably due to its uptake by various organs. The pattern of distribution of the neurotoxin is quite different from that of cardiotoxin. The concentrations of the neurotoxin in various organs are rather uniformly low, except in kidney, where a very high amount is found. Radioautography shows that the neurotoxin, like *d*-tubocurarine (Waser and Lüthi, 1957) and α-bungarotoxin (Lee and Tseng, 1966), localizes in the motor endplate zone of the diaphragm, whereas cardiotoxin spreads widely over the whole diaphragm. The brain and cerebrospinal fluid levels of both toxins are extremely low, probably as a result of the blood–brain barrier (Tseng *et al.*, 1968).

3. Fate and Excretion

Although no information is yet available as to the metabolic changes of cobra venom and its components, there is some indication that the neurotoxin may be partly metabolized in the body. Shü *et al* (1968) showed that most of the radioactivity excreted in the urine 20 min post-injection is in the intact cobrotoxin fraction, whereas half of the radioactivity appears in the free iodine fraction in the urine collected 4 hr after injection. The excretion of the neurotoxin, either unchanged or metabolized, appears to be quite fast; about 30% within 2 hr (Tseng *et al.*, 1968) and 70% within 5 hr (Shü *et al.*, 1968). The excretion of cardiotoxin is much slower, probably as a result of its fixation by various tissues (Tseng *et al.*, 1968).

C. Actions on Neuromuscular Junction, Skeletal Muscle, and Nerve

1. Action on Neuromuscular Junction

Although it had been known for many decades that cobra venom had a curare-like action (for references, *see* Meldrum, 1965a), the precise mode of action of the venom has not been elucidated until recent years, largely because of complexity of the venom compositions. Thanks to recent advances in separation methods, it became possible to use purified neurotoxin, cardiotoxin, and certain enzymes such as phospholipase A, to study their effects on neuromuscular transmission.

As summarized by Jiménez-Porras in his recent review (1968), the neuromuscular blocking action of cobra venom differs from that of curare in its slowness of onset, in the absence (or slowness) of reversibility, in the imperfect or transient antagonism by anticholinesterases, and in eliciting no or a nontypical Wedensky inhibition. High concentrations of cobra venom also depress the contraction of directly stimulated muscles and evoke a contracture on isolated preparations, probably as a result of depolarization of muscle membrane (Meldrum, 1965b; Chang and Lee, 1966). Despite all of these differences, several authors have presented evidence that cobra venom induces a neuromuscular block of the nondepolarizing type just like that of curare.

Formosan cobra (*Naja naja atra*) venom reduces the endplate depolarization by acetylcholine in the toad sartorius muscle, while leaving the depolarization by KCl unaffected. This antidepolarizing effect is additive to that of curare and is antagonized by anticholinesterase agents (Peng, 1960). The same venom blocks the contracture of frog rectus abdominis produced by acetylcholine but does not affect the contracture by KCl. Saturation with curare can protect frog rectus muscle from irreversible paralysis by this venom (Su, 1960). *Naja naja* venom blocks the depolarizing action of carbachol in the rat diaphragm (Meldrum, 1965b). The same venom, as well as venoms of *Naja haje* and *Naja nigricollis*, depresses the contracture of the denervated rat hemidiaphragm produced by acetylcholine without affecting the contractions due to direct stimulations (Cheymol *et al.*, 1966, 1967).

The consensus that cobra venom has a postsynaptic site of action has been further supported by experiments with purified cobra neurotoxin (Lee, 1963; Chang and Lee, 1966; Su *et al.*, 1967). Unlike the crude venom, cobra neurotoxin isolated from the venom of *Naja naja atra* blocks neuromuscular transmission without causing muscle contracture or inhibition of the muscle response to direct stimulation, even with high concentrations. The blockade produced by the neurotoxin can be reversed by neostigmine or repeated washing. Wedensky inhibition is observed after partial recovery of the muscle twitches from prolonged contact with and subsequent removal of the neurotoxin. Unlike the crude venom, it does not inhibit the acetylcholine release from motor nerve endings. Whereas the crude venom shifts the acetylcholine dose-response curve of the frog rectus abdominis to the right with the slope declined, and anticholinesterase agents antagonize its effect only partially (Su, 1960), the neurotoxin shifts the curve in parallel to the right without any changes in its slope, and the shift is completely reversed by neostigmine (Su *et al.*, 1967). These results are essentially similar to those obtained with *d*-tubocurarine, suggesting a competition for the acetylcholine receptor site. Pretreatment with *d*-tubocurarine can protect the chick biventer cervicis muscle from the neuromuscular blocking action of cobra neurotoxin. This protection also suggests that the same receptor sites in the subsynaptic membrane are involved in the action of curare and cobra neurotoxin.

The results of electrophysiological studies by Chang and Lee (1966) further indicate that the effect of cobra neurotoxin on neuromuscular junctions is essentially the same as that of *d*-tubocurarine. The neurotoxin depresses endplate potentials (epps) without affecting the terminal nerve spike, resting membrane potential, and action potential of the muscle. The epps of the neurotoxin-paralyzed muscles are increased in their size and prolonged in their time-course by neostigmine. The amplitude of successive epps on repetitive stimulation declines rapidly, as in the curarized muscle (Wedensky inhibition).

The similarity between the actions of cobra neurotoxin and those of *d*-tubocurarine is further observed in their inhibitory effect on the antidromic activities of motor nerve fibers in the presence of anticholinesterase agents (Chang and Lee, 1966). The significance of this presynaptic site of action in the mechanism of neuromuscular block by d-tubocurarine has been disputed (*see* Karczmar, 1967), but since the orthodromic neuromuscular transmission remains unaffected when antidromic discharges are abolished (Feng and Li, 1941; Riker *et al.*, 1959; Chang and Lee, 1966), it is unlikely that this presynaptic action is the major mechanism of neuromuscular block by cobra neurotoxin or by d-tubocurarine.

Russell (1967) concluded that the major mechanism of blocking activity of the venoms of three cobras (*Naja nigricollis*, *Naja naja*, and *Ophiophagus hannah*) is presynaptic rather than postsynaptic, since following a complete block of the indirectly stimulated spikes, the crustacean muscle still responds to glutamate (Parnas and Russell, 1967). However, their findings simply indicate that the receptor site sensitive to glutamate in the crustacean muscle is not blocked by cobra venom, and this is not surprising since, as discussed above, the receptor site which cobra neurotoxin blocks is cholinoceptive and the mode of neuromuscular transmission of the crustacean muscle is quite different from that of other species; in the crustacean muscle the neuromuscular transmission is possibly mediated by glutamate (Takeuchi and Takeuchi, 1964). Indeed, the crustacean muscle is apparently quite resistant to "neurotoxic" effects of cobra and other elapid venoms, judging from the experimental results. The block of the indirectly stimulated spikes observed in the crustacean muscle preparation might be due to conduction block of the motor nerve, probably due to component(s) other than neurotoxin, since the compound action potential of the limb nerve was also blocked by the same concentration of the venom tested (Parnas and Russell, 1967).

While it has been shown that β-bungarotoxin isolated from the venom of *Bungarus multicinctus* acts presynaptically, reducing the acetylcholine output from the nerve endings and leaving the sensitivity of the endplate to acetylcholine unaffected (Chang and Lee, 1963, Lee and Chang, 1966), so far no neurotoxin with similar mode of action has been isolated from any cobra venom. Although high concentrations of crude cobra venom diminish the acetylcholine output of rat diaphragm, the purified neurotoxin does not (Lee, 1963; Su *et al.*, 1967). Recent work by Lee *et al.* (to be published) reveals that the diminution of acetylcholine output is due to conduction block of the phrenic nerve caused by both phospholipase A and cardiotoxin.

The species difference in lethality to cobra venom has been attributed to different susceptibility of the skeletal muscle to cobra neurotoxin (Lee and Tseng, 1969). Cats are very resistant to cobra venom if given subcutaneously, since the skeletal muscle of cats is highly resistant to the neuromuscular blocking action of cobra neurotoxin. Cats are also more resistant to d-tubocurarine than other mammals (Zaimis, 1957), although the difference appears not as great as in the case of cobra venom.

It is interesting from the pharmacological point of view that *d*-tubocurarine and cobra neurotoxin have so many actions in common, although their chemical structures are quite different. Cobra neurotoxin is a basic polypeptide, having a molecular weight of about 7000 (*see* Sec. II A). The slowness of onset and the lesser reversibility of the paralysis by cobra neurotoxin as compared with *d*-tubocurarine can be accounted for by its large molecular size. It has four disulfide linkages which are essential for the polypeptide to be active (Slotta and Fraenkel-Conrat, 1938; Lee *et al.*, 1960; Yang, 1967). High contents of basic amino acids in the molecule and loss of activity after masking either amino groups or guanidyl groups (Lee *et al.*, 1960) are suggestive of the participation of these basic groups in the neuromuscular blocking action of cobra neurotoxin.

2. *Direct Action on Skeletal Muscle*

High concentrations of cobra venom produce muscle fibrillation and contractures, and depress direct excitability of the skeletal muscle (Cushny and Yagi, 1918; Houssay and Pavé, 1922; Houssay *et al.*, 1922; Epstein, 1930; Kellaway and Holden, 1932; Sarkar and Maitra, 1950; Su, 1960). Houssay and his collaborators (1922, 1925) found that cobra venom or lysolecithin applied to frog skeletal muscle produced contractures, loss of excitability, muscle swelling, and release of potassium and inorganic phossphate. A compound resembling lysolecithin could be prepared from muscle treated with venom. On the basis of these findings, Houssay (1930) concluded that phospholipase A was responsible for the direct action of cobra venom on muscle. Tobias (1955), from experiments with cobra venom that had been heated at low pH, also claimed that phospholipase A depolarizes frog skeletal muscle and lobster giant axons. However, subsequent authors (Meldrum, 1965b; Chang and Lee, 1966) have shown that the depolarization of skeletal muscle produced by whole cobra venom is primarily attributable to a basic polypeptide and not to the phospholipase A. Tobias (1955) interpreted the work of Braganca and Quastel (1953) as showing that cobra venom that has been heated to 100°C for 10 to 15 min at pH 5 contains phospholipase A, free from other activity, and, therefore, erroneously attributed effects of "acid-heated" venom to phospholipase A. Whereas the basic toxins isolated from *Naja naja* venom by Meldrum (1965b) act both at the neuromuscular junction (producing a postsynaptic block) and on the muscle cell membrane (producing depolarization), Lee and his collaborators (Chang and Lee, 1966; Su *et al.*, 1967; Lee *et al.*, 1968) have clearly shown that the component in the venom of *Naja naja atra* that causes depolarization and contracture of skeletal muscle is found in the cardiotoxic fractions and not in the neurotoxic ones. Apparently the basic toxins isolated by Meldrum (1965b) may contain both neurotoxic and cardiotoxic components. The direct effect on skeletal and cardiac muscles of the toxin isolated by Detrait and Boquet (1958) may also be due to contamination with cardiotoxic component.

Although the fraction with high phospholipase A activity (10^{-5} g/ml) does not depolarize the rat diaphragm by itself, it potentiates the depolarizing effect of the cardiotoxic fraction (Chang and Lee, 1966). In line with this finding is the observation that pancreatic phospholipase A does not release fatty acids from intact muscle cells, whereas the partially purified phospholipase A from cobra venom does (Ibrahim et al., 1964). Apparently, some component(s) in cobra venom may act as cofactor(s) with the venom phospholipase A. On the other hand, Albuquerque and Thesleff (1968) have shown that immuno-electrophoretically pure phospholipase A from bee venom and lysolecithin in sufficient doses depolarize the muscle membrane with little effect on membrane excitability. Their findings are not necessarily contradictory to those of aforementioned workers (Meldrum, 1965b; Chang and Lee, 1966), since the doses of bee venom phospholipase A and lysolecithin needed for depolarization of muscle membrane were higher and the onset of action was slower as compared with cobra venom or its cardiotoxic fraction. Recently, Chang and Lee (unpublished) have found that one of the phospholipase-A-rich fractions from Formosan cobra venom depolarizes the muscle membrane if higher concentrations (10^{-4} g/ml) are applied.

The depolarization of muscle membrane by cardiotoxin appears to be the cause of contracture and loss of excitability of the muscle. In the absence of calcium no contracture can be produced by cardiotoxin, whereas its depolarizing effect remains unaffected (Lee et al., 1968).

3. Action on Peripheral Nerve

Although cobra venom does not block conduction in mammalian nerve trunks in vivo even with supralethal doses, it can depress the excitability of isolated nerves if high concentrations are applied (Houssay et al., 1922; Gautrelet and Halpern, 1933; Cicardo, 1935; Tobias, 1955; Nelson, 1958; Rosenberg, 1966; Parnas and Russell, 1967; Condrea et al., 1967; Condrea and Rosenberg, 1968). In isolated single fibers of the frog sciatic nerve, excitability can be abolished, without any alterations in the fine structures, by high concentrations of crude or acid-heated cobra venom (Nelson, 1958). Lobster giant axons can be depolarized by 30–500 μg/ml of crude or acid-heated cobra venom (Tobias, 1955, 1960), and conduction is blocked when the resting potentials falls to two-thirds of normal (Narahashi and Tobias, 1964). The electrical activity of the squid giant axon can also be irreversibly blocked by high concentrations of Naja naja or ringhals venom, provided the preparation contained adherent nerve fibers. After pretreatment with a lower concentration which has no effect on conduction, the squid axon can be rendered sensitive to curare and acetylcholine (Rosenberg and Podleski, 1962, 1963; also *see* Chap. 5). This venom action on the squid axon, as well as on the lobster axon, was interpreted as being due to a reduction of the permeability barrier, which prevents lipid-insoluble compounds from reaching the conducting membrane, and phospholipid splitting by phospholipase A was considered the factor responsible for inducing increased permeability and block of axonal conduction (Rosenberg, 1966; Condrea *et al.*, 1967; Condrea and Rosenberg, 1968). However, subsequent studies by the same authors revealed that extensive splitting of axonal phospholipids by phospholipase C, from *Clostridium welchii*, did not block axonal conduction nor increase the penetration of lipid-insoluble compounds into the axoplasma of squid axons (Rosenberg and Condrea, 1968). They observed that both purified lysolecithin and a mixture of lysophosphatides, prepared by the action of venom phospholipase A on the phospholipids of squid axons, blocked conduction and increased penetration into giant axons. In contrast to phospholipase A, which affects giant axons only if surrounded by adherent small nerve fibers, lysolecithin and the lysophosphatide mixture acted equally well on giant axons with or without adherant small nerve fibers. On the basis of these findings, they concluded that the actions of phospholipase A on the squid giant axon are due to evolved lysophosphatides and not to phospholipid splitting *per se*. However, since the concentration of purified lysolecithin or the lysophosphatide mixture required to block conduction and increase penetration of acetylcholine was as high as 0.5 mg/ml and the total lipid phosphorus in squid axons was less than 0.5 μg/mg wet wt (Rosenberg and Condrea, 1968), it is questionable whether the hydrolysis of axonal phospholipids by phospholipase A can yield sufficient lysophosphatides to account for the block of axonal conduction and increased penetration of acetylcholine, even if the endogenous lysophosphatides might be much more effective than if they were added externally.

On the other hand, it has recently been found that the compound action potential of the isolated phrenic nerve of the rat is irreversibly blocked by 0.1 mg/ml of the phospholipase-A-rich fraction from *Naja naja atra* venom as well as by 0.2 mg/ml of cardiotoxin, whereas neither cobra neurotoxin nor purified lysolecithin up to 0.5 mg/ml has any blocking effect (Chang and Lee, unpublished). This is in marked contrast to the finding that direct lytic factor from the ringhals venom in concentrations as high as 0.25–1.2 mg/ml had no effect on axonal conduction of nerves from the walking legs of lobster (Condrea *et al.*, 1967). The terminal nerve spike recorded extracellularly in the frog nerve–sartorius muscle preparation is also abolished by cardiotoxin but not by cobra neurotoxin (Chang and Lee, 1966). Inability of cobra neurotoxin in blocking nerve conduction has been frequently reported (Chang and Lee, 1966; Rosenberg, 1965; Su *et al.*, 1967). A recent report by Bicher (1966) that conduction through the isolated frog sciatic nerve is blocked by all the three neurotoxic fractions isolated from *Naja naja* venom is rather surprising, and this is most probably due to coexistance of either phospholipase A or cardiotoxin in incompletely separated neurotoxic fractions.

D. Action on Smooth Muscle

Cobra venom, like most other snake venoms, produces a stimulant effect on various smooth muscle organs at low concentrations and a paralytic effect preceded by a stimulation at high concentrations (Cushny and Yagi, 1918; Iwase, 1933; Gautrelet *et al.*, 1934). Marked tachyphylaxis is always observed for the stimulant effect but not for the paralytic one. Recent investigations (Lee *et al.*, unpublished) have shown that both phospholipase A and cardiotoxin are responsible for the stimulant effect, while the paralysis of the muscle is caused by high concentrations of cardiotoxin, probably as a result of irreversible depolarization of the muscle membrane (Lee *et al.*, 1968). In contrast, cobra neurotoxin exerts no appreciable effects on the smooth muscle even with high concentrations.

The mechanism by which phospholipase A produces a stimulant effect on smooth muscles is not well understood. It is not yet known whether the stimulant effect is due to a direct action of the enzyme or mediated by compound(s) liberated in the course of the enzymic reaction. Two groups of pharmacologically active lipids are released by the hydrolytic action of phospholipase A on phosphatides: lysophosphatides (e.g., lysolecithin) and unsaturated fatty acids. In addition, histamine and 5-hydroxytryptamine are released by phospholipase A through formation of lysolecithin (Feldberg and Kellaway, 1938; Feldberg *et al.*, 1938; Habermann, 1957; Moran *et al.*, 1962). Although all of these events are relevant to an action on smooth muscle, their effects differ in various ways on different muscle preparations. Lysolecithin, for example, cannot explain the venom-induced contraction of the guinea-pig ileum since "purified" lysolecithin lacks the stimulant action on gut. Conversely, it reduces the spontaneous activity of the intestine of several species of animals, and also reduces the excitability to several agents, e.g., histamine and acetylcholine (Feldberg *et al.*, 1938; Rocha e Silva and Beraldo, 1948; Habermann and Neumann, 1954; Vogt, 1957). Neither can histamine release explain the venom-induced contraction of the virgin rat uterus, since this organ relaxes with histamine (Kellaway, 1929). Moreover, the time-course of the histamine-induced contraction of the guinea pig ileum is quite different from that induced by phospholipase A. On the other hand, the constriction of lung or liver vessels produced by phospholipase A or lysolecithin in cats and dogs is most probably mediated by the release of histamine and also possibly of 5-hydroxytryptamine (Moran *et al.*, 1962; Markwardt *et al.*, 1966; Lee *et al.*, unpublished).

The characteristic features of the contraction produced by cobra venom or phospholipase A, that is to say the latency and the slowness of the contraction as well as of the relaxation after changing the bath fluid, can be reproduced by the slow reacting substance (SRS-C) which is released by phospholipase A from perfused tissues or purified lecithin (Feldberg and Kellaway, 1938; Feldberg *et al.*, 1938; Vogt, 1957). SRS-C is a mixture of polyunsaturated fatty acids (Vogt, 1957) and has recently been shown to contain a hydroxy acid related to the prostaglandin group (Babilli and Vogt, 1965; Vogt *et al.*, 1966, 1969). Whereas most of the free fatty acids released by phospholipase A are devoid of smooth-muscle-stimulating activity (Feldberg *et al.*, 1938; Vogt, 1957) and become gut-stimulating agents only after formation of hydroperoxides (Dakhil and Vogt, 1962), prostaglandins are among the most active, naturally occurring hydroxy acids known to contract smooth muscle (Bergström *et al.*, 1968). Since the presence of prostaglandins has been demonstrated in almost every tissue, including lung, stomach, intestines, and nervous system, it is tempting to assume that the smooth-muscle-stimulating action of phospholipase A is predominantly, if not entirely, due to the release of prostaglandins from the tissue affected by the enzyme. Further research in this field is required for a better understanding of the complicated mode of action of phospholipase A on smooth muscle.

The mode of action of cardiotoxin on smooth muscle organs is also complex (Chiu, 1966; Lee *et al.*, 1968). The minimal effective concentration of cardiotoxin to induce contraction of the guinea pig ileum is higher than that of phospholipase A, and the muscle tone usually returns to the normal level within several minutes without washing. The stimulant effect can be partially inhibited by atropine, procaine, or morphine, but not by pyribenzamine or hexamethonium. The responses of the gut to nicotine as well as to transmural electrical stimulations are first enhanced and then depressed by cardiotoxin (10 μg/ml). In muscle preparations depolarized by KCl no response to cardiotoxin is observed (Lee and Wei, unpublished). All of these findings suggest the involvement of nervous elements of the gut in the stimulant effect of cardiotoxin, in addition to its direct action on muscle membrane.

E. Action on Sympathetic Ganglionic Transmission

Cobra venom, if administered directly into the arterial supply of the superior cervical ganglion of the cat, produces a complete ganglionic blockade after a transient phase of stimulation (Chou and Lee, 1969). Cardiotoxin is responsible for this effect; neither cobra neurotoxin nor phospholipase A exerts any appreciable effect on the ganglionic transmission.

The mechanism of ganglionic blockade by cardiotoxin is apparently different from that by *d*-tubocurarine. After blockade by *d*-tubocurarine, ganglion cells are still capable of being discharged by KCl, whereas they no longer respond to KCl after blockade by cardiotoxin. The latter effect appears to be due to nonspecific irreversible depolarization of the ganglion cells by cardiotoxin.

It is unlikely, however, that the systemic toxicity of cobra venom entails any significant element of autonomic ganglionic blockade, inasmuch as a lethal dose of the venom administered intravenously does not produce any significant effect on the ganglionic transmission.

F. Action on the Cardiovascular System

1. Action on the Heart

Cobra venom at low concentrations causes an augmentation of systole of isolated frog heart. This is followed by a diminution of diastole, sometimes accompanied by arrhythmia, and finally the heart stops altogether in systolic contracture if high concentrations are applied (Elliot, 1905; Fraser and Gunn, 1909; Cushny and Yagi, 1918; Epstein, 1930; Iwase, 1933; Nakamura, 1933; Gautrelet *et al.*, 1934; Meurling, 1935; Gottdenker and Wachstein, 1940; Sarkar *et al.*, 1942; Peng, 1951; Zaki *et al.*, 1967).

Cobra venom has a marked effect on the mammalian heart; in the animals examined (dog, cat, rabbit, etc.), this effect has been accompanied by electrocardiographic changes, such as ST depression, inverted T-wave, nodal rhythm, A-V dissociation, complete A-V block with aberrant QRS-T complex and idioventricular rhythm, although the changes may be somewhat different from one species to another (Gautrelet *et al.*, 1934; Beerens and Cuypers, 1935; Feldberg and Kellaway, 1937a,b; Kellaway and Trethewie, 1940; Amuchastegui, 1940; Lee *et al.*, 1968).

The action of cardiotoxin on the isolated frog heart resembles that of the whole cobra venom. It causes augmentation of systole at low concentrations and systolic contracture at high concentrations (Sarkar, 1951; Devi and Sarkar, 1966; Lee *et al.*, 1968). It has, therefore, been suggested that cardiotoxin has a digitalis-like action (Sarkar, 1951). However, in the rat atrium, the positive inotropic effect of cardiotoxin is quite transient and soon followed by depression. In cats, neither consistent enhancement of contractility of the heart nor a shortening of Q-T interval is observed with cardiotoxin (Lee *et al.*, 1968). Recent experiments by Chiu and Lee (unpublished) show that the transmembrane potential of the guinea pig ventricular muscle cell is irreversibly reduced by cardiotoxin. Thus, it is evident that cardiotoxin acts on the heart by an entirely different mechanism from that of digitalis.

Although Sarkar *et al.* (1942) reported that purified neurotoxin as well as hemolysin (phospholipase A) separated from *Naja naja* venom causes an augmentation followed by depression and irregularity with ventricular block in the isolated toad heart, recent studies by Tseng (1964) and Lee *et al.* (1968) demonstrate that neither cobra neurotoxin nor phospholipase A separated from *Naja naja atra* venom produces any cardiotoxic effects on the frog heart with concentrations up to 10^{-4} g/ml. Most probably, the neurotoxin and hemolysin obtained by Sarkar *et al.* (1942) were incompletely separated from cardiotoxic component(s).

2. Hemodynamic Effects

The most conspicuous and consistent cardiovascular change produced by cobra venom is an immediate fall in systemic arterial pressure, if the venom is administered intravenously (Chopra and Iswariah, 1931; Iwase, 1933; Gautrelet and Halpern, 1934; Gautrelet *et al.*, 1934; Feldberg and Kellaway, 1937a,b, 1938; Peng, 1952; Westermann and Klapper, 1960; Lee and Peng, 1961; Bicher *et al.*, 1965; Cohen and Sumyk, 1966; Vick *et al.*, 1967). The animals may die of circulatory failure within several minutes if the dose is large enough, or the pressure may return to normal and remain steady until an asphyxial increase in blood pressure occurs immediately before death. If asphyxia is prevented by artificial respiration, a secondary fall in blood pressure may be observed which persists until death. Apart from the asphyxial increase in blood pressure before death, a slight rise in blood pressure has also been reported in cats and rabbits during the initial stage after injection of cobra venom (Rogers, 1905; Elliot, 1905; Cushny and Yagi, 1918; Epstein, 1930; Chopra and Iswariah, 1931; Venkatacholam and Ratnagiriswaran, 1934; Gottdenker and Wachstein, 1940; Sarkar *et al.*, 1942).

The primary hypotensive effect of cobra venom is peripheral in nature (Gautrelet *et al.*, 1934; Peng, 1952; Bhanganada and Perry, 1963). It is not affected by atropine or bilateral vagotomy, nor is it affected by the elimination of brain circulation, nor by the destruction of both carotid sinuses and cutting of the depressor nerves. The experiments carried out in dogs with crossed cephalic circulation also underlined the absence of a central effect (Gautrelet *et al.*, 1934; Bhanganada and Perry, unpublished). The initial precipitous fall in systemic arterial pressure produced by cobra venom has been differently attributed either to vasodilatation in the periphery (Gautrelet and Halpern, 1934; Gautrelet *et al.*, 1934; Peng, 1952; Bhanganada and Perry, 1963; Morales *et al.*, 1963), combined with constriction of the hepatic veins, especially in dogs (Feldberg and Kellaway, 1937b), or to a pronounced pulmonary vasoconstriction, especially in cats (Feldberg and Kellaway, 1937a; Chiu *et al.*, 1968), or to a direct venom action on the heart (Amuchastegui, 1940; Devi and Sarkar, 1966). The vascular effects are largely explained by a liberation of histamine in the body by the action of phospholipase A, present in the venom (Feldberg and Kellaway, 1938; Feldberg *et al.*, 1938), but cannot be prevented by antihistamine drugs (Devi and Sarkar, 1966). There is evidence, however, that not only histamine but also 5-hydroxytryptamine and other vasoactive substance(s) are released from the tissues by phospholipase A (Moran *et al.*, 1962; Markwardt *et al.*, 1966; Lee *et al.*, unpublished). Recent experiments in cats carried out by Chiu *et al.* (1968) demonstrated that the initial pressure fall is chiefly, if not entirely, caused by phospholipase A, possibly intensified by cardiotoxin, producing an increase in the resistance within the pulmonary circuit, with a subsequent deficit in left heart output and changes in the ECG. Cardiotoxin is responsible for the initial pressor response, followed by more sustained hypotensive effect leading to cardiac arrest. The initial pressor response is due to peripheral vasoconstriction, which is usually masked by the more pronounced hypotensive effect produced by phospholipase A. In contrast, cobra neurotoxin is devoid of any appreciable effect on systemic blood pressure, except the asphyxial rise before death.

G. Local Action

1. Local Irritant Action

Pain, then variable swelling, and later necrosis, are the outstanding features of local effects of cobra bite in human beings (Reid, 1964). The likelihood of bacterial infection being important as a primary factor in necrosis has been excluded, since severe necrosis has resulted in dogs from subcutaneous injection of sterile venom from Malayan cobra (Reid, 1964). Experimentally, the local irritant action of cobra venom has also been observed on the conjunctiva of rabbit's eye (Peng, 1951). Marked congestion and edema of conjunctiva are produced by instillation of one drop of 0.01–0.1 % venom solution into the eye.

Cardiotoxin has been found to be responsible for the local irritant action of cobra venom (Lee *et al.*, 1968), whereas the neurotoxin has been shown to be devoid of this action (Peng, 1951). The local irritant action of cardiotoxin has also been demonstrated by the rat paw edema test (Lee *et al.*, 1968). The cytotoxic effect of cardiotoxin (Lee and Lin, unpublished) may account for the irritation and subsequent necrosis of the tissue.

2. Actions on Sensory Receptors

Cobra venom applied to the tongue produces a loss of sensation (Fontana, 1787). The venom has been shown to block tactile receptors in frog skin at a concentration of 10^{-5} g/ml and to block the responses of the frog muscle spindle at higher concentrations (Kellaway, 1934). Most probably, cardiotoxin may be responsible for these effects.

H.   Actions on the Central Nervous System

1.   Central Actions when Systemically Applied

Although the early claims that the respiratory paralysis produced by elapid venoms is central in origin have been refuted (see Sec. III A), there are still some observations supposedly demonstrating a direct action of cobra venom on the central nervous system. Macht (1935, 1943) stated that a "neurotoxic" preparation from cobra venom tends to antagonize the cerebral convulsions produced by camphor in mice, raises the pain threshold in guinea pigs, and produces sedation, ataxia, and miosis of central origin in cats. However, D'Amour and Smith (1941) were unable to detect any analgesic action in rats. Probably, most of Macht's observations may be interpreted as the result of peripheral muscular paralysis.

A recent report by Vick et al. (1964) that 0.5 mg/kg of Naja naja venom given intravenously to anesthetized dogs or monkeys produces a complete and irreversible loss of cortical electrical activity within 30–60 sec is rather surprising since unanesthetized animals injected intravenously with doses of this order exhibit organized behavior for more than 10 min after the injection until respiration starts to fail. After chromatographic separation of the venom on a CM-Sephadex C-25 column, Vick et al. (1966) obtained three physiologically identifiable components: the first one (Fr. 1) produces a loss of cortical electrical activity when injected intravenously into the dog; the second one (Frs. 5–8) causes respiratory paralysis; and the third one (Fr. 12) affects the cardiovascular system, ultimately producing irreversible hypotension. Although the first component contained phospholipase A, they felt that the change in EEG might not be due to phospholipase A activity, since the removal of the enzyme from Fr. 1 did not alter its EEG-suppressing activity. Nevertheless, Slotta and Vick (1969) stated that the most remarkable effect of phospholipase A in dogs was the dramatic loss of all cortical electrical activity within 30–60 sec after injection, and Currie et al. (1968) also reported that a very potent central nervous system toxin (corticotoxin I) from cobra venom is associated with a high phospholipase A activity. Bicher (1966) believes that the early depression of cerebral cortical activity produced by Naja naja venom is likely due to a direct central action of phospholipase A. Among the four toxic fractions obtained from this venom by paper electrophoresis, only the fraction containing phospholipase A causes the same effects as the whole or boiled venom, i.e., a diphasic circulatory shock with early depression of cerebral cortical activity in the anesthetized cat (Bicher *et al.*, 1965; Krupnick *et al.*, 1968). Although they called this fraction "neurotoxin," it was not toxic to mice, even at a dose of five mg/kg. Apparently it is quite different from "cobra neurotoxin," which is very toxic to most animals including mice, and was apparently contained in the second component (Frs. 5–8) of Vick *et al.* (1966) and probably in Fr. 3 of Bicher *et al.* (1965). Interestingly enough, neither the second component of Vick *et al.* nor Fr. 3 of Bicher *et al.* produced early depression of cerebral cortical activity. Nevertheless, Bicher (1966) assumed that Fr. 3 acted particularly on the reticular formation, as the arousal response disappeared long before the depression of cortical electrical activity became apparent. It remains to be elucidated, however, whether these central effects of cobra venom are primary results of a direct central action of venom component(s), or are secondary to other physiological changes. Since it has been shown that cobra venom labeled with ^{131}I passes into the cerebrospinal fluid (CSF) of rabbits very slowly and the brain levels are extremely low even two hr after the injection (Tseng *et al.*, 1968), it is doubtful whether cobra venom can penetrate into the brain in sufficient amounts within a short period to account for such central effects.

2. *Actions when Applied Directly to the Central Nervous System*

Pacella (1923) reported that injection of cobra venom into the subarachnoid space in dogs produces a rapid rise in arterial blood pressure, slowing of the pulse, and later diminution in and arrest of respiration. Peng (1952) observed that Formosan cobra venom injected into the cerebellomedullary cistern in the rabbit causes a rise of blood pressure and a transient stimulation of respiration followed by a depression. Additionally, he found that the MLD of this venom by cisternal application was much smaller than that by peripheral application, the ratio being 1:10–14. However, death caused by central application took place in 14–32 hr, while that by peripheral application within a few hours. To shorten the time to death by central application, doses near the intravenous MLD were required. On the other hand, Guyot and Boquet (1960) reported that the lethal dose of *Naja nigricollis* venom injected into rabbits in the region of Ammon's horn was one-hundredth of the lethal dose injected intravenously, 3.5 μg/kg producing recurrent bouts of severe motor excitement and death within a few hours.

Recent experiments by Lee and Chen (unpublished) reveal that cardiotoxin as well as phospholipase A, but not cobra neurotoxin, is responsible for the lethal effects when applied directly to the central nervous system. They observed that intracisternal injection of 0.2 mg of either cardiotoxin or phospholipase A fraction in cats produced various neurologic signs and death within a few hours, while cats injected with 0.5–1.0 mg of cobra neurotoxin into the same site showed only minor neurologic signs and all of them survived.

3. Neuropathological Changes

Neuropathological changes in rabbits and monkeys have been demonstrated after the systemic injection of cobra venom (Lamb and Hunter, 1904a,b; Hunter, 1909; Sanders et al., 1954). The most constantly observed change is in the anterior horn cells, which show every stage of acute chromatolysis with ultimately cell vacuolation and nuclear degeneration. Similar changes are also found in the cranial nerve nuclei. These morphological changes have been attributed to anoxia or ischemia rather than to a direct action of the venom on the nerve cells (Kellaway et al., 1932). Anoxic or ischemic cell damage, however, usually does not involve the anterior horn cells (Hoff et al., 1945; Meyer, 1963), and there is a delay of several hours between the anoxic episode and the appearance of ischemic cell changes; yet Lamb and Hunter saw changes within a few hours after giving the venom. On the other hand, the morphological changes described by early workers could possibly be due to postmortem lesion, since no such changes could be detected in the anterior horn cells following injection of 0.2–1.0 mg of *Naja naja atra* venom into the subarachnoid space in cats (Lee and Chen, unpublished).

I. Actions on Blood

1. Hemolytic Effects

Since the classical work by Delezenne and Ledebt (1911a,b,c; 1912), there has been widespread acceptance of the view that hemolysis by snake venoms is due to the action of phospholipase A, by producing lysophosphatides from serum or added phospholipids. Without the addition of lecithin, however, phospholipase A does not hemolyze washed red blood cells, due to its incapability to attack the phospholipids of the intact erythrocyte membrane. Besides phospholipase A, cobra venom contains a so-called direct lytic factor (DLF) which can lyse washed erythrocytes of several animal species (Grassmann and Hannig, 1954; Habermann and Neumann, 1954; Condrea et al., 1964a; Slotta et al., 1967). The DLF is, by itself, only weakly hemolytic, but acts synergistically with phospholipase A (Condrea et al., 1964a,b; Wille and Vogt, 1965; Patzer and Vogt, 1967; Slotta and Vick, 1969; Lee et al., 1970). It is believed that DLF can make phospholipids in the red cell membrane accessible to phospholipase A, as also can surface active agents such as digitonin and saponin. Erythrocytes of different animal species show striking variations in their susceptibility to hemolysis by cobra venom. This has been attributed to the difference in susceptibility of the various erythrocytes to the action of DLF (Condrea *et al.*, 1964b).

The precise mode of action of DLF on the red cells is not known, and neither is the specific structure of the red cell membrane which determines susceptibility to the action of DLF. It is noteworthy that the sequence of red cell sensitivity to the hemolytic action of DLF is in good agreement with the sequence of red cell permeability for other agents, such as glycerol, ethylene glycol, urea, and thiourea, which has been related to the variation in the red cell phospholipid composition (*see* Condrea *et al.*, 1964b). Since DLF is a strongly basic polypeptide and, moreover, its hemolytic effect can be prevented by acidic substances, such as gangliosides, RNA, and heparin (Lee *et al.*, 1970), one can envisage a role of the acidic groups in the cell membrane in determining the interaction between DLF and cell membrane.

The physicochemical and biological properties of DLF closely resemble those of cardiotoxin (Lee *et al.*, 1968; Slotta and Vick, 1969). The recent findings (Lee *et al.*, 1970) that both the contracture-inducing and direct-hemolytic activities of cardiotoxin can be prevented by gangliosides, RNA, and heparin strongly support the suggested identity of cardiotoxin with DLF (*see* Sec. II B).

Despite the presence of plasma phospholipids, hemolysis is rarely observed with cobra venom *in vivo*. Although cobra venom lowers plasma phospholipids and raises plasma lysolecithin levels, the associated sphering and crenellation of red blood cells are spontaneously reversed, since the lysolecithin attachment to the cells is temporary, due to its clearance from the circulation (De Vries *et al.*, 1962; Klibansky *et al.*, 1962, 1966). Hence, intravascular hemolysis does not occur or is inconstant.

2. *Action on Blood Coagulation*

The effect of cobra venom on blood coagulation has recently been reviewed (Meaume, 1966). Although it is generally accepted that the anticoagulant action of cobra venom is chiefly due to its antithromboplastin activity, the intimate mechanism has not been fully elucidated. While the destruction of tissue thromboplastin by cobra venom has been demonstrated by many investigators (Morawitz, 1905; Mellanby, 1909; Hirschfeld and Klinger, 1915; Link, 1935; Kruse and Dam, 1950; Fleckenstein and Fettig, 1952; Habermann, 1954; Ouyang, 1957; Lee and Ouyang, 1958), the inactivation of other clotting factors has also been reported: Factor V (Ouyang, 1957; Lee and Ouyang, 1958; De Nicola and Cappelletti, 1959), Factor VII (De Nicola and Cappelletti, 1959), Factor VIII (Marcacci and Bruzzese, 1959), Factor IX (O'Brien, 1956a,b; Mitel'man, 1966), and coagulant factors of platelets (O'Brien, 1956a,b). Unlike many crotalid venoms, cobra venom does neither affect prothrombin itself appreciably, nor affect fibrinogen

(Ouyang, 1957; De Nicola and Cappelletti, 1959; Marcacci and Bruzzese, 1959), nor has it any antithrombin effect (Ouyang, 1957; Mitel'man, 1966). These observations are in good accord with the findings that cobra venom has no or only feeble proteolytic activity (*see* Sec. II C).

On the other hand, the relationship between phospholipase A and the anticoagulant action of cobra venom has been the subject of considerable dispute. Since phospholipids are not only the constituents of thromboplastin but also required in blood clotting at stages prior to the prothrombinase (autoprothrombin C) formation, it has been suggested that phospholipase A, through phospholipid destruction, is probably the main causative agent responsible for the anticoagulant action of cobra venom (O'Brien, 1956a,b). In line with this hypothesis are the observations that phospholipase A and the anticoagulant activity of cobra venom are located in the same fraction after chromatographic separation (Boquet *et al.*, 1967b; Brisbois *et al.*, 1968). In contrast, Kruse and Dam (1950) have opposed the hypothesis of destruction of thromboplastin by phospholipase A, on the ground that phospholipase A is more heat-resistant than the anticoagulant activity of cobra venom. However, the reported heat sensitivity of the anticoagulant factor of cobra venom differs from one report to another. Thus, while Kruse and Dam (1950) stated that only a slight anticoagulant effect remains after 72°C for an hr, Boquet *et al.* (1966a, 1967b) showed that the anticoagulant factor can resist 96°C for 45 min. Apparently, the experimental conditions such as pH and concentration of the solution may affect the results. Hughes (1935) has shown that phospholipase A in cobra venom is not affected by boiling for 15 min at a pH below 5.9, but that heating at pH 7 or above destroys it. Whether the same is true for the anticoagulant factor of cobra venom remains to be demonstrated.

Besides the anticoagulant action, a coagulant effect of cobra venom has also been described (Brazil and Vellard, 1928; Taylor *et al.*, 1935). Recently, Meaume *et al.* (1966) have isolated a coagulant fraction from *Naja nigricollis* venom, which acts like prothrombinase as a direct activator of prothrombin. The exact chemical nature of this coagulant factor is still unknown.

J. Biochemical Effects

1. *Effects on Oxidative Metabolism*

Inhibition of glycolysis and of oxygen uptake by cobra venom was first demonstrated in cancer cells by Mellanby (1934–1936). Chain (1937, 1938) observed that many venoms inhibit glycolysis by muscle extracts, and from a study of the effect of black tiger snake venom on various oxidases and dehydrogenases he concluded that only those dehydrogenases which require NAD for their action are inhibited by this venom, whereas others are very little affected (Chain, 1939). Therefore, he suggested that inactivation of NAD by a nucleotidase is responsible. On the other hand, Ghosh and Chatterjee (1948) and Chatterjee (1949) demonstrated that Indian cobra venom inhibits selectively cytochrome oxidase in pigeon brain homogenate. Fleckenstein *et al.* (1951) showed that the venoms of *Naja naja, Hemachatus haemachatus*, and other species strongly inhibit the ulilization of citric acid by muscle cells of the frog. Subsequently, Braganca and Quastel (1953) found that heated cobra venom inhibits oxygen uptake of brain slices and concluded that the venom attacks phospholipids of mitochondria and thus destroys the structure required for their activity. Nygaard and Sumner (1953) reported that phospholipase A preparations abolish the succinoxidase activity of rat liver mitochondria. The factor most sensitive to phospholipase A was found to be located between cytochromes b and c (Nygaard, 1953). Yang and Tung (1953) found that Formosan cobra venom inhibits succinate-cytochrome c reductase more selectively than either succinic dehydrogenase or cytochrome oxidase. However, they concluded that the inhibitory action of cobra venom is not due to phospholipase A, because heat treatment and reduced glutathione do not affect the inhibitory potency and the phospholipase A activity to the same extent (Yang *et al.*, 1954; Yang and Tung, 1954). Lin *et al.*, (1957) suggested that the inhibitory action of cobra venom is probably attributable to free or protein-bound zinc, since ashed cobra venom still retains 60% of its inhibitory action, and EDTA can abolish this inhibition. Nevertheless, recent investigation by Lee and Lin (unpublished) revealed that among the fractions of Formosan cobra venom separated by CM-Sephadex column chromatography, the fraction with the highest phospholipase A activity exhibits the highest inhibitory effect on the succinate-cytochrome c reductase, whereas neither cobra neurotoxin nor cardiotoxin inhibits the enzyme activity significantly. The same conclusion has been reached by Habermann (1954) and Radomski and Deichmann (1958) who found that the effects on oxidative phosphorylation of fractions from *Naja flava* venom vary much more closely with their phospholipase A activity than with their toxicity. Edwards and Ball (1954) showed that exposure of a succinoxidase preparation to *Naja naja* venom produces an inhibition of succinate oxidation which is proportional to the fatty acid released by the venom and that unsaturated fatty acid added as the sodium salt causes a similar inhibition. The importance of phospholipids in mitochondrial respiration has been demonstrated; indeed extracting phospholipids from mitochondrial preparations with acetone–water destroys their capacity to carry out electron transfer, and this capacity can be restored by the addition of the appropriate phospholipids (Green and Fleischer, 1963). The uncoupling of mitochondria induced by heated cobra venom is reversed by various phospholipids (Petrushka *et al.*, 1959a,b; Elliott *et al.*, 1966; Ziegler *et al.*, 1967). Morphological studies showed a characteristic disruption of the mitochondrial membrane following phospholipase A treatment (Nygaard *et al.*, 1954; Witter and Cottone, 1956; Taub and Elliott; 1964). The swelling of mitochondria by phospholipase A was correlated with the phospholipid-splitting activity, and EDTA was found to suppress in a parallel manner both the swelling and phospholipid-splitting activity (Condrea *et al.*, 1965). Thus, there appears to be little doubt that phospholipase A plays an important role in the inhibition of mitochondrial and tissue respirations by cobra venom.

While the importance of intact phospholipids to succinate oxidase activity has been stressed by several authors (Braganca and Quastel, 1953; Nygaard and Sumner, 1953; Edwards and Ball, 1954), it has also been suggested that fatty acids released from phospholipids by phospholipase A may be responsible for the inhibitory action, since fatty acids mimic the action of snake venoms on mitochondrial systems (Vázquez-Colón *et al.*, 1966). Though lysolecithin induces disruption of mitochondrial membrane and inhibition of energy transformations (Nygaard *et al.*, 1954; Aravindakshan and Braganca, 1961b; Honjo and Ozawa, 1968), there are calculations showing that total hydrolysis of mitochondrial phospholipids would not yield sufficient lysolecithin to account for the uncoupling action (Witter and Cottone, 1956; Witter *et al.*, 1957).

It has been claimed that the inhibitory action of cobra venom on respiratory enzymes can be demonstrated *in vivo*. Aravindakshan and Braganca (1959, 1961a,b) reported that mitochondrial preparations from brain or liver of mice injected with lethal doses of heated cobra venom and "crystalline phospholipase A" show a preferential inactivation of the phosphorylation located in the cytochrome oxidase system. A fall in respiratory activity of spinal cord slices following treatment with heated cobra venom has also been reported (Hudson *et al.*, 1960). On the other hand, Huang (1954a) observed that the succinate cytochrome *c* reductase activity of brain homogenates of mice injected with lethal doses of Formosan cobra venom was partially inhibited, whereas no significant inhibition could be demonstrated in other organs, such as liver, spleen, kidney, lung, heart, and muscle. He attributed the failure to demonstrate the inhibitory action of the venom on the respiratory enzymes of various organs *in vivo* to the protective action by plasma proteins (Huang, 1954b). However, before accepting the inhibition of respiratory enzymes of the central nervous system by cobra venom or phospholipase A *in vivo* as a primary direct effect of phospholipase A, the following two questions should be first answered: (1) Can cobra venom or phospholipase A pass through the blood–brain barrier in sufficient quantity to produce such an effect? (2) Can phospholipase A gain access to the interior of brain cells, in order to act on mitochondria? For the latter question, answers differ. Ibrahim *et al.*

(1964) observed the splitting of phospholipids of rat brain slices by cobra venom and also found that the release of fatty acids is proportional to the outflow of transaminase from brain slices. However, Klibansky *et al.* (1964) failed to find any significant hydrolysis of phospholipids from rat brain slices incubated with whole cobra venom or purified phospholipase A, even in the presence of DLF. Yet a rapid conversion of phospholipids to lysophosphatides was found in brain homogenates incubated with whole venom or purified phospholipase A. For the first question, Sumyk *et al.* (1963) and Tseng *et al.* (1968) have demonstrated that there is no or very little radioactivity in brains of the animals injected with radioiodine-labeled cobra venom, indicating the presence of the blood–brain barrier. Therefore, the alleged effect of cobra venom or phospholipase A on the brain respiration *in vivo* might be possibly due to secondary effects resulted from respiratory and/or circulatory failure.

2. Biochemical Effects of Cobramines A and B

In search of factor(s) in snake venom responsible for the inhibition of iodide accumulation by thyroid slices, two basic polypeptides, named cobramines A and B, have been isolated from *Naja naja* venom (Larsen and Wolff, 1968b). Cobramines inhibit the accumulation in various tissues of four different classes of compounds: (1) small anions (I^-, TcO_4^-, ReO_4^-); (2) amino acids (both utilizable and nonutilizable); (3) the nonmetabolized hexose, 3-O-methyl glucose; and (4) the organic anion p-aminohippurate (Larsen and Wolff, 1967a,b). The transport inhibition produced by cobramines appears to be of a general nature. Although accumulation of these substances is thought to be linked to cation concentration or movement, Na^+ efflux from human erythrocytes or the inhibition of this process by ouabain is unaffected by cobramines (Larsen and Wolff, 1967b). However, the Na^+ pump of the isolated toad bladder is inhibited by cobramine B, 10 μg/ml, as is the resting potential difference (Mendoza, unpublished). Further studies on the mechanism of action of cobramine B revealed that the major portion of the inhibition of I^- accumulation by thyroid slices is due to increase I^- efflux from the tissue (Wolff *et al.*, 1968). The inhibitory effect on the accumulation of anions has a rapid onset, is temperature-dependent, and is prevented by polyanions (heparin, RNA, gangliosides, and suramin) or antivenom, but it is reversed with great difficulty, presumably because of very firm binding to tissue. Cobramine B also leads to K^+ loss from cells and increases the rate of equilibration of the sucrose or inulin spaces.

The basicity of cobramine B seems to be important in its action, since the effect is mimicked by a number of basic proteins or polyamino acids such as protamine, histone, poly-L-lysine, poly-L-ornithine, and poly-L-arginine and seems to require a minimum molecular weight of several thousands.

However, basicity alone is not sufficient for inhibition of iodide accumulation, and cobramines differ in some respects from polylysine or protamine: (1) Polylysine and polyornithine are washed off the thyroid slices more easily than these; (2) Cobramines render red cell and mitochondrial membrane phospholipids susceptible to phospholipase A hydrolysis, whereas other bases do not have this effect. Although the presence in cobramine B of some as yet undiscovered enzymatic activity has not been ruled out, it is suggested that the membrane leaks produced by cobramine B occur, at least in part, through an interaction with the fixed negative charges of the cell surface (Wolff *et al.*, 1968).

Despite the marked permeability changes produced by cobramine B, thyroid slices treated with cobramine B respond normally to thyrotropin with an increase in $^{32}P_i$ incorporation into thyroidal phospholipids (Larsen and Wolff, 1967a). This finding suggests that at least some portions of the membrane can function normally after considerable alteration in membrane integrity has been produced.

3. Miscellaneous Effects

It was reported that cobra venom causes hyperglycemia in rabbits or guinea pigs (Houssay *et al.*, 1921; Epstein, 1930; Bertrand and Vladesco, 1940a,b; Grasset and Goldstein, 1947). Feldberg (1940) showed that injection of cobra venom or lysophosphatides causes a long-sustained liberation of adrenaline. Thus, hyperglycemia induced by cobra venom was attributed to the release of adrenaline from adrenal medulla. On the other hand, Ri (1939) reported that unlike other crotalid venoms, Formosan cobra venom does not affect blood sugar levels in rabbits unless supralethal doses are given. Mebs (1968) was also unable to find any changes of blood glucose or liver and muscle glycogen in rats injected with a lethal dose of cobra venom subcutaneously. He suggested that hyperglycemia in rabbits induced by the venom might result from the stress reaction provoked by collecting blood samples continuously.

Peron (1964) found that heated cobra venom inhibits biosynthesis of corticoids from endogenous cholesterol or other intermediates by rat adrenal homogenates. This inhibitory effect is probably due to destruction of the spatial relationship of the corticosteroidogenic enzymes in the particulate fragments by phospholipase A.

K. Cytotoxic Effects

1. Cytopathic Effects on Cell Cultures

It has been repeatedly shown that snake venoms exert cytopathic effects on animal cells in culture. Levaditi and Mutermilch (1913) first demonstrated that less than 10 μg/ml crude or heated cobra venom inhibits the multiplication of chicken embryo heart cells. Subsequent studies by various authors indicate that various snake venoms differ markedly in the degree of cytopathic activity and that different kinds of cells in culture vary in their susceptibility to venom action (Ishii, 1929; Edlinger and Dietel, 1959; Gaertner *et al.*, 1962; Sato *et al.*, 1964). Experiments with chromatographic fractions of *Vipera palestinae* and *Echis colorata* venoms showed a definite correlation between the cytopathic and protease activities of the venom fractions. Heating these venoms destroyed the cytopathic activity (Gaertner *et al.*, 1962). The cytotoxicity of *Trimeresurus flavoviridis* venom could be also abolished by heating the venom solution to 100°C at pH 5.6 (Sato *et al.*, 1964). Thus, the cytopathic action of these viperid or crotalid venoms in tissue cultures may be attributable primarily to their protease and not to their phospholipase A activity. However, cobra venom contains no or little protease and its cytotoxic activity appears to be rather heat resistant (Levaditi and Mutermilch, 1913; Ishii, 1929; Braganca *et al.*, 1967). Recent experiments with chromatographic fractions of *Naja naja atra* venom demonstrated that cytopathic effects on stable tumor cell cultures (HeLa, KB) are found in three cardiotoxic fractions but in neither neurotoxic nor phospholipase A fractions (Lee and Lin, unpublished).

2. Antitumor Activity

Recently, a cytotoxic protein, which is relatively nontoxic to animals and shows selective cytotoxicity to Yoshida sarcoma ascites cells *in vitro* and *in vivo* as compared with its effects on some species of normal cells, has been isolated from *Naja naja* venom (Braganca *et al.*, 1965, 1967). This factor prevented growth of Yoshida sarcoma in rats in 1/7 of the LD_{50} dose. Most of the enzymes and other biologically active components known to be present in cobra venom were absent in the purified factor. Evidence obtained by thin-layer chromatography (Braganca and Khandeparkar, 1966) has demonstrated the presence of phospholipase C, with affinity for phosphatidyl ethanolamine and phosphatidyl serine. The cytotoxic effects were shown to be temperature- and pH-dependent. Competitive experiments using phospholipids suggested combination of the cytotoxin with the more acid phospholipids. Experiments with the cytotoxin made fluorescent by combination with Dansyl demonstrated that the cytotoxin combines initially with surface membrane components of the cell (Patel *et al.*, 1969). However, a recent observation by Lee and Lin (unpublished) that phospholipase C from *Clostridium welchii* does not inhibit the growth of HeLa cell cultures up to 500 μg/ml raises the question of the role played by phospholipase C in the cytotoxic effects of cobra venom. Moreover, the claim that cobra venom cytotoxin is different from DLF or cardiotoxin (Braganca *et al.*, 1967) remains to be confirmed in view of the finding that rat or human erythrocytes are also rather resistant to cardiotoxin (Lee *et al.*, 1970).

3. Teratogenic Effects

Ruch and Gabriel-Robez-Kremer (1962, 1963) reported that injection of 2 μg cobra venom into the developing Leghorn eggs leads to a high incidence (15%) of malformations of several organ systems, especially the heart. Although the factor responsible has not been identified, cardiotoxin is most probably responsible for such effects. Similar cardiac malformations are caused by various substances, such as bee venom, dexamethasone phosphate, cyclophosphamide, diethylstilbestrol, and hydroxy-3-butyl oxide (Ruch *et al.*, 1965).

IV. CONCLUDING REMARKS

The pharmacological properties of cobra venom, as represented by the venom of *Naja naja atra*, and of its principal components are summarized in Table V.

It is well established that the primary cause of death due to cobra venom is peripheral respiratory paralysis in most animal species. However, cobra venom also produces profound cardiovascular changes, and the envenomed animals eventually die of circulatory failure, even under artificial respiration, if larger doses are given. Besides the systemic effects, the venom often provokes local necrotic lesions in humans. Several active components, such as neurotoxin (cobrotoxin, toxin *a*), cardiotoxin, DLF, cobramines, cytotoxin, phospholipase A, and some proteins having other enzymatic activities, have been separated from cobra venom. Among them, the neurotoxin has been considered as the major toxic component of cobra venom, which is responsible for the peripheral respiratory paralysis.

Cobra neurotoxin combines firmly with the acetylcholine receptor on the motor endplate and produces "nondepolarizing" block of neuromuscular transmission. It depresses the epp without affecting resting membrane potential, muscle action potential, and terminal nerve spike. The amplitude of successive epps on repetitive stimulation declines markedly as in the curarized muscle (Wedensky inhibition). The amplitude of epp is increased and its time-course prolonged by neostigmine. Thus, the mode of neuromuscular blocking action of cobra neurotoxin is essentially similar to that of *d*-tubocurarine. The action of cobra neurotoxin is highly selective, judging from its lack of effect on the cardiovascular system, smooth muscle organs, and sympathetic ganglia, and also from its lower toxicity when applied directly to the central nervous system. The amino acid sequence of

Table V.
Pharmacological Effects of Formosan Cobra Venom and Its Components

	Cobra venom	Cobra neurotoxin	Cardiotoxin	Phospholipase A
LD$_{50}$ mouse γ/g, ip	0.44	0.074	1.48	>5
Toxicity ratio in mouse	1	6	0.3	<0.09
MLD in cat				
mg/kg, iv	1.0	0.5	1.0	1.0
mg/Animal, intracisternal	0.2	2.0	0.2	0.2
Neuromuscular block				
Rat diaphragm (γ/ml)[a]	0.5	0.1	10	?
Potency ratio	1	5	0.05	
Site of action	Endplate and muscle fiber	Endplate	Motor nerve and muscle fiber	Motor nerve and muscle fiber (?)
Acetylcholine output	Decrease	No effect	Decrease	Decrease (?)
Reversibility	−	+	−	?
Antagonism by neostigmine	±	+	−	−
Contracture of skeletal muscle	++	−	++	±
Conduction block of nerve (mg/ml)	0.2	−	0.2	0.1
Ganglionic blockade	+	−	+	−
Circulatory effects				
Cardiotoxic effect	++	−	++	±
Systemic blood pressure	Both fall and rise	No effect	Rise followed by fall	Fall
Pulmonary arterial pressure	Rise	No effect	Slight rise	Rise
Histamine release	+	−	?	++
Stimulation of smooth muscle	++	−	++	++
Local irritation	+	−		−
Hemolytic effect				
Direct lytic effect	++	−	+	−
Indirect hemolysis	+++	−	−	+++
Anticoagulant action	+++	−	−	+(?)
Cytotoxic effect	+	−	+	−
Inhibition of respiratory enzymes	+	−	−	+

[a] Complete block within 200 min.

neurotoxins from three different species has recently been determined, and the "active site" of the neurotoxin molecules has been postulated.

Cardiotoxin affects various kinds of cells, causing irreversible depolarization of cell membrane. It causes contracture of skeletal muscle as well as neuromuscular block by depolarizing both the muscle and nerve fibers; the nerve action potential is abolished and direct stimulation of the muscle fiber also fails to evoke an action potential. Cardiotoxin causes systolic arrest of the isolated heart, constriction of blood vessels, and a rise followed by a gradual fall in systemic arterial pressure, accompanied by various ECG changes. It is also responsible for the local necrotic lesions. Besides, it produces contraction of smooth muscle, stimulation followed by paralysis of sympathetic ganglia, direct hemolytic effect, and cytotoxic effects. DLF, cobramines toxin γ, and possibly cytotoxin are all closely related to cardiotoxin, if not entirely identical.

Among various enzymes present in cobra venom, only phospholipase A has been definitely shown to contribute to the overall toxicity of the venom. The toxic effects of phospholipase A are most probably due to autopharmacological reactions, liberating histamine and other vasoactive substances in the animal body. Thus, it produces a precipitous fall in systemic arterial pressure and a marked rise in pulmonary arterial pressure in the cat. *In vitro*, it produces hemolysis of washed erythrocytes if supplemented with lecithin, contraction of smooth muscle, and possibly blockage of nerve conduction. It also causes disruption of mitochondria and is probably responsible for the inhibition of tissue respiration by cobra venom. The claim that phospholipase A produces a loss of cortical electrical activity needs further confirmation. There are widespread but imprecise indications that cobra venom has other central actions that are mainly depressant in nature. Here also the venom components and pharmacological mechanisms concerned remain obscure.

The role played by enzymes other than phospholipase A in the overall toxicity of cobra venom appears to be negligible, if not entirely absent. Many of them, such as acetylcholinesterase, 5'-nucleotidase, ATPase, L-amino acid oxidase, hyaluronidase, etc., have been shown to be nontoxic or nearly so. The claim that phosphodiesterase may be responsible for the immediate fall in blood pressure following intravenous injection of cobra venom remains to be proved.

ACKNOWLEDGMENTS

Much of the work reported here was carried out with the collaboration of Drs. M. T. Peng, C. C. Chang, C. Su, C. Ouyang, T. B. Lo, S. Y. Lee, J. S. Lin, and graduate students L. F. Tseng, T. H. Chiu, P. J. S. Chiu, T. C.

Tseng, T. C. Chou, and J. W. Wei. I wish to express my appreciation for their contributions to these studies. The skillful technical assistance of Mr. Y. M. Chen is also gratefully acknowledged.

I am indebted to Drs. C. Ouyang and S. Y. Shiau Lin for their help in preparation of the sections on "Action on Blood Coagulation" and "Biochemical Effects," respectively. I am also grateful to Drs. P. Boquet, L. Grotto, and J. A. Vick for permission to include their unpublished data in Table IV.

Various aspects of the work reported here were supported by the U.S. Army Medical Research Development Command Research Grant DA-MD-49-193-64-G108, DA-MD-49-193-66-G182, DA-CRD-AFE-S92-544-67-G-89, DA-CRD-AFE-S92-544-69-G138, and by the National Council on Science Development, Republic of China.

NOTE ADDED IN PROOF

Recently Botes (1970) isolated three neurotoxins, designated α, β and δ, from the venom of the cape cobra (*Naja nivea*) by gradient chromatography on Amberlite CG-50 and CM-cellulose and gel filtration on Sephadex G-50. Neurotoxins β and δ resemble other cobra neurotoxins in consisting of 61 amino acid residues with four intramolecular disulfide bridges. Neurotoxin α, on the other hand, is a 71-residue polypeptide chain, cross-linked intramolecularly by five disulfide bridges.

V. REFERENCES

Albuquerque, E. X. and S. Thesleff (1967), *J. Physiol. (London)*, **190**:123.
Albuquerque, E. X. and S. Thesleff (1968), *Acta Physiol. Scand.*, **72**:248.
Aloof-Hirsch, S., A. De Vries, and A. Berger (1968), *Biochim. Biophys. Acta*, **154**:53.
Amuchastegui, S. R. (1940), *C. R. Soc. Biol. (Paris)*, **133**:318.
Angelakos, E. T. and P. M. Glassman (1965), *Arch. Int. Pharmacodyn.*, **154**:82.
Aravindakshan, I. and B. M. Braganca (1959), *Biochim. Biophys. Acta,* **31**:463.
Aravindakshan, I. and B. M. Braganca (1961a), *Biochem. J.*, **79**:80.
Aravindakshan, I. and B. M. Braganca (1961b), *Biochem. J.*, **79**:84.
Arthus, M. (1910), *Arch. Int. Physiol.*, **10**:161.
Augustinsson, K. B. (1951), *Acta Chem. Scand.*, **5**:699, 712.
Babilli, S. and W. Vogt (1965), *J. Physiol. (London)*, **177**:31P.
Barnes, J. M. and J. Trueta (1941), *Lancet*, **1**:623.
Beerens, J. and H. Cuypers (1935), *Brux. Méd.*, **15**:757.
Bergström, S., L. A. Carlson, and G. R. Weeks (1968), *Pharmacol. Reviews*, **20**:1.
Bertrand, G. and R. Vladesco (1940a), *Ann. Inst. Pasteur*, **64**:344.
Bertrand, G. and R. Vladesco (1940b), *Ann. Inst. Pasteur*, **65**:5.
Bhanganada, K. and J. F. Perry (1963), *J. Amer. Med. Assn.*, **183**:257.
Bicher, H. I. (1966), *Mem. Inst. Butantan, Simp. Int.*, **33**(2):523.
Bicher, H. I., C. Klibansky, J. Shiloah, S. Gitter, and A. De Vries (1965), *Biochem. Pharmacol.*, **14**:1779.
Bjork, W. (1961), *Biochim. Biophys. Acta*, **49**:195.

Bjork, W. (1964), *Biochim. Biophys. Acta*, **89**:483.

Bjork, W. and H. G. Boman (1959), *Biochim. Biophys. Acta*, **34**:503.

Boquet, P. (1964), *Toxicon*, **2**:5.

Boquet, P. (1966), *Toxicon*, **3**:243.

Boquet, P., Y. Izard, M. Jouannet, and J. Meaume (1966a), *Ann. Inst. Pasteur*, **111**:719.

Boquet, P., Y. Izard, M. Jouannet, and J. Meaume (1966b), *C. R. Acad. Sci. (Paris)*, **262**:1134.

Boquet, P., Y. Izard, M. Jouannet, and J. Meaume (1967a), Studies on some antigenic proteins and polypeptides from *Naja nigricollis* venom, *in* "Animal Toxins" (F. E. Russell and P. R. Saunders, eds.), Pergamon Press, Oxford and New York, pp. 293–298.

Boquet, P., Y. Izard, J. Meaume, and M. Jouannet (1967b), *Ann. Inst. Pasteur*, **112**:213.

Botes, D. P. (1970), Purification and amino acid sequence of three neurotoxins from the cape cobra (*Naja nivea*). 2nd Int. Symp. Animal and Plant Toxins, Israel, Abstracts, p. 33.

Botes, D., P. and D. J. Strydom (1969), *J. Biol. Chem.*, **244**:4147.

Bovet-Nitti, F. (1947), *Experientia*, **3**:283.

Braganca, B. M. and V. G. Khandeparkar (1966), *Life Sci.*, **5**:1911.

Braganca, B. M. and N. T. Patel (1965), *Canad. J. Biochem.*, **43**:915.

Braganca, B. M. and J. H. Quastel (1953), *Biochem. J.*, **53**:88.

Braganca, B. M. and Y. M. Sambray (1967), *Nature (London)*, **216**:1210.

Braganca, B. M., P. G. Badrinath, and E. J. Ambrose (1965), *Nature (London)*, **207**:534.

Braganca, B. M., N. T. Patel, and P. G. Badrinath (1967), *Biochim. Biophys. Acta*, **136**:508.

Brazil, V. and J. Vellard (1928), *Ann. Inst. Pasteur*, **42**:403.

Brisbois, L., N. Rabinovitch-Mahler, P. Delori, and L. Gillo (1968), *J. Chromatography*, **37**:463.

Brunton, T. L. and J. Fayrer (1873), *Proc. Roy. Soc.*, **21**:358.

Brunton, T. L. and J. Fayrer (1874), *Proc. Roy. Soc.*, **22**:68.

Brunton, T. L. and J. Fayrer (1875), *Proc. Roy. Soc.*, **23**:261.

Buglia, G. and G. Barbieri (1923), *Arch. Ital. Biol.*, **72**:116.

Calmette, A. (1907), "Les venins, les animaux venimeux et la sérothérapie anti-venimeuse," Masson, Paris, pp. 1–396.

Césari, E. and P. Boquet (1936), *Ann. Inst. Pasteur*, **56**:511.

Césari, E. and P. Boquet (1937), *Ann. Inst. Pasteur*, **58**:6.

Chain, E. (1937), *Quart. J. Exp. Physiol.*, **26**:299.

Chain, E. (1938), *Quart. J. Exp. Physiol.*, **27**:49.

Chain, E. (1939), *Biochem. J.*, **33**:407.

Chang, C. C. and C. Y. Lee (1955), *J. Formosan Med. Assn.*, **54**:103.

Chang, C. C. and C. Y. Lee (1963), *Arch. Int. Pharmacodyn.*, **144**:241.

Chang, C. C. and C. Y. Lee (1966), *Brit. J. Pharmacol.*, **28**:172.

Chaudhuri, D. K. (1949), *Ann. Biochem. Exp. Med.*, **9**:67, 73, 79, 85.

Chatterjee, A. K. (1949), *Indian J. Med. Res.*, **37**:241.

Chen, Y. H. and T. B. Lo (1968), *J. Chinese Chem. Soc. Ser. II*, **15**:84.

Cheymol, J., F. Bourillet, and M. Roch (1966), *Mem. Inst. Butantan, Simp. Int.*, **33**(2):541.

Cheymol, J., F. Bourillet, and M. Roch-Arveiller (1967), *Arch. Int. Pharmacodyn.*, **170**:193.

Chiang, T. S., K. J. Ho, and C. Y. Lee (1964), *J. Formosan Med. Assn.*, **63**:127.

Chiu, P. J. S. (1966), Action of cardiotoxin on the isolated guinea-pig ileum. M. S. thesis, National Taiwan University.

Chiu, T. H., C. Y. Lee, and S. Y. Lee (1968), *J. Formosan Med. Assn.*, **67**:557.

Chopra, R. N. and V. Iswariah (1931), *Indian J. Med. Res.*, **18**:1113.

Chou, T. C. and C. Y. Lee (1970), *Europ. J. Pharmacol.*, **8**:326.

Christensen, P. A. (1955), South African snake venoms and antivenoms, The South African Institute for Medical Research, Johannesburg, pp. 1–129.

65

Christensen, P. A. (1966), *Mem. Inst. Butantan, Simp. Int.* **33**(1):305.

Cicardo, V. H. (1935), *C. R. Soc. Biol. (Paris)*, **120**:732.

Cohen, M. and G. B. Sumyk (1966), *Toxicon*, **3**:291.

Condrea, E. and A. De Vries (1965), *Toxicon*, **2**:261.

Condrea, E. and P. Rosenberg (1968), *Biochim. Biophys. Acta*, **150**:271.

Condrea, E., A. De Vries, and J. Mager (1964a), *Biochim. Biophys. Acta*, **84**:60.

Condrea, E., B. Mammon, S. Aloof, and A. De Vries (1964b), *Biochim. Biophys. Acta*, **84**:365.

Condrea, E., Y. Avi-Dor, and J. Mager (1965), *Biochim. Biophys. Acta*, **110**:337.

Condrea, E., P. Rosenberg, and W. D. Dettbarn (1967), *Biochim. Biophys. Acta*, **135**:669.

Currie, B. T., D. E. Oakley, and C. A. Broomfield (1968), *Nature (London)*, **220**:371.

Cushny, A. R. and S. Yagi (1918), *Trans. Roy. Soc. (London)*, Ser. B**208**:1.

Dakhil, T. and W. Vogt (1962), *Arch. Exp. Pathol. Pharmak.*, **243**:174.

D'Amour, F. E. and D. L. Smith (1941), *J. Pharmacol.*, **72**:74.

Dawson, R. M. C. (1963), *Biochem. J.*, **88**:414.

De, S. S. (1944), *J. Indian. Chem. Soc.*, **21**:292.

Delezenne, C. (1919), *Ann. Inst. Pasteur*, **33**:68.

Delezenne, C. and S. Ledebt (1911a), *C. R. Soc. Biol. (Paris)*, **71**:121.

Delezenne, C. and S. Ledebt (1911b), *C. R. Acad. Sci. (Paris)*, **152**:790.

Delezenne, C. and S. Ledebt (1911c), *C. R. Acad. Sci. (Paris)*, **153**:81.

Delezenne, C. and S. Ledebt (1912), *C. R. Acad. Sci. (Paris)*, **155**:1101.

De Nicola, P. and G. A. Cappelletti (1959), *Edizioni Haematologica (Pavia)*, **17**:173.

Detrait, J. and P. Boquet (1958), *C. R. Acad. Sci. (Paris)*, **246**:1107.

Detrait, J., Y. Izard, and P. Boquet (1959), *C. R. Soc. Biol. (Paris)*, **153**:1722.

Devi, A. and N. K. Sarkar (1966), *Mem. Inst. Butantan, Simp. Int.*, **33**(2):573.

De Vries, A., C. Kirschmann, C. Klibansky, E. Condrea, and S. Gitter (1962), *Toxicon*, **1**:19.

Doery, H. M. and J. E. Pearson (1964), *Biochem. J.*, **92**:599.

Eaker, D. L. and J. Porath (1967), The amino acid sequence of a neurotoxin from *Naja nigricollis* venom. 7th Int. Congr. Biochem. Tokyo, Col. VIII-3, Abstracts Suppl. I, p. 1087.

Edlinger, E. and B. Dietel (1959), *Naturwissenschaften*, **46**:516.

Edwards, S. W. and E. G. Ball (1954), *J. Biol. Chem.*, **209**:619.

Elliot, R. H. (1905), *Phil. Trans. Roy. Soc.*, **197**:361.

Elliott, W. B., J. M. Augustyn, and C. Gans (1966), *Mem. Inst. Butantan, Simp. Int.*, **33**(2):411.

Epstein, D. (1930), *Quart. J. Exp. Physiol.*, **20**:7.

Feldberg, W. (1940), *J. Physiol. (London)*, **99**:104.

Feldberg, W. and C. H. Kellaway (1937a), *Aust. J. Exp. Biol. Med. Sci.*, **15**:159.

Feldberg, W. and C. H. Kellaway (1937b), *Austral. J. Exp. Biol. Med. Sci.*, **15**:441.

Feldberg, W. and C. H. Kellaway (1938), *J. Physiol. (London)*, **94**:187.

Feldberg, W., H. F. Holden, and C. H. Kellaway (1938), *J. Physiol. (London)*, **94**:232.

Felix, F., J. L. Potter, and M. Laskowski (1960), *J. Biol. Chem.*, **235**:1150.

Feng, T. P. and T. H. Li (1941), *Chinese. J. Physiol.*, **16**:37.

Fischer, G. A. and J. J. Kabara (1967), Low molecular weight toxins isolated from Elapidae venoms, *in* "Animal Toxins" (F. E. Russell and P. R. Saunders eds.), Pergamon Press, Oxford and New York, pp. 283–292.

Fleckenstein, A. and O. Fettig (1952), *Arch. Exp. Pathol. Pharmak.*, **216**:415.

Fleckenstein, A. and H. Gerhardt (1952), *Arch. Exp. Pathol. Pharmak.*, **214**:135.

Fleckenstein, A. and W. Jaeger (1952), *Arch. Exp. Pathol. Pharmak.*, **215**:163.

Fleckenstein, A., G. Berg, J. Gayer, and S. Schönig (1951), *Arch. Exp. Pathol. Pharmak.*, **213**:265.

Fontana, F. (1787), Treatise on the venom of the viper, on the American poisons, and on the cherry laurel, and some other vegetable poisons, vols. I and II, J. Murray, London, pp. 1–409; 1–395.

Fraser, T. R. (1897a), *Brit. Med. J.*, **2**:595.

Fraser, T. R. (1897b), *Indian Med. Rec.*, 13:147.
Fraser, T. R. and J. A. Gunn (1909), *Phil. Trans. Roy. Soc. (London)*, B200:241.
Gaertner, C., N. Goldblum, S. Gitter, and A. De Vries (1962), *J. Immunol.*, 88:526.
Ganguly, S. N. and M. Malkana (1936), *Indian J. Med. Res.*, 24:281.
Gautrelet, J. and N. Halpern (1933), *C. R. Soc. Biol. (Paris)*, 113:1486.
Gautrelet, J. and N. Halpern (1934), *C. R. Soc. Biol. (Paris)*, 115:942.
Gautrelet, J., N. Halpern, and E. Corteggiani (1934), *Arch. Int. Physiol.*, 38:293.
Ghosh, B. N. and A. K. Chatterjee (1948), *J. Indian Chem. Soc.*, 25:359.
Ghosh, B. N., P. K. Dutt, and D. K. Chowdhury (1939), *J. Indian Chem. Soc.*, 16:75.
Gitter, S., S. Amiel, G. Gilat, T. Sonnino, and Y. Welwart (1963), *Nature (London)*, 197:383.
Gottdenker, F. and M. Wachstein (1940), *J. Pharmacol.*, 69:117.
Grasset, E. and P. A. Christensen (1947), *Trans. Roy. Soc. Trop. Med. Hyg.*, 41:207.
Grasset, E. and L. Goldstein (1947), *Trans. Roy. Soc. Trop. Med. Hyg.*, 40:771.
Grasset, E., A. Zoutendyk, and A. Schaafsma (1935), *Trans. Roy. Soc. Trop. Med. Hyg.*, 28:601.
Grassmann, W. and K. Hannig (1954), *Hoppe-Seylers Z. Physiol. Chem.*, 296:30.
Green, D. E. and S. Fleischer (1963), *Biochim. Biophys. Acta*, 70:554.
Green, H. N. and H. B. Stoner (1950), Biological actions of the adenine nucleotides, H. K. Lewis & Co., Ltd., London, pp. 1–221.
Gulland, J. M. and E. M. Jackson (1938a), *Biochem. J.*, 32:590.
Gulland, J. M. and E. M. Jackson (1938b), *Biochem. J.*, 32:597.
Guyot, P. and P. Boquet (1960), *C. R. Acad. Sci. (Paris)*, 251:1822.
Habermann, E. (1954), *Naturwissenschaften*, 41:429.
Habermann, E. (1957), *Arch. Exp. Pathol. Pharmak.*, 230:538.
Habermann, E. (1960), *Arch. Exp. Pathol. Pharmak.*, 238:502.
Habermann, E. and J. Jentsch (1967), *Hoppe-Seyler's Z. Physiol. Chem.*, 348:37.
Habermann, E. and B. Krusche (1962), *Biochem. Pharmacol.*, 11:400.
Habermann, E. and W. P. Neumann (1954), *Arch. Exp. Pathol. Pharmak.*, 223:388.
Habermann, E. and K. G. Reiz (1965), *Biochem. Z.*, 343:192.
Hirschfeld, L. and R. Klinger (1915), *Biochem. Z.*, 70:398.
Hoff, E. C., R. G. Grenell, and J. F. Fulton (1945), *Medicine*, 24:161.
Honjo, I. and K. Ozawa (1968), *Biochim. Biophys. Acta*, 162:624.
Houssay, B. A. (1930), *C. R. Soc. Biol. (Paris)*, 105:308.
Houssay, B. A. and P. Mazzocco (1925), *C. R. Soc. Biol. (Paris)*, 93:1120.
Houssay, B. A. and S. Pavé (1922), *C. R. Soc. Biol. (Paris)*, 87:821.
Houssay, B. A., N. J. Otero, J. Negrete, and P. Mazzocco (1921), *Rev. Assn. Méd. Argent.*, 34:299.
Houssay, B. A., J. Negrete, and P. Mazzocco (1922), *C. R. Soc. Biol. (Paris)*, 87:823.
Huang, P. C. (1954a), *J. Formosan Med. Assn.*, 53:128.
Huang, P. C. (1954b), *J. Formosan Med. Assn.*, 53:353.
Hughes, A. (1935), *Biochem. J.*, 29:430.
Hunter, W. K. (1909), *Proc. Roy. Soc. Med.*, 3(ii):105.
Ibrahim, S. A., H. Sanders, and R. H. S. Thompson (1964), *Biochem. J.*, 93:588.
Ishii, T. (1929), *Jap. J. Microbiol. Pathol.*, 23:1093, 1127.
Iwase, Y. (1933), *J. Formosan. Med. Assn.*, 32:624.
Iyergar, N. K., K. B. Sehra, B. Mukerji, and R. N. Chopra (1938), *Current Sci. Indian Inst. Sci.*, 7:51.
Izard, Y., M. Boquet, A. M. Rousseray, and P. Boquet (1969a), *C. R. Acad. Sci. (Paris)*, 269:96.
Izard, Y., P. Boquet, E. Golémi, and D. Goupil (1969b), *C. R. Acad. Sci. (Paris)*, 269:666.
Jiménez-Porras, J. M. (1968), *Ann. Rev. Pharmacol.*, 8:299.
Johnson, M., M. A. G. Kaye, R. Hems, and H. A. Krebs (1953), *Biochem. J.*, 54:625.
Kaiser, E. and H. Michl (1958), Die Biochemie der tierischen Gifte, Franz Deuticke, Vienna, pp. 1–258.
Karczmar, A. G. (1967), *Ann. Rev. Pharmacol.*, 7:241.

Karlsson, E., D. L. Eaker, and J. Porath (1966). *Biochim. Biophys. Acta*, **127**:505.
Kaye, M. A. G. (1955), *Biochim. Biophys. Acta*, **18**:456.
Kaye, M. A. G. (1960), *Biochim. Biophys. Acta*, **38**:34.
Kellaway, C. H. (1929), *Brit. J. Exp. Pathol.*, **10**:281.
Kellaway, C. H. (1932), *Austral. J. Exp. Biol. Med. Sci.*, **10**:195.
Kellaway, C. H. (1937), *Bull. Johns Hopkins Hosp.*, **60**:20.
Kellaway, C. H. and F. Holden (1932), *Austral. J. Exp. Biol. Med. Sci.*, **10**:167.
Kellaway, C. H. and E. R. Trethewie (1940), *Austral. J. Exp. Biol. Med. Sci.*, **18**:63.
Kellaway, C. H., R. O. Cherry, and F. E. Williams (1932), *Austral. J. Exp. Biol. Med. Sci.*, **10**:181.
Klibansky, C. and A. De Vries (1964), *Toxicon*, **2**:181.
Klibansky, C., E. Condrea, and A. De Vries (1962), *Amer. J. Physiol.*, **203**:114.
Klibansky, C., J. Shiloah, and A. De Vries (1964), *Biochem. Pharmacol.*, **13**:1107.
Klibansky, C., E. Ozcan, H. Joshua, M. Djaldetti, H. Bessler, and A. De Vries (1966), *Toxicon*, **3**:213.
Krupnick, J., H. I. Bicher, and S. Gitter (1968), *Toxicon*, **6**:11.
Kruse, I. and H. Dam (1950), *Biochem. Biophys. Acta*, **5**:268.
Lamb, G. and W. K. Hunter (1904a), *Lancet*, **1**:20.
Lamb, G. and W. K. Hunter (1904b), *Lancet*, **1**:518.
Larsen, P. R. and J. Wolff (1967a), *Science*, **155**:335.
Larsen, P. R. and J. Wolff (1967b), *Biochem. Pharmacol.*, **16**:2003.
Larsen, P. R. and J. Wolff (1968a), *Biochem. Pharmacol.*, **17**:503.
Larsen, P. R. and J. Wolff (1968b), *J. Biol. Chem.*, **243**:1283.
Lee, C. Y. (1963), *J. Showa Med. Assn.*, **23**:221.
Lee, C. Y. and C. C. Chang (1966), *Mem. Inst. Butantan, Simp. Int.*, **33**(2):555.
Lee, C. Y. and C. Ouyang (1958), *Proc. 7th Int. Congr. Int. Soc. Haematol. Rome*, **2**, 1.
Lee, C. Y. and M. T. Peng (1961), *Arch. Int. Pharmacodyn.*, **13**:180.
Lee, C. Y. and L. F. Tseng (1966), *Toxicon*, **3**:281.
Lee, C. Y. and L. F. Tseng (1969), *Toxicon*, **7**:89.
Lee, C. Y., C. C. Chang, and K. Kamijo (1956), *Biochem. J.*, **62**:582.
Lee, C. Y., C. C. Chang, and C. Su (1960), *J. Formosan Med. Assn.*, **59**:1065.
Lee, C. Y., C. C. Chang, C. Su, and Y. W. Chen (1962), *J. Formosan Med. Ass.*, **61**:239.
Lee, C. Y., C. C. Chang, T. H. Chiu, P. J. S. Chiu, T. C. Tseng, and S. Y. Lee (1968), *Arch. Exp. Pathol. Pharmak.*, **259**:360.
Lee, C. Y., J. S. Lin, and J. W. Wei (1970), Identification of cardiotoxin with cobramine B, DLF and cobra venom cytotoxin. 2nd Int. Symp. Animal and Plant Toxins, Israel, Abstracts, p. 59.
Levaditi, C. and S. Mutermilch (1913), *C. R. Soc. Biol. (Paris)*, **74**:1305.
Lin, Y. C. and L. T. Chang (1957), *J. Formosan Med. Assn.*, **56**:336.
Lin, Y. C., T. C. Su, and K. H. Ling (1957), *J. Formosan Med. Assn.*, **56**:176.
Link, T. (1935), *Z. Immun-Forsch.*, **85**:504.
Lo, T. B. and Y. H. Chen (1966), *J. Chinese Chem. Soc., Ser. II*, **13**:195.
Lo, T. B., Y. H. Chen, and C. Y. Lee (1966), *J. Chinese Chem. Soc., Ser. II*, **13**:25.
Macht, D. I. (1935), *Amer. J. Physiol.*, **113**:90.
Macht, D. I. (1936), *Proc. Soc. Exp. Biol. Med.*, **35**:316.
Macht, D. I. (1943), *Proc. Soc. Exp. Biol. Med.*, **53**:225.
Macht, D. I. and D. B. Kehoe (1943), *Fed. Proc.*, **2**:31.
Marcacci, M. and L. Bruzzese (1959), *Edizioni Haematologica, (Pavia)*, **17**:231.
Markwardt, F., W. Barthel, E. Glusa, and A. Hoffmann (1966), *Arch. Exp. Pathol. Pharmak.*, **252**:297.
Master, R. W. P. and S. S. Rao (1961), *J. Biol. Chem.*, **236**:1986.
Meaume, J. (1966), *Toxicon*, **4**:25.
Meaume, J., Y. Izard, and P. Boquet (1966), *C. R. Acad. Sci. (Paris)*, **262**:1650.
Mebs, D. (1968), *Europ. J. Pharmacol.*, **2**:403.
Meldrum, B. S. (1965a), *Pharmacol. Reviews*, **17**:393.
Meldrum, B. S. (1965b), *Brit. J. Pharmacol.*, **25**:197.

Mellanby, E. (1934–1936), *Ann. Rep. Brit. Empire Cancer Campaign*, **11**:81, **12**:99, **13**:99.
Mellanby, J. (1909), *J. Physiol. (London)*, **38**:441.
Meurling, S. (1935), *C. R. Soc. Biol. (Paris)*, **120**:1119.
Meyer, A. (1963), Anoxias, intoxication and metabolic disorders, *in* "Neuropathology" (W. Blackwood, W. H. McMenemey, A. Meyer, R. M. Norman, and D. S. Russell, eds.), Edward Arnold, London, pp. 235–287.
Mitel'man, L. S. (1966), *Byul. Eksp. Biol. Med.*, **62**:69.
Morales, F., K. Bhanganada, and J. F. Perry (1963), Effect of several agents on the lethal action of two common venoms, *in* "Venomous and Poisonous Animals and Noxious Plants of the Pacific Region" (H. L. Keegan and W. V. Macfarlane, eds.), Pergamon Press, New York, pp. 385–398.
Moran, N. C., B. Uvnös, and B. Westerholm (1962), *Acta Physiol. Scand.*, **56**:26.
Morawitz, P. (1905), *Ergebn. Physiol.*, **4**:307.
Mounter, L. A. (1951), *Biochem. J.*, **50**:122.
Nakamura, T. (1933), *J. Formosan Med. Assn.*, **32**:33.
Narahashi, T. and J. M. Tobias (1964), *Amer. J. Physiol.*, **207**:1441.
Narita, K. and C. Y. Lee (1970), The amino acid sequence of cardiotoxin from *Naja naja atra* venom, *Biochem. Biophys. Res. Comm.* (in press).
Neelin, J. M. (1963), *Canad. J. Biochem. Physiol.*, **41**:1073.
Nelson, P. G. (1958), *J. Cell. Comp. Physiol.*, **52**:127.
Nygaard, A. P. (1953), *J. Biol. Chem.*, **204**:655.
Nygaard, A. P. and J. B. Sumner (1953), *J. Biol. Chem.*, **200**:723.
Nygaard, A. P., M. U. Dianzani, and G. F. Bahr (1954), *Exp. Cell Res.*, **6**:453.
O'Brien, J. R. (1956a), *Brit. J. Haemat.*, **2**:430.
O'Brien, J. R. (1956b), *J. Clin. Pathol.*, **9**:47.
Oh, Y. (1942), *J. Formosan Med. Assn.*, **41**:1185.
Ouyang, C. (1957), *J. Formosan Med. Assn.*, **56**:435.
Pacella, G. (1923), *C. R. Soc. Biol. (Paris)*, **88**:366.
Parnas, I. and. F. E. Russell (1967), Effects of venoms on nerve, muscle and neuromuscular junction, *in* "Animal Toxins" (F. E. Russell and P. R. Saunders, eds.), Pergamon Press, Oxford and New York, pp.401–415.
Patel, T. N., B. M. Braganca, and R. A. Bellare (1969), *Exp. Cell Res.*, **57**:289.
Patzer, P. and W. Vogt (1967), *Arch. Exp. Pathol. Pharmak.*, **257**:320.
Peng, M. T. (1951), *Mem. Fac. Med. Nat'l. Taiwan Univ.*, **1**:200.
Peng, M. T. (1952), *Mem. Fac. Med. Nat'l. Taiwan Univ.*, **2**:170.
Peng, M. T. (1960), *J. Formosan Med. Assn.*, **59**:1073.
Peron, F. G. (1964), *Biochim. Biophys. Acta*, **82**:125.
Petrushka, E., J. H. Quastel, and P. G. Scholefield (1959a), *Canad. J. Biochem. Physiol.*, **37**:975.
Petrushka, E., J. H. Quastel, and P. G. Scholefield (1959b), *Canad. J. Biochem. Physiol.*, **37**:989.
Porath, J. (1966), *Mem. Inst. Butantan, Simp. Int.*, **33**:(2)379.
Radomski, J. L. and W. B. Deichmann (1958), *Biochem. J.*, **70**:293.
Ragotzi, V. (1890), *Virchows Arch. Pathol. Anat. Physiol.*, **122**:201.
Raudonat, H. W. and R. Holler (1958), *Arch. Exp. Pathol. Pharmak.*, **233**:431.
Ray, P. (1940), *J. Indian Chem. Soc.*, **17**:681.
Razzell, W. E. and H. G. Khorana (1959a), *J. Biol. Chem.*, **234**:2105.
Razzell, W. E. and H. G. Khorana (1959b), *J. Biol. Chem.*, **234**:2114.
Reid, H. A. (1964), *Brit. Med. J.*, **2**:540.
Ri, T. (1939), *Folia Pharmacol. Japonica*, **27**:13.
Richards, G. M., G. Du Vair, and M. Laskowski (1965), *Biochemistry*, **4**:501.
Riker, W. F., G. Werner, J. Roberts, and A. Kuperman (1959), *Ann. N.Y. Acad. Sci.*, **81**:328.
Rimon, A. and B. Schapiro (1959), *Biochem. J.*, **71**:620.
Rocha e Silva, M. and W. T. Beraldo (1948), *J. Pharmacol.*, **93**:457.

Rogers, L. (1905), *Phil. Trans. Roy. Soc.*, **B197**:123.
Rosenberg, P. (1965), *Toxicon*, **3**:125.
Rosenberg, P. (1966), *Mem. Inst. Butantan, Simp. Int.*, **33**(2):477.
Rosenberg, P. and E. Condrea (1968), *Biochem. Pharmacol.*, **17**:2033.
Rosenberg, P. and T. R. Podleski (1962), *J. Pharmacol.*, **137**:249.
Rosenberg, P. and T. R. Podleski (1963), *Biochim. Biophys. Acta*, **75**:104.
Ruch, J. V. and O. Gabriel-Robez-Kremer (1962), *C. R. Soc. Biol. (Paris)*, **156**:1508.
Ruch, J. V. and O. Gabriel-Robez-Kremer (1963), *C. R. Soc. Biol. (Paris)*, **157**:2291.
Ruch, J. V., M. Zahnd, O. Gabriel-Robez-Kremer, Y. Rumpler, and P. Gerlinger (1965), *Arch. Biol. (Liège)*, **76**:25.
Russell, F. E. (1967), *Federation Proc.*, **26**:1206.
Sanders, M., B. A. Arin, and M. G. Soret (1954), *Acta Neuroveg.*, **8**:362.
Sarkar, B. B., S. R. Maitra, and B. N. Ghosh (1942), *Indian J. Med. Res.*, **30**:453.
Sarkar, N. K. (1947a), *J. Indian Chem. Soc.*, **24**:227.
Sarkar, N. K. (1947b), *J. Indian Chem. Soc.*, **24**:61.
Sarkar, N. K. (1951), *Proc. Soc. Exp. Biol. Med.*, **78**:469.
Sarkar, N. K. and S. R. Maitra (1950), *Amer. J. Physiol.*, **163**:209.
Sasaki, T. (1957a), *J. Pharmaceut. Soc. Japan*, **77**:845.
Sasaki, T. (1957b), *J. Pharmaceut. Soc. Japan*, **77**:848.
Sato, I., K. W. Ryan, and S. Mitsuhashi (1964), *Jap. J. Exp. Med.*, **34**:119.
Sato, S. and N. Tamiya (1968), The primary structure of erabutoxin. *19th Seminar on Protein Structure, Tokyo, Proc.*, p. 13.
Shü, I. C., K. H. Ling, and C. C. Yang (1968), *Toxicon*, **5**:295.
Slotta, K. H. (1955), *Fortschr. Chem. Org. Naturst.*, **12**:406.
Slotta, K. H. and H. L. Fraenkel-Conrat (1938), *Ber. Deutsch. Chem. Gesellsch.*, **71A**:264.
Slotta, K. H., J. D. Gonzalez, and S. C. Roth (1967), The direct and indirect hemolytic factors from animal venoms, *in* "Animal Toxins" (F. E. Russell and P. R. Saunders, eds.), Pergamon Press, Oxford and New York, pp. 369–377.
Slotta, K. H. and J. A. Vick (1969), *Toxicon*, **6**:167.
Su, C. (1960), *J. Formosan Med. Ass.*, **59**:1083.
Su, C., C. C. Chang, and C. Y. Lee (1967), Pharmacological properties of the neurotoxin of cobra venom, *in* "Animal Toxins" (F. E. Russell and P. R. Saunders, eds.), Pergamon Press, Oxford and New York, pp. 259–267.
Sulkowski, E., W. Bjork, and M. Laskowski (1963), *J. Biol. Chem.*, **238**:2477.
Sumyk, G., H. Lal, and E. J. Hawrylewicz (1963), *Federation Proc.*, **22**:668.
Suzuki, T. (1966), *Mem. Inst. Butantan, Simp. Int.*, **33**(2):389.
Suzuki, T. and S. Iwanaga (1958), *J. Pharmaceut. Soc. Japan*, **78**:354.
Takeuchi, T. and N. Takeuchi (1964), *J. Physiol. (London)*, **170**:296.
Tamiya, N. and H. Arai (1966), *Biochem. J.*, **99**:624.
Tamiya, N. and S. Sato (1967), *7th Int. Congr. Biochem., Tokyo, Col. VIII*-2, *Abstracts III*, p. 497.
Taub, A. M. and W. B. Elliott (1964), *Toxicon*, **2**:87.
Taylor, J., S. M. K. Mallick, and M. L. Ahuja (1935), *Indian J. Med. Res.* **23**:131.
Tobias, J. M. (1955), *J. Cell. Comp. Physiol.*, **46**:183.
Tobias, J. M. (1960), *J. Gen. Physiol.*, **43**:57.
Tseng, L. F., T. H. Chiu, and C. Y. Lee (1968), *Toxicol. Appl. Pharmacol.*, **12**:526.
Tseng, T. C. (1964), A study on cardiotoxin isolated from Formosan cobra venom, M. S. thesis, National Taiwan University.
Tu, A. T., G. P. James, and A. Chua (1965), *Toxicon*, **3**:5.
Ueda, E., T. Sasaki, and M. T. Peng (1951), A chemical study on Formosan cobra venom, *Mem. Fac. Med. National Taiwan Univ.*, **1**:194.
Vázquez-Colón, L., F. D. Ziegler, and W. B. Elliott (1966), *Biochemistry*, **5**:1134.
Ventakachalam, K. and A. M. Ratnagiriswaran (1934), *Indian J. Med. Res.*, **22**:289.
Vick, J. A., H. P. Ciuchta, and E. H. Polley (1964), *Nature (London)*, **203**:1387.
Vick, J. A., H. P. Ciuchta, and E. H. Polley (1965), *Arch. Int. Pharmacodyn.*, **153**:424.

Vick, J. A., H. P. Ciuchta, and J. H. Manthei (1967), Pathophysiological studies of ten snake venoms, *in* "Animal Toxins" (F. E. Russell and P. R. Saunders, eds.), Pergamon Press, Oxford and New York, pp. 269–282.

Vogt, W. (1957), *J. Physiol. (London)*, **136**:131.

Vogt, W., T. Suzuki, and S. Babilli (1966), *Mem. Soc. Endocrinol.*, **14**:137.

Vogt, W., U. Meyer, H. Kunze, E. Lufft, and S. Babilli (1969), *Arch. Exp. Pathol. Pharmak.*, **262**:124.

Vollmer, E. (1893), *Arch. Exp. Pathol. Pharmak.*, **31**:1.

Wakui, K. and S. Kawachi (1961), *J. Pharmaceut. Soc. Japan*, **81**:1394.

Waser, P. G. and U. Lüthi (1957), *Arch. Inst. Pharmacodyn.*, **112**:272.

Westermann, E. and W. Klapper (1960), *Arch. Exp. Pathol. Pharmak.*, **239**:68.

Wille, G. and W. Vogt (1965), *Arch. Exp. Pathol. Pharmak.*, **251**:193.

Williams, E. J., S. C. Sung, and M. Laskowski (1960), *J. Biol. Chem.*, **236**:1130.

Witter, R. F. and M. A. Cottone (1956), *Biochim. Biophys. Acta*, **22**:364.

Witter, R. F., A. Morrison, and G. R. Shepardson (1957), *Biochim. Biophys. Acta*, **26**:120.

Wolff, J., H. Salabé, M. Ambrose, and P. R. Larsen (1968), *J. Biol. Chem.*, **243**:1290.

Yamaguti, K. (1923), *Z. Hyg. Infektionskrank.*, **100**:182.

Yang, C. C. (1965), *J. Biol. Chem.*, **240**:1616.

Yang, C. C. (1967), *Biochim. Biophys. Acta*, **133**:346.

Yang, C. C. and L. T. Chang (1954), *J. Formosan Med. Assn.*, **53**:609.

Yang, C. C. and T. C. Tung (1953), *J. Formosan Med. Assn.*, **52**:83.

Yang, C. C. and T. C. Tung (1954), *J. Formosan Med. Assn.*, **53**:123.

Yang, C. C., L. C. Huang, and T. C. Tung (1954), *J. Formosan Med. Assn.*, **53**:1.

Yang, C. C., C. J. Chen, and C. C. Su (1959), *J. Biochem. (Tokyo)*, **46**:1201.

Yang, C. C., C. C., Chang, K. Hayashi, and T. Suzuki (1969a), *Toxicon*, **7**:43.

Yang, C. C., H. J. Yang, and J. S. Huang (1969b), *Biochim. Biophys. Acta*, **188**:65.

Zaimis, E. J. (1957), Factors influencing the action of neuromuscular blocking substances, *in* "Lectures on the Scientific Basis of Medicine," John de Graif, Inc., New York, p. 208.

Zaki, O. A., A. Khogali, D. Petkovic, and S. A. Ibrahim (1967), *Toxicon*, **5**:91.

Zeller, E. A. (1947), *Experientia*, **3**:375.

Zeller, E. A. (1948), *Advan. Enzymol.*, **8**:459.

Zeller, E. A. (1950), *Arch. Biochem.*, **28**:138.

Zeller, E. A. (1951), Enzymes as essential components of bacterial and animal toxins, *in* "The Enzymes" (J. B. Summer and K. Myrback, eds.) Vol. 1, Pt. 2, Academic Press, New York, pp. 986–1013.

Ziegler, F. D., L. Vázquez-Colón, W. B. Elliott, C. Gans, and A. Taub (1967), Production by snake venoms of uncoupling activity and reverse acceptor control in rat liver mitochondrial preparations. Part II. Studies on energy metabolism following treatment of mitochondria with several snake venoms. In "Animal Toxins" (F. E. Russell and P. R. Saunders, eds.), Pergamon Press, Oxford and New York, pp. 236–243.

Chapter 3

Symptomatology of Experimental and Clinical Crotalid Envenomation

James A. Vick

Walter Reed Army Institute of Research
Walter Reed Army Medical Center
Washington, D.C., U.S.A.

I. THE RATTLESNAKE

Rattlesnakes, indigenous to the North American continent, are all members of the family of poisonous snakes called Crotalidae (*see* Fig. 1). This family, Crotalidae, is one of the four major families of poisonous snakes. The other three are: Elapidae, Viperidae, and Hydrophiidae. A fifth group of rear-fanged poisonous snakes has been described and is usually classified as Boiginae, a subfamily of Colubridae (Conant, 1958; Klauber, 1956; Stebbeirs, 1954).

By comparison with other areas of the world, North America has a comparatively small but extremely well-known selection of poisonous snakes. In addition to 15 species of rattlesnakes, the North American continent harbors copperheads, water mocassins, and two species of coral snakes (Department of the Navy, 1968; Stebbeirs, 1954; Wright and Wright, 1957). All of these snakes, with the exception of the coral snakes, are members of the family of pit vipers, Crotalidae.

Basically, rattlesnakes are unique to the American continent and can be identified readily by the presence of a jointed rattle located at the tip of the tail. The facial pits of the rattlesnake, which account for the origin of the name "pit viper," are heat-sensitive organs located just forward of the eye on either side of the head. These, in addition to the rattle, distinguish the North American rattlesnake. The fangs of the rattlesnake are usually quite

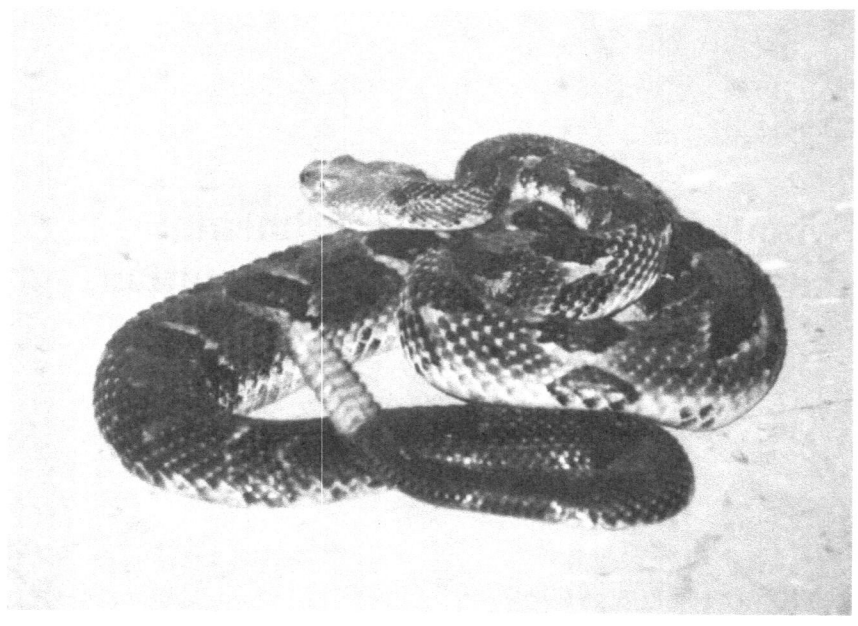

Fig. 1. *Crotalus horridus horridus* (timber rattlesnake).

long when compared to those of the family Elapidae and are hinged rather than fixed. It is interesting to note that poisonous snakes have voluntary control over the discharge of venom from fangs and can, during biting, release venom from either fang, both, or, in rare instances, neither (Conant 1958; Department of the Navy, 1968). Rattlesnakes usually discharge $\frac{1}{4} - \frac{3}{4}$ of the venom content of their modified salivary gland when they envenomate or bite a victim. Effects of envenomation are, therefore, directly proportional not only to the potency of the venom, but also to the actual amount received at time of bite.

Incidence of rattlesnake bite in the United States has been estimated at from 700 to 1000 per year, with approximately 20 deaths (Department of the Navy, 1968). Typical of the bite of the Crotalidae family of snakes is the presence of one or more deep fang marks due to the rather long, jointed nature of the fangs of these pit vipers. In most cases there is immediate pain in the area of the bite with progressive swelling and edema taking place over the first 10 min. If untreated, swelling, edema, and pain progress rapidly and soon involve a large area adjacent to the bite. Maximum swelling usually occurs at from 24 to 36 hr following envenomation. Hemorrhagic vesiculations and petechiae are usually seen at approximately this same period of time, with or without the presence of shiny, smooth skin vesicles.

Associated with the rather intense pain that follows crotolid envenomation is a generalized feeling of weakness, faintness, and nausea. Lymph nodes enlarge in the area of the bite and are usually quite tender. Numbness has been reported in the region of the head, usually about the scalp and mouth (Deichman et al., 1958; Gennaro, 1963; McCollough and Gennaro, 1963).

If untreated, the bite of certain rattlesnakes can result in death in from 48 to 96 hr. Current approaches to the treatment of crotalid bite will be discussed under Sec. IV.

Many of the known symptoms of rattlesnake envenomation have been gleaned from clinical observation of bite victims (Russell, 1967; Russell and Emery, 1961). Such observations are often inconsistent for at least two reasons. First, the interval between patient envenomation and patient care under a physician varies widely. Never is a full spectrum of symptomology witnessed because of the unlikeliness of bite taking place in close proximity to medical or laboratory apparatus. Second, the physician ordinarily attends to those symptoms most conspicuous in contributing to victim peril, and subleties may escape notice.

For these reasons, efforts in our laboratory have been directed toward assessing the full pathophysiology of rattlesnake envenomation. We have attempted to monitor the full complement of body reactions to snake bite. What follows is a resume of our observations. The primary purpose of the first portion of this chapter is to evaluate the actual venom potency of the more widely distributed North American rattlesnakes and to characterize, if possible, the primary mechanism by which each or all of these venoms kill. Secondly, a comparison is made between the potency and effects of re-constituted dry venom and that of venom obtained from an actual snake bite. Finally, the more interesting aspects of rattlesnake venom are briefly contrasted with those venoms obtained from the other three families of poisonous snakes.

II. RATTLESNAKE VENOM POTENCY

A. Mouse

A total of 600 mice have been used to establish the LD_{100} dose of the six rattlesnake venoms described in this portion of the chapter. An LD_{100} dose of venom is that amount of venom that, when injected into a group of experimental animals, will kill 100% in 72 hr. Venoms were obtained in a dried lyophilyzed form from the Miami Serpentarium, Miami, Florida. Prior to injection, all venoms were reconstituted with normal saline to a final concentration of 1 mg/cc. Mice were injected intravenously with varying amounts of each venom to establish a statistically significant LD_{100}

Table I.

Establishment of LD100 Doses of Each of Six Rattlesnake Venoms in the Mouse, Anesthetized Dog, and Monkey

Experimental animal	Scientific name of venom source	Common name	Distribution	Dose, mg/kg
Mouse	Crotalus d. durissus	Tropical rattlesnake	N., C., and S. America	0.10
	Crotalus adamanteus	Eastern diamondback	N. America	1.58
	Crotalus cerostes	Sidewinder	N. America	1.95
	Crotalus horridus horridus	Timber rattler	N. America	2.82
	Crotalus atrox	Western diamondback	N. America	3.03
	Sistrurus miliarius barbouri	Pigmy rattlesnake	N. America	4.47
			Average	2.36
Dog	Crotalus d. durissus	Tropical rattlesnake	N., C., and S. America	0.25
	Crotalus adamanteus	Eastern diamondback	N. America	0.50
	Crotalus cerostes	Sidewinder	N. America	0.30
	Crotalus horridus horridus	Timber rattler	N. America	0.38
	Crotalus atrox	Western diamondback	N. America	0.50
	Sistrurus miliarius barbouri	Pigmy rattlesnake	N. America	0.75
			Average	0.45
Monkey	Crotalus d. durissus	Tropical rattlesnake	N., C., and S. America	0.05
	Crotalus adamanteus	Eastern diamondback	N. America	0.25
	Crotalus cerostes	Sidewinder	N. America	0.30
	Crotalus horridus horridus	Timber rattler	N. America	0.125
	Crotalus atrox	Western diamondback	N. America	4.00
	Sistrurus miliarius barbouri	Pigmy rattlesnake	N. America	5.00
			Average	1.65

dose. All mice were followed for 72 hr or until death. Results as shown in Table I indicate that the six rattlesnake venoms vary widely as to their potency in mice. By far the more potent venom appears to be that obtained from the tropical rattlesnake; and the least potent that of the pigmy rattlesnake. The average lethal dose of all venoms studied in the mouse was 2.36 mg/kg of body weight.

B. Dog

On hundred twenty adult mongrel dogs anesthetized with sodium pentobarbital have been used to study the effects of a single intravenous dose of each of the six venoms. Each venom was given in graded doses to groups of 20 dogs to determine the LD_{100} dose in dogs and to characterize, if possible, the changes in vital function that follow envenomation with a lethal dose of each of the venoms. Data presented in Table I show that the same relative potency of venom exists in the dog as in the mouse, with the important exception that an anesthetized dog is approximately five times more susceptible than a mouse to all venoms. As with the mouse, the venom of the tropical rattlesnake appears to be the more potent, while that of the pigmy rattlesnake is the least potent. There is, however, much less variation between potencies of venom in the dog as opposed to the mouse.

C. Monkey

Thirty adult rhesus monkeys have been placed in restraining chairs and injected with varying doses of each of the six venoms. It is important to note that in these experiments the venom was administered intramuscularly rather than intravenously. All animals were followed until death or survival, which was established at 72 hr post-injection. One monkey from each group of five was autopsied for gross and microscopic tissue changes. Table I presents the data obtained from these studies. The unanesthetized monkey appears to respond to snake venom in much the same manner and dose as the unanesthetized mouse. The difference in venom dose noted in the dog may be due in part to the influence of barbiturate anesthesia.

D. Averaged Potency

A further comparison of the venoms of the six rattlesnakes studied has been obtained by averaging the LD_{100} dose in the mouse, the dog, and the monkey. The average lethal dose of venom for the tropical rattlesnake was 0.13 mg/kg; the eastern diamondback, 0.78 mg/kg; the sidewinder, 0.85 mg/kg; the timber rattler, 1.11 mg/kg; the western diamondback, 2.51 mg/kg; and the pigmy rattlesnake, 3.40 mg/kg. There appears to be a 30-fold difference in potency of venom obtained from the 6 rattlesnakes.

III. PHYSIOLOGICAL EFFECTS OF VENOM

In addition to determining the lethal dose of venom in mice, dogs and monkeys, we have obtained certain critical physiological measurements from time of injection until death. In the dog, arterial blood pressure was recorded via a Statham strain gauge and a Hewlett–Packard polyviso recorder. ECG, heart rate, and respiration were monitored with needle-tipped electrodes placed in either side of the chest wall. Cortical electrical activity (EEG) was continuously followed using silver wire electrodes placed directly on the dura of each hemisphere of the brain. The typical response of the anesthetized dog to a single intravenous dose of rattlesnake venom is shown in Fig. 2. The initial response is characterized by an immediate and precipituous fall in arterial blood pressere and a marked decrease in heart rate. This fall in pressure and heart rate persists for from 10 to 30 min and is due to pooling in the hepatosplanchnic bed (Russell, 1968; Vick *et al.*, 1966; Vick and Ciuchta, 1965). At approximately 30–60 min post injection, both parameters return toward control or near control values. These cardiovascular functions then remain unchanged until the onset of respiratory difficulties, at which time blood pressure decreases abruptly terminating in profound hypotension and finally, death. Shortly after injection of venom, the ECG pattern of the dog shows abnormalties characterized as extrasystoles, bigeminal pulses,

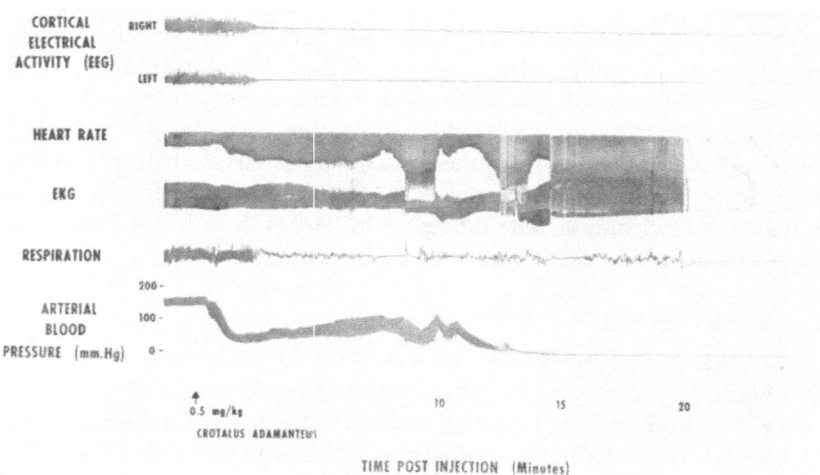

Fig. 2. Effect of a lethal dose of *Crotalus adamanteus* venom (eastern diamondback rattlesnake) on cortical activity, heart rate, ECG, respiration, and arterial blood pressure in the anesthetized dog.

depressed S-T segments, arrhythmias, and premature ventricular beats. These changes persist in certain animals and may play a role in the observed action of the venom on heart rate and blood pressure. All parameters considered, however, the primary mechanism of death in the dog is most likely respiratory in nature, and appears to be due to blockade of neuromuscular transmission at the level of the diaphragm (Deichman et al., 1958; Vick and Ciuchta, 1965; Vick et al., 1966, 1968). It must be noted, however, that artifical ventilation alone is not successful in preventing ultimate death (Russell, 1968). Secondary complications which may lead to death will be described in later paragraphs.

A. Effects of Venom on Cortical Electrical Activity

1. EEG—Dog, Anesthetized

We have frequently seen a unique and dramatic loss of cortical electrical activity within 30–60 sec after intravenous injection of certain snake venoms (Vick et al., 1966, 1968; Slotta and Vick, 1969). This decrease in activity following the intravenous injection of eastern diamondback rattlesnake

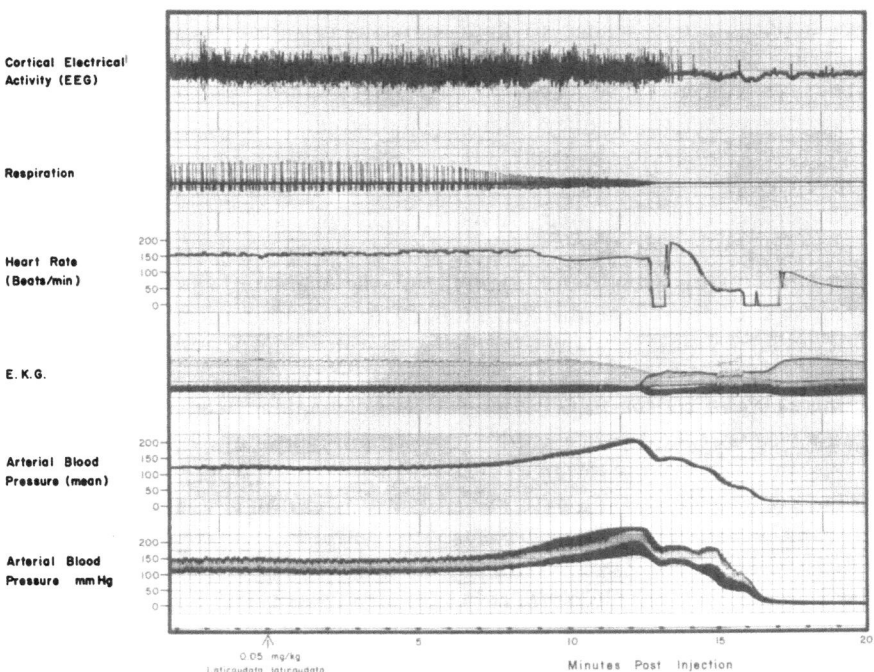

Fig. 3. Effect of a lethal dose of *Laticauda laticaudata* venom (sea snake) on cortical activity, respiration, heart rate, ECG, and arterial blood pressure in the anesthetized dog.

venom was of an irreversible nature and was not related to the previously reported changes in cardiovascular function (Fig. 2). None of the other rattlesnake venoms when administered to the dog produced this devastating effect on EEG activity (Vick, unpublished observations). This phenomenon is unexplained at the present time, but it is interesting to compare this effect of rattlesnake venom on EEG with that produced by the injection of sea-snake venom (Fig. 3). Cardiovascular changes much like those observed after rattlesnake venom are noted; however, cortical electrical activity is relatively unaffected by the venom of the sea snake *Laticauda laticaudata*. It is only after several minutes of complete respiratory arrest that the EEG trace eventually becomes isoelectric and remains so until death of the animal. This effect is undoubtedly related to brain hypoxia and not to any direct action of sea snake venom on brain function *per se* (Russell, 1962).

2. EEG—Monkey, Unanesthetized

The effects of a lethal intravenous dose of rattlesnake venom on the cortical electrical activity of the anesthetized dog have been described (Vick *et al.*, 1964). The loss of EEG activity, as produced by the venom of the eastern diamondback rattlesnake, may be a unique response of the dog, or a phenomenon related to the conditions of injection. With these perplexing possibilities in mind, both eastern and western diamondback rattlesnake venoms have been injected intravenously and intramuscularly into unanesthetized monkeys that were monitored primarly for EEG change. Two weeks prior to challenge, dural electrodes were implanted bilaterally over the superior frontal, precentral, and postcentral gyri of the monkey. Subcortical electrodes were stereotactically placed in the mesencephalic reticular formation (MRF) amygdala, globus pallidus, caudate nucleus, and the nucleus centrum medianum of the thalamus (SM). The typical response of the unanesthetized monkey to an intramuscular injection of rattlesnake venom is shown in Fig. 4. Results show a rather sudden appearance of high-voltage, slow-wave activity indicative of cerebral depression. This pattern appeared about 3 hr following intramuscular injection and was associated with cardiac arrhythmias and dyspnea. The cortex exhibited this change prior to the subcortical areas, which in some cases showed no change until just prior to death. During the terminal phase, cortical activity exhibited a generalized dyssynchrony and eventual flattening of the EEG trace. The exact relationship between the effect of venom on respiratory function and cortical activity is not clear; but it is interesting to note that some respiratory distress always preceeded the changes in cortical activity in these studies.

The effect of rattlesnake venom on EEG when administered intravenously to monkeys is identical to that following intramuscular injection,

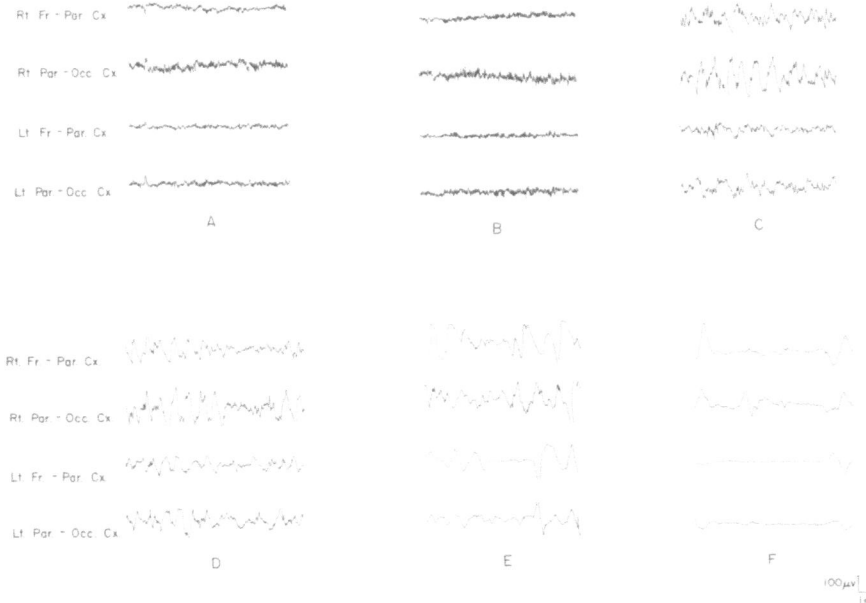

Fig. 4. Effect of a lethal dose of *Crotalus adamanteus* venom (eastern diamondback rattlesnake) on cortical activity in the unanesthetized monkey. A. Control. B. 1 hr after intramuscular injection of venom, some respiratory difficulties. C. 3 hr after injection; monkey somnolent, progressive dyspnea. D. 3 hr, 5 min after injection; monkey stuporous, no response to stimulation, severe dyspnea. E. 3 hr, 10 min after injection; monkey unconscious. F. 3 hr, 15 min after injection; respiratory paralysis, death.

with the important exception that both onset of action and time-to-death were accelerated (3.5 hr *vs* 1.5 hr).

B. Effects of Venom on Plasma Factors

In addition to measurement of physiological function and cortical activity following envenomation, serial blood samples have been drawn for determination of hematocrit, fibrinogen, platelets, hemolysis, and each of the plasma clotting factors. In general, all members of the Crotalidae family induced hemolysis, formation of microthrombi, thrombocytopenia, and marked coagulation defects (*see* Chap. 4, Sec. II). As an example, timber rattlesnake venom causes decreases in fibrinogen from a control value of 200 mg % to less than 75 mg %. Platelets simultaneously decrease from 431,000 to less than 2000. Clotting factor VIII decreases sharply after venom, indicating the possible formation of disseminating intravascular clots.

Table II.
Effect of Rattlesnake Venom on Plasma

Venom	Fibrinogen	Platelets	Hematocrit	Hemolysis	Clothing factors in monkey
Timber rattlesnake	Severely depressed Pre: 200–280 μg % Post: 75–147 μg %	Severely depressed Pre: 431,000–563,000 Post: 2,000– 64,000	Unchanged	None	No significant changes
Eastern diamondback rattlesnake	Severely depressed Pre: 270–300 μg % Post: 4– 93 μg %	Severely depressed Pre: 390,000–620,000 Post: 4,000– 20,000	Unchanged	None	Inhibition with some clotting

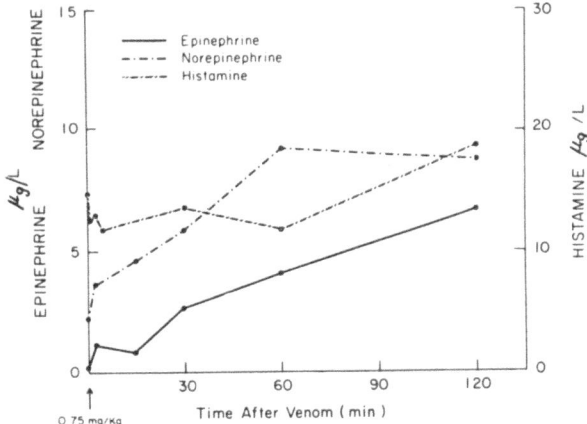

Fig. 5. Effect of a lethal dose of *Crotalus horridus horridus* venom (timber rattlesnake) on plasma levels of epinephrine, norepinephrine, and histamine.

Figure 5 shows the effect of timber rattlesnake venom on plasma epinephrine, norepinephrine, and histamine. Following the administration of 0.75 mg/kg of *Crotalus horridus horridus*, there is a slow gradual increase in both catecholamines reaching a maximum of 5–10 μg/liter in 120 min. Plasma histamine does not increase significantly from time of injection until death of the monkey. The increased catecholamine levels are most probably associated with generalized "stress reaction" following envenomation (Rosenberg *et al.*, 1961).

C. Effects of Actual Snake Bite

The effect of an actual snake bite has been compared with that produced by injecting reconstituted lyophilyzed venom. Studies have been carried out in a series of 13 adult mongrel dogs anesthetized with sodium pentobarbital and monitored for changes in blood pressure, ECG, heart rate, and respiration. Envenomation was accomplished by grasping the head of the poisonous reptile and allowing the snake to strike the shaved exposed thigh muscle of the dog. Estimates of venom content per bite were made by averaging the volume of venom obtained from numerous and periodic "milkings" of the same snake.

The snake, the time-to-death, the approximate dose of venom, and the tissue damage noted following envenomation are shown in Table III.

Results indicate that envenomation by members of the Crotalid family produce death at from 8 to 24 hr. Immediately following the bite there is a significant increase in both heart rate and blood pressure. This is quite unlike the effect of rattlesnake venom when injected intravenously, which

Table III.
Effect of Actual Rattlesnake Bite on Survival Time and Tissue Damage in the Dog

Snake	Survival time	Approximate dose of venom	Tissue damage
Crotalus durissus terrificus (tropical rattlesnake)	<24 hr	150 mg	None
Crotalus horridus atricaudatus (canebrake rattlesnake)	<24 hr	150 mg	None
Crotalus horridus horridus (timber rattlesnake)	>72 hr	150 mg	None
Crotalus lepidus klauberi (rock rattlesnake)	>72 hr	15 mg	None
Crotalus scutulatus (Mojave rattlesnake)	2 hr	50 mg	None
Crotalus oreganus (Pacific rattlesnake)	>72 hr	75 mg	None
Sistrurus miliarius barbouri (pigmy rattlesnake)	>72 hr	25 mg	Edema, necrosis, and generalized tissue breakdown

Table IV.

Effect of Actual Snake Bite on Survival Time and Tissue Damage. Major Families of Snakes

Family	Survival time	Approximate dose of venom	Tissue damage
Crotalidae			
Crotalus rhodostoma	<24 hr	50 mg	Local hemorrhage; generalized bleeding
Trimeresurus popeorum	>72 hr	50 mg	Massive tissue damage at site of bite
Trimeresurus purpureomaculatus	>72 hr	50 mg	Massive tissue damage at site of bite
Agkistrodon piscivorus	<8 hr	150 mg	Massive tissue damage at site of bite
Agkistrodon c. mokeson	>72 hr	50 mg	Massive tissue damage at site of bite
Agkistrodon c. contorix	<24 hr	50 mg	Tissue damage
Bothrops atrox	<14 hr	200 mg	Swelling edema
Crotalus durissus terrificus	<24 hr	150 mg	No tissue damage
Crotalus horridus atricaudatus	<24 hr	150 mg	No tissue damage
Crotalus horridus horridus	>72 hr	150 mg	No tissue damage
Crotalus viridus oreganus	>72 hr	75 mg	No tissue damage
Crotalus lepidus klauberi	>72 hr	15 mg	No tissue damage
Lachesis mutus	<24 hr	250 mg	Swelling edema
Viperidae			
Bitis arietans	>72 hr	200 mg	No tissue damage
Vipera russelli	< 3 hr	200 mg	No swelling; some local hemorrhage
Elapidae			
Naja haje	< 2 hr	100 mg	No tissue damage
Naja naja	< 1 1/2 hr	25 mg	No tissue damage
Bungarus caeruleus	< 4 hr	35 mg	No tissue damage
Naja naja kaouthia	< 2 hr	200 mg	No tissue damage
Ophiophagus hannah	28 min	500 mg	No tissue damage
Naja nivea	12 min	200 mg	No tissue damage
D. angusticeps	36 hr	100 mg	No tissue damage
D. polylepis	40 min	75 mg	No tissue damage
Hydrophiidae			
Laticauda semifasciata	>72 hr	10 mg	No tissue damage
Boiginae			
B. dendrophila	>72 hr	20 mg	Slight edema and hemorrhage at site of bite
D. typus	24 hr	25 mg	No tissue damage

produces a fall in both heart rate and blood pressure. Death, however, appeared to be similiar to that produced by the reconstituted venom and was primarily respiratory in nature. It is evident that many of the changes produced by actual envenomation are similar to those previously described following intravenous or intramuscular injection of dry venom.

A comparison of the effects of actual snake bite on survival times among the four families of poisonous snakes is shown in Table IV. The true vipers and members of the Elapidae appear to kill much more quickly than either Crotalidae or Hydrophiidae. The number of snakes studied in each family is small however, and data presented may not be true for the entire spectrum of poisonous snakes.

IV. TREATMENT OF SNAKE BITE

Proper treatment of snake bite has been and remains an extremely controversial subject. Much folklore has been generated in areas of the Unites States where human envenomation is most common. In an effort to dissect the most medically sound approachs to the treatment of snake envenomation from those which appear to have little scientific basis, experts such as Russell (1967), Gennaro (1963), Buckley and Parges (1956), and Keegan and Macfarlane (1963) have outlined specific steps for the treatment of snake bite. The following is a summary, of most important aspects of this problem.

Basically, treatment can be divided into five categories:

1. Immediate attempts to stop or slow the absorption of the toxin from the site of the bite.
2. Removal of as much unabsorbed venom as is possible in the shortest period of time.
3. Administration of a specific substance (antisera) to neutralize or inactivate the remaining venom.
4. Prevention of the more deleterious effects of the toxin at its specific effector site.
5. Good nursing care to reduce the possibilities of secondary infection and/or other complications.

Russell defines the treatment of snake bite more specifically:

Step one: Capture and kill the snake, if possible.
Step two: Apply a constricting band or venous tourniquet above the first joint proximal to the bite. Release every 90 sec. for 10 min.
Step three: Apply incision and suction (of particular value in cases of North American rattlesnake bites).

Step four: Immobilize the injured part and keep patient quiet.
Step five: Transport the patient to definitive medical care. Keep
             warm and avoid walking.
Step six: Antivenin—given only after appropriate sensitivity tests.

Gennaro reports excellent success in experimental animals given a lethal dose of rattlesnake venom followed by antivenin. Local hemorrhage, tissue necrosis, and death all appear to be prevented by timely (up to 4 hr) and appropriate dosages of the antivenin (usually 2–5 units).

Wyeth Laboratories recommends that their antivenin, Crotaline, polyvalent USP, be given intramuscularly unless early severe symptoms are present or a delay of 4 hr or more is anticipated from time of bite until definitive care is afforded the patient (Russell, 1967). Russell (1967) routinely administers the antivenin intravenously during hospital treatment of envenomation in children, because the amount of venom on a mg/kg basis is always much higher and more devastating than in the healthy adult (Gennaro, 1963).

All things considered, it appears as though early and cautious use of antivenin is advocated following the bite of the American rattlesnake, if no sensitivity to horse serum is present.

V.   CONCLUDING REMARKS

The venom of the American rattlesnake appears to produce a variety of toxic manifestations in the experimental animal. When administered intravenously in a lethal dose, both arterial blood pressure and heart rate decrease dramatically. With some venoms (eastern diamondback rattlesnake) a dramatic and irreversible loss of cortical activity is observed. Death is due primarily to a blockade of nerve impulse transmission at the level of the diaphragm. Where death is not immediate, changes in plasma factors are noted. Potency of venoms obtained from various rattlesnakes differ widely as to lethal dose and time-to-death, depending on the experimental animal used in the test.

It is extremely interesting to note that the effects of lyophilyzed venom and that venom obtained by direct bite are remarkably similiar. Drying of the venom does not appear to alter markedly either the enzymatic activity of the venom or its potency.

It is the author's opinion that the most remarkable observation made concerning the action of rattlesnake venom is that each venom possesses a wide spectrum of activities each of which partially dictates the proper course of treatment in cases of envenomation.

VI. REFERENCES

Buckley, E. and N. Parges (1956), "Venoms," American Association for the Advancement of Science, Wash., D.C.

Conant, R. (1958), "A Fieldguide to Reptiles and Amphibians of the United States and Canada," Houghton Mifflin, Boston.

Deichman, W. B., J. L. Radomski, J. J. Farrell, W. E. MacDonald, and M. L. Keplinger (1958), *Amer. J. Med. Sci.*, **326**:204.

Gennaro, J. F., Jr. (1963), "Venoms and Poisonous Animals and Noxious Plants of the Pacific," Pergamon, Oxford.

Keegan, H. L. and W. V. Macfarlane, "Venoms and Poisonous Animals and Noxious Plants of the Pacific Region," Pergamon, Oxford.

Klauber, L. M. (1956), "Rattlesnakes; Their Habits, Life Histories, and Influence on Mankind," vol. 1, Univ. of Calif. Press, Berkeley, Calif.

McCollough, N. C. and J. F. Gennaro, Jr. (1963), *J. Fla. Med. Assn.*, **49**:959.

National Academy of Sciences, National Research Council, Committee on Snakebite Therapy (1963), *Toxicon*, **1**:81.

Poisonous Snakes of the World, 1968, Department of the Navy, Bureau of Medicine and Surgery, U.S. Government Printing Office, Washington, D.C.

Rosenberg, J. C., R. Lillehei, J. Longerbeam, and B. Zimmerman (1961), *Ann. Surg.*, **154**:611.

Russell, F. E. (1961), *Cur. Therapy Res.*, **3**:438.

Russell, F. E. (1962), "Cyclopedia of Medicine, Surgery and the Specialties," vol. II, F. A. Davis, Philadelphia.

Russell, F. E. (1967), *Toxicon*, **4**:285.

Russell, F. E. and J. A. Emery (1961), *Amer. J. Med. Sci.*, **241**:160.

Russell, F. E. (1968), *Clin. Pharmacol. Therap.*, **8**:849.

Slotta, K. H. and J. A. Vick (1969), *Toxicon* **6**:167.

Stebbeirs, R. C. (1954), "Amphibians and Reptiles of Western North America," McGraw-Hill, New York.

Vick, J. A. and H. P. Ciuchta (1965), *Arch. Intern. Pharmacodyn.*, **153**:424.

Vick, J. A., H. P. Ciuchta, and J. H. Manthei, "Animal Toxins," Pergamon Press.

Vick, J. A., H. P. Ciuchta, and E. H. Polley (1964), *Nature*, **203**:1387.

Vick, J. A., C. R. Roberts, and M. N. Heiffer (1968), *Fed. Proc.*, **27**:707.

Vick, J. A., H. P. Ciuchta, C. Broomfield, and B. Currie (1966), *Toxicon*, **3**:237.

Wright, A. H. and A. A. Wright, "Handbook of Snakes of the United States and Canada," Camstock, New York.

Chapter 4

The Mechanism of
Snake Venom Actions—Rattlesnakes
and Other Crotalids

Anthony T. Tu

Department of Biochemistry
Colorado State University
Fort Collins, Colorado, U.S.A.

I. INTRODUCTION

A. Snakes in Family Crotalidae

Of the nearly 2000 different types of snakes that exist, about 300 are known to be venomous. The venomous snakes are classified according to morphological characteristics and comprise five families: Crotalidae (crotalid), Viperidae (viperid), Elapidae (elapid), Hydrophiidae (sea-snakes), and Colubridae (colubrid).

Colubridae are rear-fanged snakes, and because of the awkward position of the fangs, they seldom envenomate victims by natural bite. In most cases, when one speaks of venomous snakes, he is referring to the first four families.

In this chapter, the discussion will be limited to the family of Crotalidae, which includes rattlesnakes. Snakes of Crotalidae are distributed in North, Central, and South America, and in most parts of Asia. They are not found in Western Europe, Africa, or Australia. The Crotalidae comprises of six genera, which include *Crotalus*, *Sistrurus*, *Agkistrodon*, *Bothrops*, *Lachesis*, and *Trimeresurus*. The *Crotalus* is found in North, Central, and South America. The *Crotalus* and *Sistrurus* genera are the rattlesnakes. *Bothrops* is found only in Central and South America. *Agkistrodon* includes the copperheads and moccasins. There are nine species in Asia and three in North and Central America. *Lachesis* has only one species and is distributed from Central to South America. *Trimeresurus* is the Asiatic pit viper which lives only in Asia; there are 31 species in this genus.

B. Components of Snake Venoms

Snake venom expelled from a venom gland is generally a yellow, viscous liquid, 80–90% of which is water, the remainder consisting of proteins, protein derivatives, small organic compounds, and inorganic salts. On a dry-weight basis, proteins account for approximately 90% of the total weight. Venom is not composed of a single substance common to all venomous snakes. The proportions of the different substances in venom and their specific pharmacological actions may vary among individual snakes. The differences are most noticeable at the family level and less pronounced at genus and species levels.

There are many different types of proteins in a venom, some being enzymes and some being nonenzymatic (*see* review by Devi, 1968). At one time it was considered that venom toxicity was due to enzymatic actions of venoms (Zeller, 1951). However, recent studies by a number of investigators indicate that lethal action can be separated from many enzyme activities. This is particularly true of neurotoxins which are devoid of enzymatic activity. This does not mean that the enzymes are unrelated to venom actions. The various enzymes may participate in blood coagulation, anticoagulation, hemorrhage, necrosis, hemolysis, and autopharmacological action due to snake envenomation.

Any given snake venom usually contains more than one toxic principle, and these tend to act in combination. Therefore, we may say, in a broad sense, that toxicity is due to enzymes as well as to nonenzymatic proteins.

Venom proteins can be divided into simple proteins and conjugated proteins. Among the conjugated proteins, the presence of flavoprotein is well recognized. Many snake venoms possess a slightly yellow color due to the presence of L-amino acid oxidase, and riboflavin occurs as a prosthetic group of this oxidase. Glycoprotein has also been found in snake venoms. One proteolytic enzyme isolated from *Agkistrodon halys blomhoffii* venom is a glycoprotein containing galactose, mannose, glucosamine, and sialic acid (Oshima *et al.*, 1968). Many venom enzymes lose activity in the presence of EDTA, suggesting that some of the enzymes may be metalloproteins or may require metals for their enzyme action.

Serotonin is present in venoms of certain snakes such as *Sistrurus miliarius barbouri*, *Agkistodon contortrix*, *Agkistrodon piscivorus*, and *Bothrops atrox* (Welsh, 1966).

Agkistrodon halys blomhoffii venom contains two tripeptides with the following structures: pyroglutamic acid-Asp(NH_2)-Trp, and pyroglutamic acid-Glu(NH_2)-Trp (Kato *et al.*, 1965).

II. ACTION OF SNAKE VENOMS

A. Local Actions

On occasion, snake bite victims who survive sustain permanent tissue damage that may extend into the muscle, tendons, and cartilage (Emery and Russell, 1963; McCollough and Gennaro, 1963). In relatively light cases of poisoning, tissue damage is generally limited to cutaneous areas. Local tissue damage is a typical finding in cases due to crotalid and viperid envenomations. Because of the extensive use of antivenin in the United States and in other countries, mortality has been reduced considerably. The real problem resulting from snake bite is the destruction of tissue and possible dysfunction or complete loss of a finger, hand, arm, or other limb, since, in many cases, histolysis is not prevented by the use of antivenin (Stahnke, 1966). Practically all Crotalidae simultaneously cause hemorrhagic and necrotic effects by envenomation.

Many investigators (Flowers, 1963; Goucher and Flowers, 1964; Emery and Russell, 1963) use the terms hemorrhage and myonecrosis interchangeably. This is because most of the crotalid venoms, including those from rattlesnakes, cause both effects. However, these two effects can be distinguished by histologic study. Tu *et al.* (1969) investigated five venoms of Viperidae and found that some venoms elicit a hemorrhagic effect but not a myonecrotic effect. Some venoms cause a more pronounced myonecrotic effect with little hemorrhage. All five *Bothrops* venoms investigated in our laboratory induced both effects (Tu and Homma, 1970). Uncomplicated myonecrosis can be detected only by histological observation. Apparently, myonecrotic and hemorrhagic actions are initiated by two different toxins present in snake venoms.

1. *Myonecrosis*

One of the most pronounced local effects of envenomation is myonecrosis, destruction of muscle bundles. An example of myonecrosis due to *Crotalus adamanteus* envenomation is shown in Fig. 1.

A characteristic symptom of *Trimeresurus flavoviridis* envenomation is severe local tissue damage such as myolysis, hemorrhage, and edema. In this venom, the necrotic toxin is more stable to heat treatment than the hemorrhagic toxin. When this venom is heated at 100°C for 10 min the venom causes only myolysis at the site of injection without causing hemorrhage (Okonogi *et al.*, 1962).

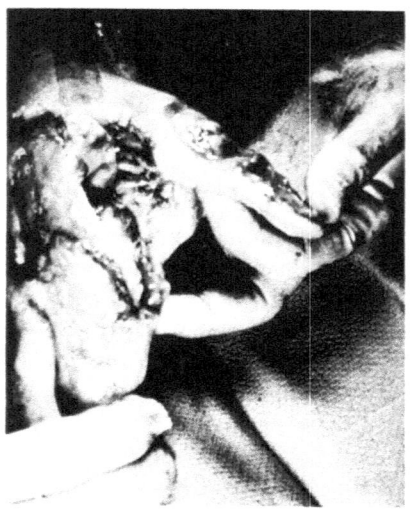

Fig. 1. Necrosis due to *Crotalus adamanteus* (eastern diamondback rattlesnake) envenomation. A male, 23 years old, was bitten by the rattlesnake on the dorsum of the right thumb web. The photograph was taken one month after the bite by Dr. John H. Tenery. (Reproduced from "The Treatment of Venomous Bites and Stings," by the permission of the author, Dr. Herbert L. Stahnke of Arizona State University.)

Venoms of *Bothrops* possess profound histolytic activity. Venoms of *Bothrops atrox*, *Bothrops schlegelii*, and *Bothrops nummifera* produce pronounced myolytic necrosis, while those from *Bothrops picadoi* and *Bothrops nasuta* produce hyaline degeneration (Tu and Homma, 1970). Edema, hyperemia, and necrosis occur in rabbits nine days after they receive *Bothrops jararaca* venom subcutaneously (Saliba, 1965).

There was considerable speculation that necrosis is caused by venom protease (Stahnke *et al.*, 1957; Ohsaka *et al.*, 1960). Okonogi *et al.* (1960) isolated protease from *Trimeresurus flavoviridis* venom and found that the enzyme caused myonecrosis similar to that produced by crude venom. However, the hemorrhagic action was rather slight as compared with crude venom. The chemical nature of venom proteases has been studied extensively by a number of investigators. The enzymes are somewhat similar to trypsin but can be distinguished from trypsin in the presence of trypsin inhibitors (Tu *et al.*, 1966a). In order to clarify whether other proteolytic enzymes would cause tissue damage, Okonogi *et al.* (1960) injected various proteases. By intradermal injection, pronase and trypsin produced subcutaneous hemorrhage. Following intramuscular injection, nagase and pronase produced necrosis, edema, and hemorrhage in muscle, but no change was observed following injection of trypsin. This is further evidence that venom protease is different from trypsin.

Maeno *et al.* (1959) isolated two proteolytic enzymes from the same venom and found that one of the proteolytic enzymes caused necrosis with hemorrhage. Maeno *et al.* (1962) isolated a heat-stable factor which had phospholipase A activity 20 times higher than crude venom. This factor had myolytic activity when 1 μg was injected into the leg of a mouse. Kurashige *et al.* (1966) further purified *Trimeresurus flavoviridis* venom until they were able to obtain phospholipase A and two synergistic proteins, either of which, when added to the phospholipase A fraction, caused myolysis when injected into mice. None of these fractions alone caused myolysis. The purified factors showed no proteolytic enzyme, RNase, or esterase activities. Kurashige *et al.* isolated a heat-labile fraction that possesses lytic activity without addition of phospholipase A. Apparently there are two distinct myolytic factors in the one venom.

2. Hemorrhage

Another important local tissue damage due to crotalid and viperid venoms is hemorrhage at the vicinity of the bite. Examples of hemorrhage due to different rattlesnake venoms are shown in Fig. 2. Most of the rattlesnake and *Bothrops* venoms from the American continents produce strong hemorrhagic effects with accompanying myonecrotic action. Many investigators (Gaertner *et al.*, 1962) suggest that the venom proteolytic

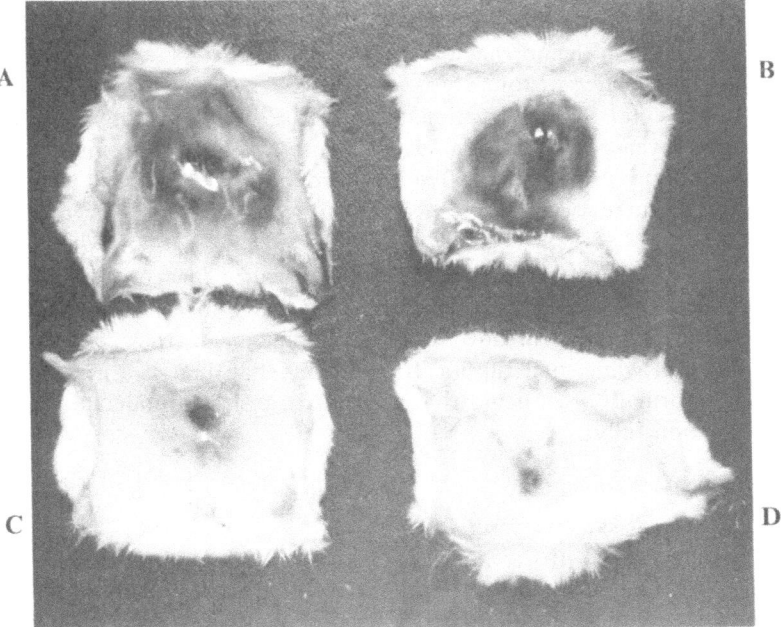

Fig. 2. Local hemorrhage caused by the venoms of A. *Crotalus adamanteus*; B. *Crotalus durissus totonocus*; C. *Crotalus basiliscus*; D. *Crotalus durissus terrificus*. In each case, 50 μg venom was injected into mice intradermally.

enzymes are factors for local histolysis. This assumption may be an over-simplification. It is quite common that one venom contains more than two hemorrhagic toxins. Ohsaka *et al.* (1960) isolated two hemorrhagic factors from *Trimeresurus flavoviridis* venom. The first hemorrhagic factor, HR-1, was unrelated to proteolytic activity on casein, while HR-2 did have proteolytic activity on casein. The hemorrhagic factor is not necessarily identical to the lethal toxin, because HR-2 and lethality can be separated. The HR-1 and HR-2 can be distinguished immunologically. These are two distinct toxins exerting the same pathological effect (Ohsaka *et al.*, 1966).

Maeno *et al.* (1959) isolated two proteolytic enzymes from the same venom. The Hα-proteinase caused necrosis with hemorrhage histologically identical to that caused by crude venom. The fraction also contained lethal toxicity. On the other hand, the Hβ-proteinase caused necrosis with hemorrhage, but the actions were milder than those of crude venom (Maeno and Mitsuhashi, 1961).

In the case of *Agkistrodon halys blomhoffii* venom there are two hemorrhagic toxins which possess lethal activity (Omori *et al.*, 1964). Proteolytic activity was observed in one of the hemorrhagic toxins by Suzuki (1966). Proteinase b, one of the two hemorrhagic factors, has been isolated. It is a glycoprotein (Oshima *et al.*, 1968) with a molecular weight of 95,000. Suzuki (1966) isolated a hemorrhagic factor with no proteinase activity from *Crotalus adamanteus* venom.

Toom *et al.* (1969) fractionated by isoelectric focusing *Agkistrodon rhodostoma* venom. They isolated two hemorrhagic factors with no lethal action and no proteolytic activity toward casein. However, one of the hemorrhagic toxins exerted esterase activity on *N*-benzoyl-L-arginine ethyl ester.

From these examples one can easily visualize the complex nature of hemorrhagic toxins. Some toxins are apparently identical to proteolytic enzymes and others are not. Moreover, some hemorrhagic toxins show lethal actions while some do not. It is obvious that there is a need for more precise information on hemorrhagic toxins in order to understand hemorrhagic action fully.

B. Systemic Action

1. Effect on Nervous System

In contrast to the venoms of Elapidae and Hydrophiidae, not all crotalid venoms are neurotoxic. Venom of *Crotalus durissus terrificus*, commonly found in South America, is notably neurotoxic. Therefore, the neurotoxic action of this venom has been the subject of extensive study.

The first isolation of a neurotoxin from snake venoms was achieved by Slotta and Fraenkel-Conrat (1938a,b; 1939) using *Crotalus aurissus terri-*

ficus venom. The toxin was named "crotoxin" and was homogeneous in electrophoresis. Combined sedimentation and diffusion values suggested a molecular weight of 30,000. Crotoxin possesses lethal action as well as hemolytic and smooth-muscle-stimulating activities, phospholipase A, and hyaluronidase. Crotoxin was further separated into different fractions: crotamin, neurotoxin, and proteolytic enzyme (Goncalves, 1956). Neumann and Habermann (1955) separated a toxic fraction and phospholipase A from crotoxin. Although crotoxin is not a pure toxin, its isolation marked a great achievement in the field of venoms. The techniques available for protein fractionation were very limited in the 1930s. The discovery of crotoxin stimulated many investigators to isolate other toxins from snake venoms.

Crotoxin evokes paralysis similar to that caused by curare in dogs, cats, monkeys, mice, rats, pigeons, guinea pigs, and rabbits (Brazil *et al.*, 1966). The neurotoxic action of crotoxin is believed to be due to neuromuscular blockade (Brazil, 1966). The blockade is of the nondepolarizing type and is caused by a decrease in the sensitiveness of the endplate to the depolarizing action of acetylcholine.

Crotamin, a toxic component of *Crotalus durissus terrificus* venom, provokes extension and paralysis of the hindlegs of mice when injected intravenously (Cheymol *et al.*, 1963). Crotamin-containing rattlesnake venoms and crotamin itself cause contraction, an effect on skeletal muscles which can be observed on intact and conscious animals as well as on *in situ* and isolated preparations.

The noncrotaminic rattlesnake venoms elicit a weak and slowly induced paralytic effect. Paralysis is due to a direct action on the muscle fiber without desensitization of endplate receptors. Prado-Franceschi and Brazil (1969) isolated from *Crotalus durissus terrificus* venom a new neurotoxic factor, convulsin, which was different from crotoxin and crotamin. Mice injected with convulsin show tachypnea within 20 sec, followed by apnea of short duration. Large doses cause convulsions that end, as a general rule, in death of the animal. Neither crotoxin nor crotamin produce such convulsions (Brazil *et al.*, 1969).

Injections of *Crotalus adamanteus* venom (Russell and Bohr, 1962) produce changes in behavior, motor, and parasympathetic functions. In these studies, intraventricular injections of *Crotalus adamanteus* venom in cats failed to produce the typical cardiovascular responses observed following intravenous injection of *Crotalus* venoms. Therefore, the amount of venom that passes through the blood–brain barrier is very small.

At one time, it was believed that phospholipase A was identical to neurotoxin (Braganca and Quastel, 1952, 1953). However, separation of phospholipase A from the toxic fraction has been accomplished by a number of workers (Master and Rae, 1961; Neumann and Habermann, 1955). Evidently phospholipase A is not a neurotoxin *per se*, but the enzyme does facilitate penetration of neuropharmacologically active substances into nervous tissue (Rosenberg and Ng, 1963). Venom of *Agkistrodon piscivorus piscivorus*, at low concentrations, does not block the action potential; nevertheless, it does render the squid axon sensitive to curare and acetylcholine. Membrane permeability is markedly increased. A much higher concentration of *Crotalus adamanteus* venom is required to produce the same effect (Condrea and Rosenberg, 1968; *see* Chap. 5).

Phopholipase A and lysolecithin *in vitro* can cause demyelination and can clear brain honogenates (Deuch, 1957; Webster, 1957). It is doubtful that such phenomena take place in actual envenomation, because injected venom hardly reaches nerve cells located in the interior of the body.

Cottonmouth moccasin and eastern diamondback rattlesnake venoms increase the cholinesterase activity observed on intact squid and lobster nerves and single electroplax (Rosenberg and Dettbarn, 1964).

2. Effect on Respiratory System

Death due to respiratory failure is common in snake bite poisoning. The mechanism of respiratory failure is unclear and complicated.

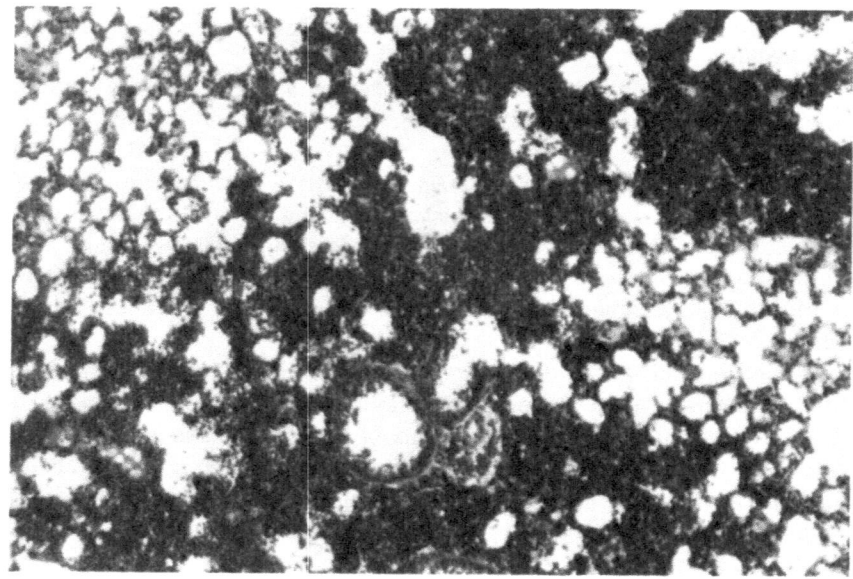

Fig. 3. Pulmonary hemorrhage caused after 30 min by i.m. injection of *Bothrops nasuta* venom (150 μg), into mouse. H and E stain. × 50.

When *Agkistrodon piscivorus* venom labeled with ^{131}I is injected into mice, the most striking early concentration of the iodine is in the lungs, the concentration being 10 times greater than in the liver (Gennaro and Ramsey, 1959). Crotoxin, a main toxin of *Crotalus durissus terrificus* venom, was labeled with radioactive iodine and injected intravenously into mice. The crotoxin accumulated mainly in the kidneys, liver, lungs, and spleen. In cases of *Bothrops* venoms from Costa Rica, hemorrhages were observed in the heart, lungs, mesentery, and small intestine of mice. The hemorrhagic effects of *Bothrops picadoi* and *Bothrops nasuta* venoms are especially pronounced in heart and lungs (Tu and Homma, 1970). An example of pulmonary hemorrhage due to *Bothrops nasuta* venom is shown in Fig. 3. Therefore, respiratory failure secondary to hemorrhage can be a direct action of snake venoms.

A brief period of apnea and a long-lasting period of tachypnea were noted in dogs within a few seconds after administration of *Crotalus durissus terrificus* venom (the variety devoid of crotamine). The brief period of apnea originated from stimulation of receptors in the lungs, while the respiratory stimulation is due to an activation of chemoreceptors in the aortic and carotid sinus bodies and to a direct action on the respiratory centers (Brazil *et al.*, 1966).

While crude venom causes respiratory disturbance, crotoxin does not cause respiratory failure (Brazil *et al.*, 1966b). The neurotoxin which causes respiratory disturbance has been isolated and was different from crotoxin and crotamin. The toxin responsible for the respiratory effects acts on the pulmonary vagus receptors whose stimulation generates inhibiting impulses for the respiratory centers (Brazil *et al.*, 1967).

Respiration is not significantly modified by crotoxin, so acute disturbances elicited by the *Crotalus durissus terrificus* venom on respiration cannot be due to crotoxin or to crotamine. There are other venom components whose pharmacological actions must play an important role in *Crotalus durissus terrificus* envenomation, especially in the genesis of shock (Brazil *et al.*, 1966).

3. Effect on Kidney

According to Raab and Kaiser (1966a), snake venoms cause three types of renal damage. There are glomerular alterations (nephritis), tubular alterations (nephrosis), and renal infarction. Significant increase in urinary alkaline phosphatase and leucine aminopeptidase activities are observed after rats receive *Agkistrodon piscivorus* venom. The increase in enzyme activity is due to tubular damage by the venom, and activation of renal plasminogen causes a further increase in leucine aminopeptidase activity (Raab and Kaiser, 1966a,b). Tubular casts of hemoglobin and degenerative changes in the tubular epithelium can be observed under the microscope after injection of *Crotalus terrificus* venom. These lesions resemble those observed in the kidneys of human cases of fatal envenomation (Amorim *et al.*, 1960). Renal lesions identical to those originally found in crush syndrome, hemoglobinuric nephrosis, lower nephron nephrosis or tubulorhexis have been described in autopsy and biopsy tissue from human cases of snake bite caused by *Crotalus durissus terrificus* (Amorim and Mello, 1952, 1954).

Crotoxin isolated from *Crotalus durissus terrificus* venom causes kidney damage when injected intraveneously into dogs (Hadler and Brazil, 1966). In early lesions produced within the first 4 days following crotoxin injection, the renal tubules are altered less than the glomeruli, which show congestion, thickness of the basement membrane, deposit of PAS (periodic acid-Schiff reaction)—positive material between the capillary loops, and nuclear pycnosis of some glomerular cells. In late lesions, tubular damage predominates with the proximal segment altered the most. There is intense microvascular degeneration as well as nuclearpycnosis and necrosis of many epithelial cells. Crotoxin concentrates in the kidneys, liver, lungs, and spleen in that order, when administered intraveneously into mice.

4. Effect on Circulatory System

a. Hypotensive Action. One of the most common effects due to crotalid envenomation is fall in blood pressure. Russell *et al.* (1962) observed an immediate and profound fall in systemic right arterial pressure when a cat or a dog received intravenous injections of *Crotalus atrox* venom. The hypotensive response occured whether or not there was an increase or decrease in cardiac rate. Therefore, the hypotensive action was not due to a decrease in heart rate or contractile force. Studies with the isolated heart demonstrated that when normal arterial pressure is maintained by an exogenous source, decrease in contractile force and cardiac output was not great enough to produce the sudden and precipitous fall in systemic arterial pressure. Using *Crotalus atrox* venom in sheep, Halmagyi *et al.* (1965) observed a fall in arterial blood pressure in 5 min. They also observed a fall in cardiac output and systemic arterial resistance; a stable shock was observed at higher doses. Crotoxin isolated from *Crotalus durissus terrificus* venom is much less active than the original venom in producing hypotension and in increasing the hematocrit value (Brazil *et al.*, 1966).

The exact mechanism of the hypotensive effect is not yet clear, but a number of possible factors might be considered. Several physiologically active substances are released due to autopharmacological actions provoked by venoms. For instance, bradykinin is released by the action of crotalid venoms. Bradykinin is known to cause a marked fall in systemic arterial pressure. Histamine, another hypotensive agent, is also released by auto-pharmacological actions after snake envenomation. Bradykinin- and histamine-releasing factors will be discussed in detail in later sections.

L-Amino acid oxidase present in venom is excluded as a hypotensive factor. Russell *et al.* (1963b) isolated the enzyme from *Crotalus adamanteus* venom and found that the enzyme did not contribute to the production of the profound fall in systemic arterial pressure usually seen following injection of crude rattlesnake venoms. The hypotensive effect of venom phosphodiesterase was also tested (Russell *et al.*, 1963a). The enzyme isolated from *Crotalus atrox, Crotalus adamanteus, Crotalus viridis helleri*, and *Crotalus horridus horridus* venoms produced an immediate and profound fall in systemic arterial pressure of cats. However, the enzyme preparations showed several fractions in disc electrophoresis. Consequently, it still is not clear whether the effect was due to the enzyme or to a contaminant (Russell, 1967). Lysolecithin derived from lecithin by the action of snake venom phospholipase A causes positive inotropic and chronotropic effects in isolated preparations of guinea pig, rat, and rabbit heart (Govier and Boadle, 1967). Reid (1968) observed that patients of *Agkistrodon rhodostoma* bite usually have normal electocardiograms, but sometimes the electrocardiograms show marked inverted T-waves.

b. Hemolysis. It has been known that some snake venoms hemolyze erythrocytes readily, while other venoms can hemolyze erythrocytes only when serum is added. This eventually led to the conclusion that there are two types of hemolysis due to snake venom actions. These are frequently referred to as direct hemolysis and indirect hemolysis. Direct hemolysin in snake venoms can hemolyze erythrocytes directly; the indirect hemolysin causes hemolysis only when serum or lecithin is added to the reaction mixture (Condrea and de Vries, 1965). It was Delezenne and Ledebt (1911a, b) who demonstrated that lysolecithin is the causative agent of hemolysis.

In general, venoms of Crotalidae require a cofactor or activator (lecithin), while those of Elapidae contain a direct lytic factor, thereby causing direct hemolysis (Slotta and Borchert, 1954; Condrea *et al.*, 1964; *see* Chap. 2, Sec. II). The direct lytic factor has been isolated and purified from *Hemachatus haemachatus* venom (Aloof-Hirsch *et al.*, 1968). It is a basic polypeptide with a molecular weight of 7000. The direct lytic factor alone is moderately hemolytic. In combination with venom phospholipase A, hemolytic activity is greatly increased. Apparently, phospholipase A and direct lytic factor act synergistically, producing hemolysis of a much greater degree than either alone (Habermann and Neumann, 1954; Condrea *et al.*, 1964).

Unlike cobra venoms, most rattlesnake and other crotalid venoms do not contain direct lytic factor. Addition of serum or lecithin to the erythrocyte suspension is needed to cause hemolysis. Lysolecithin produced by the action of phospholipase A on lecithin is the actual causative agent of hemolysis (Levene and Rolf, 1923). Therefore, direct lytic factor and lysolecithin act similarly. Certain natural and synthetic basic polypeptides such as gramicidin S and poly (ornithine–leucine), poly (ornithine–leucine–alanine), and poly (lysine–leucine) can replace the direct lytic factor or lysolecithin (Klibansky et al., 1968).

Hemolytic action can be explained using unit membrane hypothesis. The basic, hydrophilic, direct lytic factor can cause a rearrangement of the surface proteins of the erythrocyte membrane so that the underlying phospholipids can be attacked by phospholipase A. Lysolecithin can also act as a surface active agent. An erythrocyte membrane weakened in this manner can undergo lysis by an osmotic flow of water or by loss of structural integrity.

Venom phospholipase A is one venom component that has been studied extensively. Most snake venoms contain more than two forms of phospholipase A. The venom of *Agkistrodon halys* contains two phospholipase A fractions; one is basic and the other is nearly neutral (Iwanaga and Kawachi, 1959). *Crotalus adamanteus* venom has two phospholipase A components which are very similar except for their electrophoretic mobilities (Saito and Hanahan, 1962; Wells and Hanahan, 1969). They both have a molecular weight of 30,000 as determined by sedimentation and diffusion, sedimentation equilibrium, and amino acid composition data.

Hemolytic activity can be separated from crotactin, the major protein fraction of *Crotalus durissus terrificus* venom, and from the protein fraction which carries the histamine-releasing activity (Rothschild, 1966). The phospholipase A itself is nonlethal and devoid of hemorrhagic and neurotoxic action (de Vries et al., 1962). Hemolytic activity is separated from the toxic fraction of *Trimeresurus flavoviridis* venom (Ohsaka, 1958). Hemolytic activity is distinct from coagulant and fibrinolytic fractions (Rosenfeld et al., 1960–62).

Classification of venom hemolysins into two groups, namely direct hemolysin and indirect hemolysin, is actually an oversimplification. Whether hemolysis takes place or not depends upon the animal species tested (Rosenfeld et al., 1968). For instance, the venom of *Bothrops cotiara* is not readily hemolytic toward the erythrocytes of dog, horse, rat, and mouse. This is probably due to the difference in erythrocyte membrane structure.

Some attempts were made to correlate hemolytic action with snake classification; however, there is no definite relationship between them.

c. *Blood Coagulation.* The effect of snake venoms on blood coagulation is extraordinarily complicated. For the purpose of simplicity, two types of action are considered—promotion of coagulation and anticoagulation. The situation is more complex when both factors are present, as in the venoms of *Agkistrodon acutus, Bothrops atrox, Crotalus horridus, Lachesis mutus,* and *Trimeresurus gramineus.* If anticoagulant activity is stronger than coagulant activity, a fibrin clot is not observed since fibrin is hydrolyzed as soon as it is formed. When coagulant action is stronger than anticoagulant action, a fibrin clot is first formed and then slowly disappears. If one uses separated fractions, both coagulant and anticoagulant actions can be observed separately. Occasionally coagulation or anticoagulation vary with venom concentration.

Promotion of Coagulation. The ability of snake venoms to convert fibrinogen to a fibrin clot was observed by Eagle (1937). This thrombinlike activity may not be identical to thrombin since it is not subject to heparin antagonism.

There are several different mechanisms even among the venoms which contain coagulant activity. Different results may be obtained depending on the system used. One should note whether results were obtained using whole blood, plasma, fibrinogen only, or fibrinogen with other blood coagulation factors.

Venoms of *Trimeresurus okinavenisis* coagulate whole blood and plasma. Calcium is not required for clot formation. A high concentration of venom inhibits coagulation of plasma (Klose and Summary, 1964). This is an example of coagulation and anticoagulation depending on venom concentration. On the other hand, venoms of *Agkistrodon acutus* and *Trimeresurus gramineus* have coagulant action at high concentrations and an anticoagulant action at low concentrations (Ouyang, 1957). Coagulation is due to a thrombinlike action.

Agkistrodon rhodostoma venom also contains a clotting enzyme as well as a lytic enzyme. The clotting enzyme produces stable clots *in vitro,* which are indistinguishable from normal fibrin clots (Regoeczi, 1966).

Conversion of fibrinogen to fibrin can be made directly with *Akgistrodon rhodostoma* venom in the absence of other clotting factors. This activity is not inhibited by heparin. The venom acelerates formation of prothrombin activator in thromboplastin generation test and in Hicks–Pitney screening test (Chan *et al.,* 1965). A clot formed by a coagulation enzyme obtained from *Bothrops jararaca* is more readily dissolved in 30% urea solution than a fibrin clot caused by thrombin (Conner and Houskova, 1967).

The coagulant and anticoagulant principles of the venom of *Agkistrodon acutus* can be separated. Both coagulant and esterase activities are found in the same fraction, so the thrombinlike activity of this venom is esterase in nature (Cheng and Ouyang, 1967). Lake and Gladner (1964) demonstrated

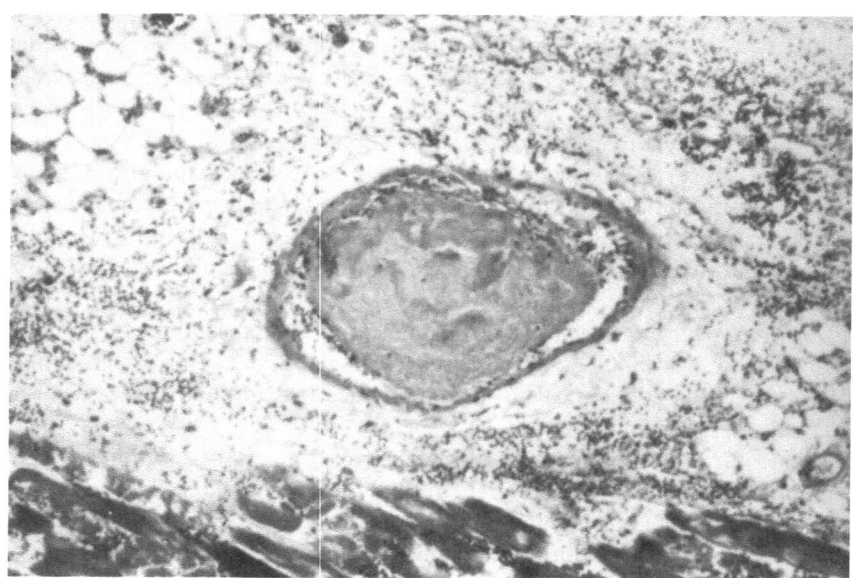

Fig. 4. Thrombus formation in the vein due to *Bothrops atrox* venom (150 μg), 24 hr after i. m. injection. H and E stain. × 50.

that, during the inactivation of thrombin with DFP (diisopropyl phosphofluoridate), the loss of clotting activity was proportional to the loss of esterase activity.

The coagulant principle of *Trimeresurus gramineus* venom can be separated from the anticoagulant principle (Shiau and Ouyang, 1965). The thrombinlike activity has been separated from the bradykinin-releasing enzyme (Holtz *et al.*, 1960).

The coagulant principle has been partially purified from the venom of *Bothrops jararaca* (Banerjee *et al.*, 1960). The fraction is capable of converting fibrinogen to fibrin, of hydrolozying *p*-toluene–arginine methyl ester, but not of proteolyzing activity.

Coagulation of blood in snakebite victims may cause serious disturbances. Thrombosis may cause death or secondary necrosis several days after snake bite. Thrombus formation in the vein due to *Bothrops atrox* venom is illustrated in Fig. 4.

Anticoagulation. It has been shown by clinical observations that a patient who has suffered from *Agkistrodon rhodostoma* poisoning suffers a prolonged coagulation defect due to defibrination syndrome (Reid *et al.*, 1963). A striking characteristic effect of this venom is that the condition of poor or no blood clotting persists over a prolonged period of 6–15 days

(Chan, 1963). Unusual prolonged fibrinogen deficiency is not due to suppression of fibrinogen production in the liver but is due to fibrinogenolysis (Chan, 1963). Intravenous injection of *Agkistrodon rhodostoma* venom into rabbits 24–48 hr after the injection of ^{131}I-labeled fibrinogen causes conversion of the fibrinogen into microclots which are trapped in the smaller vessels of various organs (Regoezi *et al.*, 1966). The microclots are rapidly lysed by the fibrinolytic action of venom components present in the blood, but their presence can be demonstrated histologically by autoradiography and by a double-isotope technique in the early stages of the poisoning.

The anticoagulant activity of *Agkistrodon rhodostoma* venom has been a subject of intensive study, because it has potential therapeutic use in cardiovascular disease. The venom of *Agkistrodon rhodostoma* proved to be highly effective in preventing experimental thrombosis (Marsten *et al.*, 1966).

The anticoagulant activity of *Agkistrodon rhodostoma* venom is frequently described as thrombinlike activity (Esnouf and Tunnah, 1967). This is rather confusing and misleading. When fibrinogen is mixed together with *Agkistrodon rhodostoma* venom, a fine suspension is formed which is generally called a microclot. The microclot formation may be due to the breakdown of fibrinogen or to breakdown products of fibrin. The fraction which converts fibrinogen to the so-called microclot has been isolated from *Agkistrodon rhodostoma* venom (Esnouf and Tunnah, 1967). The molecular weight is 30,000, as calculated from sedimentation data and from amino acid analysis. The fraction has enzymatic activity and hydrolyzes arginine esters, carbobenzoxy-tryptophane, carbobenzoxy-phenylalanine, and carbobenzoxytyrosine. Microclot formation is quite common among other snake venoms (Tu *et al.*, 1966a,b).

Although the venom of *Agkistrodon rhodostoma* venom causes a prolonged defibrination state on envenomation, thromboplastin generation tests carried out on the blood of a fibrinogenopenic subject are normal. This suggests that there is no loss of activity of the factors necessary for thromboplastin formation. By using this property, it is possible to prepare plasma deficient in fibrinogen but containing Factor VIII, antihemophilic factor. Rizza *et al.* (1965) thus separated Factor VIII from fibrinogen by means of a snake venom.

The venom of *Agkistrodon acutus* contains three anticoagulant principles in addition to coagulation principles. All three anticoagulant principles prolong plasma prothrombin time (Chen and Ouyang, 1967). One of the anticoagulant principles contains proteolytic activity. Anticoagulant activity of the venom of *Agkistrodon acutus* is believed to be due to the destruction of prothrombin, thromboplastin, and Ac-globulin (Ouyang, 1957).

Lee and Ouyang (1958) consider that there are five mechanisms for anticoagulation action of Formosan cobra and habu venoms: digestion of

Table I.
Mechanism of Blood Coagulation and the Site of Inhibition due to Snake Venom Action

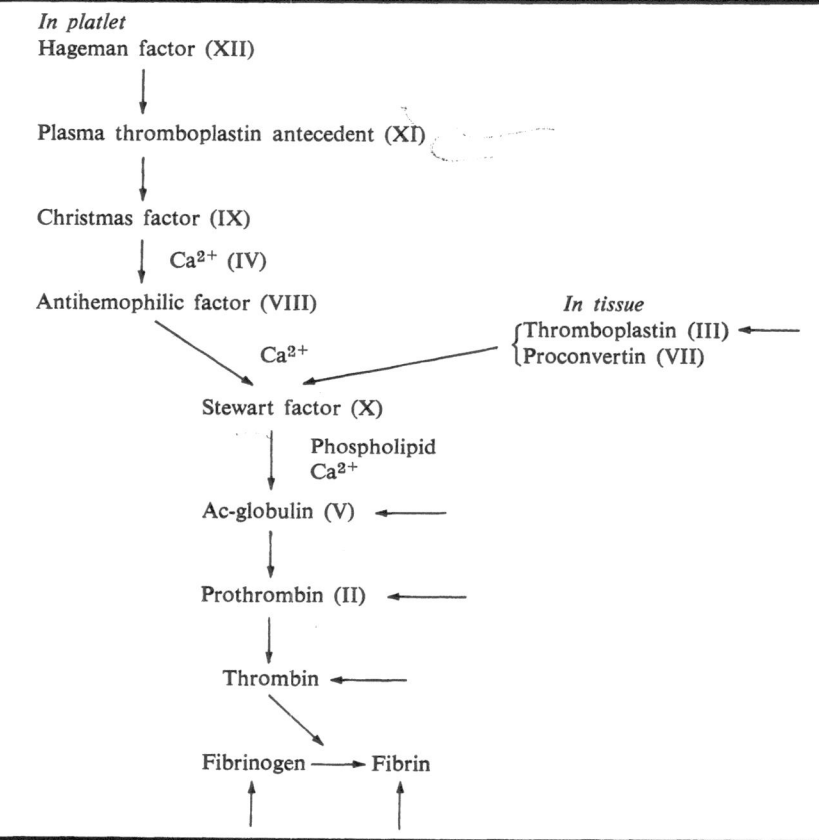

fibrinogen: destruction of prothrombin; antithromboplastin action; antithrombic activity; and inactivation of Ac-globulin. The amount of clottable fibrinogen is decreased markedly after incubation of fibrinogen with *Trimeresurus mucrosquamatus* venom. The venom also destroys prothrombin and thromboplastin.

Fibrinolytic properties of venoms from *Agkistrodon piscivorus* and *Agkistrodon contortrix* are associated with proteolytic activities (Kornalik, 1966).

In order to visualize the mechanism of venom anticoagulant actions, normal blood mechanisms and sites of inhibition are summarized in Table I. The site of inhibition is pointed out by a large arrow. For clarity, the mechanism of blood coagulation is simplified. Many factors actually have both inactive forms and active forms. These are all combined as one factor. For instance, inactive and active Hageman factors as a Hageman factor; inactive and active plasma thromboplastin antecedents as a plasma thromboplastin antecedent; inactive and active Christmas factors as a Christmas factor; inactive and active antihemophilic factors as an antihemophilic factor; and inactive and active accelerator globulins as an Ac-globulin.

5. *Effect on Cell Respiration*

It has been known for a number of years that snake venoms have the ability to inhibit enzymes involved in cell respiration. The factor responsible for inhibition of mitochondrial respiration may be due to phospholipase A.

Purified phospholipase A isolated from *Bothrops neuwidii* venom inhibits NADH oxidase and succinate and NADH-cytochrome with reductase activities. Menadiol oxidase, ubiquinone reductase, and cytochrome oxidase are less inhibited. NADH dehydrogenase and succinate dehydrogenase activities are not affected by the enzyme preparation (Vidal *et al.*, 1966). This inhibition is believed to be due to the hydrolysis of a phospholipid-containing factor involved in the succinate oxidase and NADH-oxidase-systems (Edward and Ball, 1954; Casu and Modena, 1963). The effect of phospholipase A is more indirect than direct. The enzyme disintegrates the mitochondrial membrane, thus inhibiting cell respiration.

Nearly all mitochondrial lipid is present in the membrane, and over 90% of this lipid is phospholipid. The membrane consists of a bimolecular layer of enzymes coated on both sides by protein films. The enzymes involved

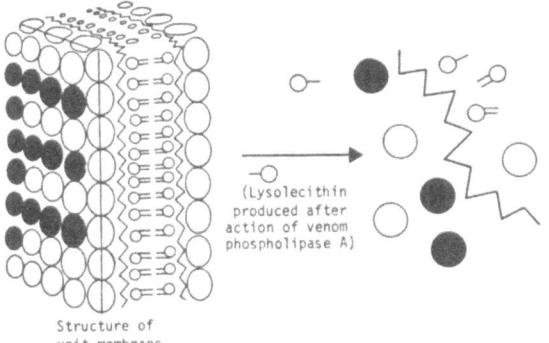

Fig. 5. Solubilization of enzyme due to disruption of mitochondrial membrane. The electron transport carriers and enzymes (dark sphere) are arranged in sequential order of electron transport. ● Respiratory enzymes; ○ functional enzymes other than respiratory enzymes; ○= membrane phospholipids; ○– lysolecithin produced after venom phospholipase A action; ∨∨∨ mitochondrial membrane structural protein.

in respiration are firmly embedded in the mitochondrial membranes. Lysolecithin is formed from lecithin by the action of venom phospholipase A. Lysolecithin attaches itself to membrane phospholipids and disorganizes the arrangement of phospholipids due to the detergent action of lysolecithin. In this process, the functional enzymes including respiratory enzymes are disintegrated. This causes the electron transport enzymes to be removed from the reaction sequence, thus uncoupling electron transport (Fig. 5).

C. Autopharmacological Effects

One complication in the study of snake venom action is the release of pharmacologically active substances from plasma proteins and platelets of victims. These substances are not originally present in the venoms, but rather, are released by the action of the venoms on tissue. These substances include serotonin, histamine, ATP, and bradykinin.

1. Bradykinin Release

Bradykinin is released by the action of snake venoms on plasma globulin. This was first observed by Rocha e Silva et al. in 1949. The factor responsible for bradykinin release is related to the hydrolytic action on arginine esters (Hambery and Roche e Silva, 1957; Iwanaga et al., 1965). It is well known that pancreatic trypsin has an ability to release bradykinin from plasma protein; however, the venom of Crotalus atrox is more potent than crystalline trypsin in liberating a bradykininlike substance in vitro from bovine and human plasma (Margolis et al., 1965).

Bovine plasma contains at least two kininogens from which bradykinin is released by the action of trypsin or snake venoms (Suzuki et al., 1966). A compound related to bradykinin, calidin, is also released from plasma by snake venoms.

The bradykinin-releasing principles of the venoms of Bothrops jararaca and Crotalus atrox are partially dialyzable through cellophane (Holtz et al., 1960). Since the fraction is free from proteolytic and coagulating principles of the venoms, it is likely that the bradykinin-releasing principle is different from the factors responsible for protein hydrolysis and blood coagulation (Holtz et al., 1960; Henriques et al., 1962). A bradykinin-releasing enzyme of the venom of Agkistrodon halys blomhoffii does not require metal ions, has a pH optimum of 8.5, and is most stable in neutral pH (Iwanaga et al., 1965).

2. Histamine Release

The histamine-releasing factor is not phospholipase A, because the enzyme is separated from a histamine-releasing principle in Crotalus durissus *terrificus* venom (Rothschild, 1967). Isolated phospholipase A fails to release histamine. Crotamin is also excluded as a possible histamine-releasing factor. The venoms of certain varieties of Brazilian rattlesnakes which do not contain crotamin have histamine-releasing activity (Rothschild, 1966). The releasing factor seems to be a proteolytic enzyme that has the ability to destroy bradykinin. Rothschild (1966) demonstrated that isolated phospholipase A released only 7.3% of isolated rat mast cell histamine.

Histamine release due to envenomation certainly has pronounced pharmacological effects, but histamine release is not the cause of death. Antihistamine does not prolong the survival time of mice given a lethal dose of *Agkistrodon piscivorus* venom (Kaiser and Raab, 1966).

D. Lethal Action of Snake Venoms

In Sec. II, each action caused by snake envenomation has been described. However, no venoms cause a single action. Any given snake venom usually contains more than one toxic principle, and these tend to act in combination. Symptoms arising in the victim of snake envenomation result from the combined effect of complex protein components present in venom.

Crotoxin, a neurotoxic component of *Crotalus durissus terrificus* venom, not only evokes paralysis but also causes many other symptoms, such as albuminuria, hemoglobinuria, oliguria, and nephrotic lesions (Brazil *et al.*, 1966a; Hadler and Brazil, 1966).

Isolation of pure lethal toxin is sometimes difficult. In some snake venoms, the fraction with hemorrhagic activity also shows lethal activity (*Agkistrodon halys blomhoffii* venom, Omori *et al.*, 1964). On other occasions, the hemorrhagic toxin is readily separated from the lethal toxin. For instance, lethal toxin is separated from hemorrhagic toxin in *Agkistrodon rhodostoma* venom, and the lethal toxin is only a small fraction of the total venom (Toom *et al.*, 1969). Although the lethal fraction represents but a small portion of the total distribution pattern, the toxicity is about twice that of crude venom. Thus, it appears likely that components other than the lethal fraction exert a synergistic effect with regards to the lethal action on the whole venom.

Identification of the lethal toxin even for one venom may be difficult. For instance, a venom may cause death due to massive hemorrhage of internal organs, while the same venom may also cause death due to thrombosis. Thus, the cause of death due to crotalid envenomation varies from case to case. Contrary to the case of crotalid venoms, the cause of death due to elapid venoms is more clear-cut. In this case, the neurotoxin effect becomes predominant.

ACKNOWLEDGMENTS

This work was supported by a U.S. Public Health Service Grants Nos. 2R01 GM15591 and 5R01 FD-00014; ONR Contract N00014-67-A-0299-0005; and NIH Career Development Award, 5-K4-GM-41, 786-02. The author thanks Mrs. Pam Watson, typist.

III. REFERENCES

Aloof-Hirsch, S., A. de Vries, and A. Berger (1968), *Biochim. Biophys. Acta*, **154**:53.
Amorium, M. F. and R. F. Mello (1952), *Mem. Inst. Butantan*, **24**:281.
Amorium, M. F. and R. F. Mello (1954), *Amer. J. Path.*, **30**:479.
Amorium, M. F., R. F. Mello, and F. Saliba (1960), *Rev. Brasil Biol.*, **20**:359.
Augustyn, J. M. and W. B. Elliott (1967), *Toxicon*, **5**:135.
Banerjee, R., A. Vevi, and N. Sarkar (1960), *Thromb. Diath. Haemorrh.*, **5**:296.
Bodano, B. N. and A. M. Stoppani (1962), *Rec. Soc. Arg. Biol.*, **38**:793.
Bodano, B. N. and A. M. Stoppani (1964), *Biochem. Pharmacol.*, **13**:793.
Braganca, B. M. and J. H. Quastel (1952), *Nature*, **169**:695.
Braganca, B. M. and J. H. Quastel (1953), *Biochem J.*, **53**:83.
Brazil, O. V. (1966), *Mem. Inst. Butantan*, **33**:981.
Brazil, O. V., R. Farina, L. Yoshida, and A. V. De Oliveira (1966), *Mem. Inst. Butantan*, **33**:993.
Brazil, O. V., J. P. Franceschi, and E. Waisbich (1966a), *Mem. Inst. Butantan*, **33**:973.
Brazil, O. V., J. P. Franceschi, and E. Waisbich (1967), *Cult. (Saõ Paulo)*, **19**:658–65.
Brazil, O. V., G. M. Laszlo, and O. A. G. B. Eugenio (1969), Origem da paralisia respiratoria dausada pela crotoxina, Abstract, *IX Congresso Latino Americano de Ciencias Fisiologicas*, Brazil.
Casu, A. and B. Modena (1963), *Biochem, J.*, **89**:65.
Chan, K. E. (1963), Regeneration of fibrinogen after defibrination with the Malayan pit viper venom, *Transactions of the Conference Held Under the Auspices of the International Committee on Blood Clotting Factors*, Gleneagles, Scotland, July 1963, F. K. Schattauer-Verlag, Stuttgart.
Chan, K. E., C. R. Rizza, and M. P. Henderson (1965), *Brit. J. Hematol.*, **11**:646.
Cheng, H. C. and C. Ouyang (1967), *Toxicon*, **4**:235.
Cheymol, J., F. Bourillet, and M. Roch-Areiller (1963), *Biochem. Pharmacol.*, **12**:126.
Cohen, S. (1959), *J. Biol. Chem.*, **234**:1129.
Condrea E. and A. de Vries (1965), *Toxicon*, **2**:261.
Condrea E., A. de Vries, and J. Mager (1964), *Biochim. Biophys. Acta*, **84**:60.
Condrea E. and P. Rosenberg (1968), *Biochim. Biophys. Acta*, **150**:271–284.
Delezenne, C. and S. Ledebt (1911a), *Compt. Rend. Acad. Sci.*, **152**:790.
Delezenne, C. and S. Ledebt (1911b), *Compt. Rend. Acad. Sci.*, **153**:81.
Deuch, H. (1957), "Cerebral lipidoses," Blackwells, London. *Toxicon*, **1**:19.
Devi, A. (1968), The protein and nonprotein constituents of snake venoms, in "Venomous Animals and Their Venoms" (W. Bücherl, E. Buckley, and V. Deulofeu, eds.), Vol. I, Academic Press, New York, pp. 119–166.
Donner, L. and Houskova (1967), *Vintr. Lek.*, **13**:647.
Eagle, H. (1937), *J. Expt. Med.*, **65**:613.
Edward, S. W. and E. G. Ball (1954), *J. Biol. Chem.*, **209**:619.
Emery, J. A. and R. E. Russell (1963), Lethal and hemorrhagic properties of some North American snake venoms, *in* "Venomous and Poisonous Animals and Noxious Plants of the Pacific Region", (H. L. Keegan and W. V. Macfarlane, eds.), The Macmillan Co., New York, pp. 409–413.
Esnouf, M. P. and G. W. Tunnah (1967), *Brit. J. Haemat.*, **13**:581.

Flowers, H. H. (1963), *Toxicon*, **1**:131.

Gaertner, C., N. Goldblum, S. Getter, and A. de Vries (1962), *J. Immunol.*, **88**:526.

Gennaro, J. F., Jr. and H. W. Ramsey (1959), *Nature*, **184**:1244.

Goncalves, J. M. (1956), Purification and properties of crotamine, *in* "Venoms" (E. E. Buckley and N. Porges, eds.), American Association for the Advancement of Science, Washington, D.C., pp. 261–274.

Goucher, C. R. and H. H. Flowers (1964), *Toxicon*, **2**:139.

Govier, W. C. and M. C. Boadle (1967), *J. Pharmacol. Exp. Ther.*, **156**:339.

Habermann, E. and W. Neumann (1954), *Arch. Exp. Pathol. Pharmacol.*, **223**:388.

Hadler, W. A. and O. V. Brazil (1966), *Mem. Inst. Butantan*, **33**:1001.

Halmagyi, D. F. J., B. Starzecki, and G. J. Hormer (1965), *J. Appl. Physiol.*, **20**:709.

Hambery, U. and M. Rocha e Silva (1957), *Experientia*, **13**:489.

Henriques, O. B., Z. P. Picarelli, and M. C. Rerraz de Oliveira (1962), *Biochem. Pharmacol.*, **11**:707.

Holtz, P., H. W. Raudonat, and C. Contzen (1960), *Arch. Exp. Pathol. Pharmak.*, **239**:54.

Iwanga, S. and S. Kawachi (1959), *J. Pharm. Sci. Japan*, **79**:582.

Iwanga, S., T. Sato, Y. Mizushima, and T. Suzuki (1965), *J. Biochem.*, **58**:123.

Kaiser, E. and W. Raab (1966), *Mem. Inst. Butantan*, **33**:461.

Kato, H., S. Iwanga, and T. Suzuki (1965), *Experientia*, **22**:49.

Klibansky, C., Y. London, A. Frenicel, and A. de Vries (1968), *Biochim. Biophys. Acta*, **150**:15.

Klose, W. and J. J. Summary (1964), *Amer. J. Med. Sci.*, **248**:189.

Kornalik, F. (1966), *Mem. Inst. Butantan*, **33**:179.

Kurashige, S., Y. Hara, M. Kawakami, and S. Mitsuhashi (1966), *Jap. J. Microbiol.*, **10**:23.

Laki, K. and J. A. Gladner (1964), *Physiol. Rev.*, **44**:127.

Lee, C. Y. and C. Ouyang (1958), Mechanism of anticoagulant action of snake venoms. A comparison of the effects of the venoms of *Naja naja atra* (cobra) and *Trimeresurus mucrosquamatus* (habu), *Proc. VIIth Intern. Cong. of the Intern. Soc. Hemat.*, Rome, Sept. 7–13, 1958, vol. 2.

Levene, P. A. and I. P. Rolf (1923), *J. Biol. Chem.*, **55**:743.

Maeno, H. and S. Mitsuhashi (1961), *J. Biochem.*, **50**:330.

Maeno, H., S. Mitsuhashi, Y. Sawai, and T. Okonogi (1959), *Jap. J. Microbiol.*, **3**:131.

Maeno, H., S. Mitsuhashi, T. Okonogi, S. Hoshi, and M. Homma (1962), *Jap. J. Exp. Med.*, **32**:55.

Margolis, J., S. Bruce, B. Starzecki, G. J. Horner, and D. F. J. Halmagyi (1965), *Austral. J. Exp. Biol. Med. Sci.*, **43**:237.

Markwardt, F., W. Barthel, E. Glusa, A. Hoffmann, and P. Walsmann (1966), *Naunyn-Schmiedebergs Arch. Exp. Pathol. Pharmak.*, **252**:297.

Marsten, J. L., K. E. Chan, J. L. Ankeney, and R. E. Botti (1966), *Circulation Research*, **19**:514.

Master, R. W. P. and S. S. Rao (1961), *J. Biol. Chem.*, **236**:1986.

McCollough, N. D. and J. F. Gennaro, Jr. (1963), *J. Ha. Med. Assoc.*, **49**:959.

Neumann, W. P. and E. Habermann (1955), *Biochem. Fr.*, **327**:170.

Ohsaka, A. (1958), *J. Biochem.*, **45**:259.

Ohsaka, A., H. Ikezawa, H. Kondo, S. Kondo, and N. Uchida (1960), *Brit. J. Exp. Pathol.*, **41**:478.

Ohsaka, A., T. Omori-Satoh, H. Kondo, S. Kondo, and R. Murata (1966), *Mem. Inst. Butantan*, **33**:193.

Okonogi, T., S. Hoshi, M. Homma, S. Mitsuhashi, H. Maeno, and Y. Sawai (1960), *Jap. J. Microbiol. Pathol.*, **4**:189.

Okonogi, T., S. Hoshi, M. Homma, K. Suto, H. Iizuka, and M. Sato (1962), *J. Kitakanto Med.*, **12**:199.

Omori, T., S. Iwanaga, and T. Suzuki (1964), *Toxicon*, **2**:1.

Oshima, G., S. Iwanaga, and T. Suzuki (1968), *J. Biochem.*, **64**:215.

Ouyang, C. (1957), *J. Formosan Med. Assn.*, **56**:19.

Prado-Franceschi, J. and O. V. Brazil (1969), Convulxina, uma nova neurotoxina da peconha da *Crotalus durissus terrificus*, Abstract, IX Congresso Latino Americano de Ciencias Fisiologicas, Brazil.

Raab, W. and E. Kaiser (1966a), *Mem. Inst. Butantan (Saõ Paulo)*, 33:1017.

Raab, W. and E. Kaiser (1966b), *Wien Z. Inn. Med. Grenzgeb.*, 47:327.

Regoeczi, E. (1966), *Z. Tropenmed. Parasitol.*, 17:114.

Regoeczi, E., J. Gergely, and A. S. McFarlan (1966), *J. Clin. Invest.*, 45:1202.

Reid, H. A. (1968), Sympomatology, pathology and treatment of land snake bite in India and Southeast Asia, in "Venomous Animals and Their Venoms" (W. Bücherl, E. Buckley, and V. Deulofeu, eds.), vol. I, Academic Press, New York, pp. 611–642.

Reid, H. A., K. E. Chang, and P. C. Thean (1963), *Lancet*, 1:621.

Rizza, C. R., K. E. Chan, and M. P. Henderson (1965), *Nature*, 207:90.

Rocha e Silva, M., W. T. Beraldo, and G. Rosenfeld (1949), *Amer. J. Physiol.*, 156:261.

Rosenberg, P. and W. D. Dettbarn (1964), *Biochem. Pharmacol.*, 13:1157.

Rosenberg, P. and K. Y. Ng (1963), Factors in venoms leading to block of axonal conduction by curare, *Biochim. Biophys. Acta*, 75:116.

Rosenfeld, G., E. M. A. Kelen, and F. Nudel (1960–62), *Mem. Inst. Butantan*, 30:103.

Rosenfeld, G., L. Nahas, and E. M. Kelen (1968), Coagulant, proteolytic properties of some snake venoms, in "Venomous Animals and Their Venoms, Venomous Vertebrates" (W. Bücherl, E. E. Buckley, V. Deulofeu, eds.), vol. I, Academic Press, New York and London, pp. 229–273.

Rothschild, A. M. (1966), *Mem. Inst. Butantan*, 33:467.

Rothschild, A. M. (1967), *Experientia*, 23:751.

Russell, F. E. (1967), *Clinical Pharmacol. Therap.*, 8:849.

Russell, F. E. and V. C. Bohr (1962), *Tox. Appl. Pharmacol.*, 4:165.

Russell, F. E., F. W. Buess, and J. Strassberg (1962), *Toxicon*, 1:5.

Russell, F. E., F. W. Buess, and M. Y. Woo (1963a), *Toxicon*, 1:99.

Russell, F. E., F. W. Buess, M. Y. Woo, and R. Eventov (1963b), *Toxicon*, 1:229.

Saito, K. and D. J. Hanahan (1962), *Biochem. J.*, 1:521.

Saliba, F. (1965), *Mem. Inst. Butantan*, 31:191.

Shiau, S. Y. and C. Ouyang (1965), *Toxicon*, 2:213.

Slotta, K. H. and P. Borchert (1954), *Mem. Inst. Butantan*, 26:297.

Slotta, K. H. and H. L. Fraenkel-Conrat (1938a), *Nature*, 142:213.

Slotta, K. H. and H. L. Fraenkel-Conrat (1938b), *Ber. Deut. Chem. Ges.*, 71:1076.

Slotta, K. H. and H. L. Fraenkel-Conrat (1939), *Nature*, 144:290.

Stahnke, H. L. (1966), "The Treatment of Venomous Bites and Stings," Bureau of Publications, Arizona State University, Tempe, Arizona.

Stahnke, H. L., F. M. Allen, R. V. Moran, and J. H. Tenery (1957), *Amer. J. Trop. Med. Hyg.*, 6:323.

Suzuki, T. (1966), *Mem. Inst. Butantan*, 33:519.

Suzuki, T., S. Iwanaga, T. Sato, S. Nagasawa, H. Kato, M. Yano, and K. Horiuchi (1966), *Int. Symp. Vasoactive Polypeptides: Bradykinin and Related Kinins*, Ribeirao Preto, Brazil, pp. 27–35.

Taub, A. and W. B. Elliott (1964), *Toxicon*, 2:87.

Toom, P. M., P. G. Squire, and A. T. Tu (1969), *Biochim. Biophys. Acta*, 181:339.

Tu, A. T. and M. Homma (1969), *Tox. Appl. Pharmacol.*, in press.

Tu, A. T., A. Chua, and G. P. James (1966a), *Tox. Appl. Pharmacol.*, 8:218.

Tu, A. T., R. B. Passey, and T. Tu (1966b), *Toxicon*, 4:59.

Tu, A. T., M. Homma, and B. Hong (1969), *Toxicon*, 6:175–178.

Vidal, J. C., B. N. Bodano, A. O. M. Stoppani, and A. A. Boveris (1966), *Mem. Inst. Butantan*, 33:913.

Webster, G. R. (1957), *Nature*, 180:660.

Wells, M. A. and D. J. Hanahan (1969), *Biochem.*, 8:414.

Welsh, J. H. (1966), *Mem. Inst. Butantan*, 33:509.

Zeller, E. A. (1951), Enzymes as essential components of toxins, in "The Enzymes"

(J. B. Sumner and K. Myrback, eds.), vol. 1, no. 2, Academic Press, New York, pp. 986–1013.

Chapter 5

The Use of Snake Venoms as Pharmacological Tools in Studying Nerve Activity

Philip Rosenberg

Division of Pharmacology
School of Pharmacy and Pharmacy Research Institute
The University of Connecticut
Storrs, Connecticut, U.S.A.

I. INTRODUCTION

Most texts and review articles on venoms have been primarily concerned with chemical properties or mechanisms of action (Bücherl *et al.*, 1968; Jiménez-Porras, 1968; Devi, 1968; Sarkar and Devi, 1968; Russell, 1967; Russell and Saunders, 1967; Condrea and de Vries, 1965; Meldrum, 1965; Braganca and Aravindakshan, 1962; Buckley and Porges, 1956; Zeller, 1951). Indeed, understanding of the pharmacological actions of venoms was greatly aided by the study of their effects on various organ systems such as nerve, muscle, and blood. It was, however, not so readily apparent that this complex, specialized saliva of snakes could be used as a tool for analysis of physiological processes. For example, by 1963 about 6000 papers on snake venoms and venomous snakes had been published (Russell and Scharfenberg, 1964), with relatively few of these having as their direct concern a better understanding of the physiological processes affected by venoms. A notable exception was the process of blood coagulation, which has been clarified by studying the action of snake venoms or venom components (Jimenez-Porras, 1968; Condrea and DeVries, 1965; Boquet, 1964). Snake venoms have also been useful as tools in general biochemical research, where

111

the primary interest has been in extracting and studying enzymes obtained from venoms (Zeller, 1966).

I shall emphasize in this chapter those studies, using snake venoms, in which prime consideration was given to obtaining a better understanding of neural activity. Other experiments using venoms will be mentioned only if we can derive information concerning the nervous system from them. I shall attempt to show that by "pouring" venoms, about which we still know relatively little, into the nervous system, about which we know less, we obtain a better understanding of both.

II. DEVELOPMENT AND DIFFERENTIATION OF THE NERVOUS SYSTEM

Just as our understanding of CNS function was aided by the availability of drugs which stimulated or depressed CNS activity, so our knowledge of growth and differentiation might be aided if we understood how specific agents stimulate or depress this property of nerve. In 1956 a potent nerve growth stimulating factor (NGF) was isolated from snake venom (Cohen and Levi-Montalcini, 1956). This component of Elapidae, Viperidae, and Crotalidae venoms (Cohen, 1959) causes a marked increase in the size and number of sensory nerve cells and an even greater increase in the sympathetic nerve cell population (Levi-Montalcini and Cohen, 1956). Similar effects are produced by an extract from mouse salivary glands (Levi-Montalcini, 1958).

The response to NGF in sympathetic ganglia of chick embryos consists of an increase in mitotic activity, acceleration of maturation processes, and hypertrophy of differentiated nerve cells. Sensitivity to NGF has been observed in newborn and adult mice; depending on stage of development, there is either hypertrophy or hyperplasia of the sympathetic ganglia (Levi-Montalcini and Booker, 1960a). NGF activity has been bioassayed by its ability to produce a fibrillar "halo effect" in cultured sympathetic or sensory chick ganglia. The size of the halo and density of the fibers surrounding the ganglia are taken as measures of activity. As with any bioassay, problems have been associated with the quantitative measurement of NGF activity (Levi-Montalcini and Angeletti, 1968a).

Cohen (1958) succeeded in effecting about a 40-fold purification of NGF from cottonmouth moccasin venom (CMV). The biological activity which appeared to be associated with a single protein (molecular weight about 20,000) was lost by incubation either with proteolytic enzymes or antiserum to snake venom. The active factor is nondialyzable, destroyed by heat at pH 7.4 and unstable in acid. No enzymatic activity was found associated with NGF, and it appears to be distinct from enzymes and toxins previously found in venoms. The NGF isolated from *Crotalus adamanteus* (eastern diamondback rattlesnake) venom appears to have a minimum molecular weight of 5000 based on its amino acid composition (Angeletti *et al.*, 1967). It is possible that NGF is a protein which exists in multiple possible aggregate states. The NGF isolated from salivary gland appears not to be identical with the snake venom factor, although its effects on growth are similar (Levi-Montalcini and Angeletti, 1968a).

Despite increasing knowledge concerning the metabolic effects of NGF, we still do not know its primary site or mechanism of action. Nevertheless, in the process of studying the action of NGF, we also study those cellular processes responsible for normal growth and cell differentiation.

III. NEURONAL DEGENERATION AND DEMYELINATION

A. Immunosympathectomy by Antibodies to Nerve Growth Factor

An antiserum to NGF was prepared by injecting a purified preparation from salivary gland into rabbits (Levi-Montalcini and Booker, 1960b). This antiserum neutralizes the *in vitro* activity of NGF derived from snake venom, thus indicating some similarity in venom and gland NGF immunological properties (Levi-Montalcini and Angeletti, 1961). Within 4 hr after the injection of antiserum into newborn mammals, marked cytolytic changes are already apparent which culminate in the selective and almost complete destruction of sympathetic nerve cells (Sabatini *et al.*, 1965). The suggestion has been made that the nucleus is the primary target of the antiserum to NGF (Levi-Montalcini and Angeletti, 1968a). However, it has not been clarified whether these changes in sympathetic tissue resemble in any manner those changes seen in clinical conditions of central nervous system degeneration or demyelination. For example, the possibility of multiple sclerosis having an immunological cause is being actively studied.

B. Neuropathological Changes Induced by Venoms

Various venoms cause pathological changes in the central nervous system of animals (Okonogi *et al.*, 1960; Morrison and Zamecnik, 1950; Hunter, 1909; Lamb and Hunter, 1904). Morrison and Zamecnik (1950) found *in vitro* demyelination of brain and spinal cord of laboratory animals induced by cobra and rattlesnake venoms as well as by *Clostridium welchii* toxin. Hudson *et al.* (1960) have reported that *Naja naja* venom, heated at an acid pH [source of phospholipase A (PhA)], when injected into the intrathecal space produces severe paralysis from which there is considerable recovery in 3–4 weeks. How closely these changes mimic demyelinating diseases, one of the major problems in neurology, has not received the attention it deserves. The suggestion has been made that free fatty acids which would be produced by the action of circulating PhA could cause an unwrapping of the myelin sheath, which in turn could be the causative factor in multiple sclerosis (Swank, 1961). Others have proposed that the demyelinating plaques seen in multiple sclerosis are due to the action of some lytic factor in the nervous system (Thompson, 1964; Adams and Richardson, 1961). Sjöstrand (1963) points out that splitting a fatty acid from lipids, as by PhA, might cause an increase in the surface area of the lipoprotein layers in myelin, one of the earliest changes observed in demyelination. It should be noted that various mammalian tissues, and especially several snake and bee venoms, are sources of PhA (Condrea and de Vries, 1965; Zeller, 1951).

Certain organophosphates, such as triorthocresyl phosphate (TOCP), induce selective degeneration of nerve fibers in the spinal cord and sciatic nerve of susceptible species such as hen and man (for references, see Morazain and Rosenberg, 1969). Interest in this condition has developed because of its possible similarities to multiple sclerosis and other clinical disorders. Much of the biochemical research has been concerned with the lipids, since in Wallerian degeneration, a condition often compared with TOCP neuropathy, extensive modifications of lipid metabolism are observed (Rossiter, 1961). It was recently found that TOCP induces marked changes in the stability of phospholipids from hen sciatic nerve as judged by sensitivity to hydrolysis by snake venom PhA (Morazain and Rosenberg, 1969). Even before the time of onset of TOCP paralysis, the phospholipid splitting induced by CMV was two to three times as great as in control tissues. This phenomenon is, interestingly enough, only observed in those tissues where lesions eventually develop. These findings might indicate a reorientation due to TOCP of the phospholipids (PL) within the membrane or a change in membrane permeability. These would allow externally applied enzyme to come into closer contact with its PL substrate. This supposition is supported by the finding that membranal PL hydrolysis induced by snake venom, or its isolated PhA, varies greatly dependent on the physical state of the PL (Condrea and DeVries, 1965; Ibraham et al., 1964; Condrea et al., 1962). Further studies will be required to determine whether in TOCP intoxication PL alterations are the cause or the result of axonal degeneration.

IV. AXONAL CONDUCTION

A. Use of Venoms as Chemical Dissectors

The electrophysiological properties of the action potential are known in considerable detail (Katz, 1966; Eccles, 1964; Hodgkin, 1964). However, no explanation of those physical and chemical events responsible for the genesis of bioelectricity is as yet widely accepted. The possible roles of PL (Goldman, 1964) and fixed charges (Tasaki, 1968) in axonal function have been discussed. Nachmansohn (1959; 1969) has attempted to explain bioelectricity as being fundamentally an enzyme–receptor–substrate inter-action between ACh, AChE, and a macromolecular protein in or near the excitable membrane.

Tobias (1958; 1955; Narahashi and Tobias, 1964) was one of the early investigators to use enzymes as chemical dissectors in order to obtain information about the structure and function of the nervous system. He compared the effects of acid-heated *Naja naja* venom (source of PhA), PhC, hyaluronidase, collagenase, chymotrypsin, papain, and ribonuclease on lobster giant axons and frog sartorius muscle. Phospholipases produced depolarization as well as block of conduction in nerve and contracture in muscle. Similar effects were found with phospholipases on nodal prepa-rations from the frog sciatic nerve (Nelson, 1958). None of the other enzymes had any effect on the action or the resting potential.

We likewise attempted to produce predetermined chemical changes in a nerve with the hope that the functional consequences observed might allow us to test the ACh theory of bioelectricity as proposed by Nachman-sohn (1959; 1969). Many investigators have not accepted the proposal that ACh is essential for axonal conduction, maintaining that it is essential only for transmission of impulses at certain junctional regions. One of their objections is based upon the failure of ACh and other quaternary nitrogen derivatives to affect conduction in nerve axons similar to their powerful actions on junctions. Experimental evidence was obtained for the existence around axons of barriers which prevent lipid insoluble compounds, like ACh and neostigmine, from penetrating, but which allow lipid soluble tertiary nitrogen derivatives, such as physostigmine, to penetrate readily (Rothenberg *et al.*, 1948; Bullock *et al.*, 1946). If ACh and *d*-tubocurarine (curare) are inactive on axons because of permeability barriers, then it might be possible by chemical treatment to decrease these barriers.

B. Effects of Cholinergic Agents on Axonal Conduction

In order to evaluate whether an axonal preparation, the squid giant axon, might have a strong permeability barrier, we compared the effects of tertiary and quaternary nitrogen compounds on the squid axon and on a synaptic preparation, the electroplax synapse, where barriers are probably minimal (Table I). The lipid soluble tertiary nitrogen derivatives were effective in similar concentrations on the two preparations, whereas the quaternary nitrogen containing compounds were inactive on control squid axons, but highly potent at the electroplax synapse. Curare and ACh were inactive both on control squid giant axon preparations, which were carefully

Table I.

Minimal Concentrations of Several Compounds Required to Block Conduction of Control and Venom-Treated Squid Giant Axons and Synaptic Transmission in the Isolated Single Electroplax[a]

Compound	[M] to Block conduction		
	Squid axon[b]		Electroplax synapse[c]
	Control	Venom treated	
Tertiary nitrogen derivatives			
Atropine	2×10^{-3}	3×10^{-4}	3×10^{-4}
Methantheline	2×10^{-3}		5×10^{-4}
Physostigmine	7×10^{-3}	1×10^{-3}	7×10^{-4}
Procaine	3×10^{-3}		1×10^{-3}
Dibucaine	3×10^{-5}		3×10^{-5}
Diphenhydramine	4×10^{-4}		2×10^{-4}
Chlorpromazine	1×10^{-4}		1×10^{-4}
Quaternary nitrogen derivatives			
Acetylcholine	$>10^{-1}$	2×10^{-4}	3×10^{-6}
Curare	$>10^{-2}$	3×10^{-5}	3×10^{-6}
Decamethonium	$>10^{-1}$	2×10^{-3}	3×10^{-6}
Benzoylcholine	$>10^{-1}$	2×10^{-2}	1×10^{-3}
Chlorisondamine	$>10^{-1}$	1×10^{-2}	2×10^{-4}
PAM	$>10^{-1}$	1×10^{-2}	
Choline	$>10^{-1}$	$>10^{-1}$	$>10^{-1}$

[a] Compounds were applied for 30 min. Venom-treated axons were pretreated for 30 min with 15 μg/ml CMV. $>$ Indicates that at concentration shown no effect on conduction was observed. Table modified from Rosenberg (1966).

[b] Data from Rosenberg and Podleski (1963, 1962); Rosenberg and Ehrenpreis (1961).

[c] Data from Rosenberg et al. (1960); Rosenberg and Higman (1960).

dissected free of all adhering small nerve fibers, as well as on preparations containing surrounding small nerve fibers (Rosenberg and Hoskin, 1965). Physostigmine, a reversible AChE inhibitor which blocks axonal conduction, was equally potent in both preparations. These results indicate that adhering small nerve fibers and associated connective tissue do not alter the effects on the squid giant axon of externally applied compounds.

In attempting to reduce possible permeability barriers surrounding the squid giant axon, various enzymes, detergents, and other compounds were applied to the axon. After removal of the pretreatment agent and rinsing of the nerve in normal sea water, curare (1.4×10^{-3} M) was applied. Curare was used as the test compound since it is highly potent at synapses and is not readily catabolized by enzymes of biological tissue. Curare had no effect on conduction following exposure of the axon to digitonin, hyaluronidase, trypsin, chymotrypsin, hydrolase mixture, lipase, lysozyme, papain, alkaline phosphatase, sodium desoxycholate, Span 20, Tween 20, neuraminidase, saponin, arsenite, dimethyl formamide, dimethyl sulfoxide, or histamine (Rosenberg and Ehrenpreis, 1961; Rosenberg, 1965). Following pretreatment with certain snake venoms, however, curare reversibly blocked conduction. An axon rendered sensitive to curare by venom remained so for the entire survival period of the preparation (4–8 hr). Of a series of 23 venoms tested, CMV was the most effective in rendering axons sensitive to curare (Table II). Examples of the effects of curare following CMV are

Table II.
Concentrations of Venom Pretreatment which Rendered the Squid Giant Axon Sensitive to Curare, and Concentrations Required to Block Directly the Conducted Action Potential (AP)[a]

Venom	μg/ml		Curare effect
	Direct block of AP	Pretreatment	
Agkistrodon piscivorus piscivorus	50	15	+++
Hemachatus hemachatus	50	15	++
Notechis scutatus	100	30	+++
Acanthophis antarcticus	100	30	++
Naja naja	100	30	++
Heloderma horridum	100	30	++
Heloderma suspectum	100	30	++
Enhydrina schistosa	100	20	−
Dendroaspis polylepis	100	30	+
Bungarus caeruleus	250	50	++
Ophiophagus hannah	400	100	++
Vipera palestinae	400	100	++
Crotalus atrox	500	150	+
Agkistrodon contortrix mokeson	1000	200	+
Bothrops atrox	1000	200	+
Bitis arietans	2000	500	++
Vipera russellii	>1000	500	+
Centruroides sculpturatus	> 100	100	−
Vespula arenaria	> 100	100	−
Latrodectus geometricus	> 100	100	−
Latrodectus varidus	> 250	250	−
Crotalus horridus horridus	> 500	500	−
Crotalus adamanteus	>2000	2000	−

[a] Venoms were applied for 30 min. > indicates that at concentration shown no effect on AP was observed. +++, ++, +, and − indicate respectively a 80–100%, 50–80%, 20–50% and 0–20% decrease in the AP produced in 30 min or less by 1.4×10^{-3} M curare after venom pretreatment. The effect of curare was readily reversible (Condrea and Rosenberg, 1968; Rosenberg, 1965; Rosenberg and Podleski, 1963; 1962; Rosenberg and Ehrenpreis, 1961). Table modified from Rosenberg (1966).

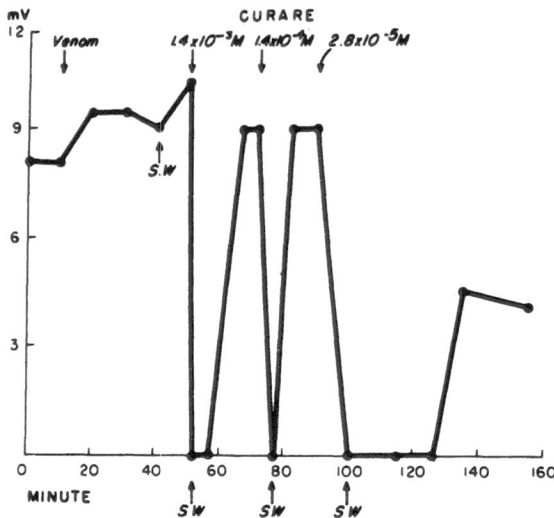

Fig. 1. Effect of curare on the giant axon of squid following pretreatment with 15 μg/ml CMV. SW indicates return to sea water (Rosenberg and Podleski, 1962).

shown in Figs. 1 and 2. In the concentrations used for pretreatment, the venoms had no effect on the action potential. Higher concentrations of CMV block conduction, after which they induce membrane depolarization (Fig. 3). In contrast to the reversible conduction block induced by curare, venom block is irreversible. Venoms do not block axonal conduction of

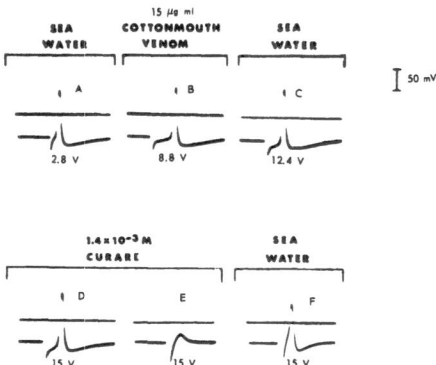

Fig. 2. Effect of curare on the resting and action potential of the squid giant axon following exposure to CMV. A, control; B, after exposure to 15 μg/ml venom for 15 min; C, 15 min after return to sea water (stimulus voltage remained constant for this period); D, E, 4 and 8 min after exposure to 1.4 mM curare; F, 22 min after return to sea water (Rosenberg and Podleski, 1963).

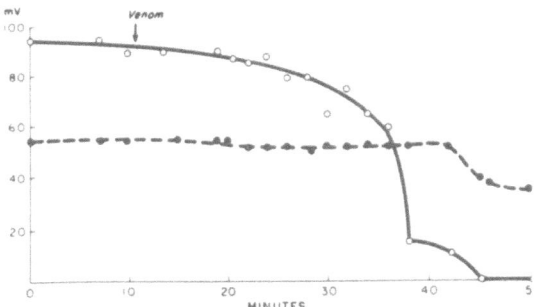

Fig. 3. Effect of 50 μg/ml of CMV on the resting potential ($\bullet$—$\bullet$) and action potential (O—O) of the giant axon of squid (Rosenberg and Podleski, 1962).

mammalian nerve preparations when tested *in vivo* (Russell, 1967; Meldrum, 1965). It is of interest that the relative potency of several of the venoms on the squid axon (Table II) agrees with their potency in blocking neuro-muscular transmission (Russell and Long, 1961; Kellaway and Holden, 1932), causing demyelination (Birkmayer and Neumayer, 1957; Morrison and Zamecnik, 1950) and inducing hemolysis or hemagglutination (Minton, 1956).

The venom-treated axon becomes sensitive not only to curare but also to several other quaternary nitrogen derivatives including ACh (Table I). The minimal concentration of ACh which blocked conduction had no effect on the resting potential, althorgh concentrations 10 times higher depolarized the membrane. The inactivity of choline even in venom treated axons indicates some specificity in the action of ACh. The results indicate that venoms expose a membranal component, perhaps the physiological ACh receptor, which reacts with externally applied quaternary nitrogen derivatives.

C. The Acetylcholine Receptor

Since the presence and chemical reactivity of the ACh receptor at so-called cholinergic junctions has been well characterized, it was of interest to compare the chemical sensitivity of the ACh receptor at junctions to that existing along the squid axon. An analysis was made possible by the availability of sulfur and selenium analogs of benzoylcholine. Benzoylcholine is similar in structure to ACh, and is thought to react at the junction with the ACh receptor. While the molecular size and shape of those isologs is similar, their electron distribution differs markedly. If the action of ACh is due to a specific effect on an ACh receptor, one might expect this receptor to be similar in all excitable membranes. We therefore compared the effects of oxygen, sulfur, and selenium isologs of benzoylcholine on the venom treated squid axon to their effects on the electroplax synapse (Rosenberg and Mautner, 1967; Rosenberg *et al.*, 1966; Webb and Mautner, 1966). Because the penetration of these compounds is poor, venom pretreatment of axons was essential. Substitution of O by S and further substitution by Se in a series of isologs resulted in a progressive increase of potency in both axon and synapse. The ACh receptor thus appears to be similar in its specific reactions, both in axons and synapses.

D. Hyperexcitability

Certain nerves when exposed to solutions deficient in Ca^{2+} or total divalent cations will develop spontaneous or repetitive electrical activity (for references, *see* Rosenberg and Bartels, 1967). The molecular mechanism of this increased irritability has not been elucidated. The study of compounds which block with some degree of specificity the effect of Ca^{2+} removal might aid our understanding of the role of Ca^{2+} in conduction. Studies of this nature might have some bearing on the genesis and possible treatment of certain convulsive disorders, especially epilepsy. It has been pointed out that the spontaneously firing, peripheral axon bears similarity to convulsive activity of brain cells (Toman, 1949). It is of interest that CMV antagonized spontaneous firing in the squid axon, whether it was induced by decreased divalent cations, by dimethylaminoethyl acetate, or by ammonia (Rosenberg and Bartels, 1967; Rosenberg and Ehrenpreis, 1961). Concentrations of CMV as low as 2 μg/ml blocked spontaneous firing induced by low Ca^{2+} and Mg^{2+}, whereas 30 μg/ml was required to block the evoked action potential (Rosenberg and Bartels, 1967). The specificity of the venoms' action resembles that observed with antiepileptic and anti-parkinsonian compounds, except that the venom block of spontaneous firings was irreversible.

V. MEMBRANE PERMEABILITY

A. Increased Permeability Induced by Venoms

Since venoms sensitize the squid axon to curare and ACh (see Sec. IV), it is important to determine whether this effect is due to reduction of the permeability barriers that prevent externally applied lipid insoluble compounds from reaching the conducting membrane. Toward this end, we have exposed axons to ^{14}C-labeled compounds, then extruded and assayed axoplasm for radioactivity. The penetration of curare and ACh was greatly increased after treatment with CMV. After eastern diamondback rattlesnake venom, curare neither penetrates nor does it affect electrical activity (Fig. 4; Table I). The control penetration of ACh, choline, and dimethylcurare is less than 1 % of that expected if no barrier were present, and even this may

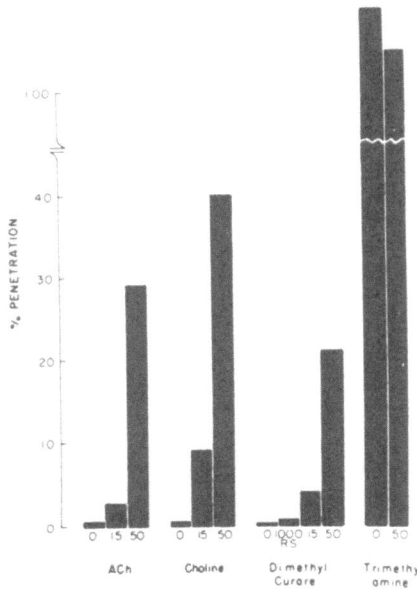

Fig. 4. Penetration of (^{14}C) labeled ACh, choline, dimethylcurare, and trimethylamine into the axoplasm of squid giant axon with and without exposure to CMV. The percentage indicates the radioactivity of the axoplasm compared to that in the outside fluid. The figures below the columns indicate the μg of venom/ml. In contrast to the moccasin venom, that of the eastern diamondback rattlesnake (RS), even in 1000 μg/ml, had no significant effect on the penetration of dimethylcurare. Trimethylamine readily penetrates with and without exposure to venom (Rosenberg and Hoskin, 1963).

be due to contemination during extrusion. The marked difference in the effects of ACh, depending on its ability to penetrate through permeability barriers surrounding the axon, is further evidence that the external concentrations required to affect electrical activity may be of little significance. CMV increased the permeability to many other poorly penetrating compounds including sucrose, glutamate, glutamine, γ-amino butyric acid (GABA), 3,4-dihydroxy phenyl alanine (DOPA), and serotonin (Hoskin and Rosenberg, 1965). Hadidian (1956) had found that CMV increased the penetration of procaine into frog sciatic nerve.

The penetration of all compounds is not markedly increased by CMV. Neostigmine does not penetrate into the axoplasm even after 25 μg/ml CMV, a concentration which increases penetration of ACh and curare (Brzin *et al.*, 1965a). These findings may explain why neostigmine has no effect on conduction even in venom treated axons (Rosenberg and Podleski, 1962).

In attempting to determine whether snake venom increased permeability to ACh in preparations other than the squid giant axon, we used techniques not requiring the extrusion of the cells contents. It has been shown that the ratio of AChE in intact and homogenized preparations, which we shall refer to as the permeability constant (PC), serves as an index of the permeability barrier (Rosenberg and Dettbarn, 1963). If the AChE of the tissue were completely accessible to ACh, which is used as substrate for the enzyme assay, then the PC would be 1, whereas complete inaccessibility would give a PC ratio of O.

The PC ratios in various biological tissues indicated that the eel electroplax has the strongest barrier to ACh, and the squid stellar nerve has the weakest (Table III). Since at least 96% of the AChE activity of the squid stellar nerve is present in the small nerve fibres, these figures would not indicate the barrier present in the giant axon (Brzin *et al.*, 1965b). CMV, and to a lesser extent rattlesnake venom, increased the AChE activity of intact axons of the squid stellar nerve, nerve fibers from the walking legs of lobster, and the isolated eel electroplax (Table III). The greater effectiveness

Table III.
Effect of Venoms on Permeability of Various Preparations as Judged by the Ability of 5×10^{-3} M Acetylcholine to Penetrate and Assay the Available AChE in Intact Biological Preparations[a]

Tissue	Venom	μg/ml	AChE Homogenized	AChE Intact	PC
Squid stellar nerve			57	42	0.74
	CMV	15	57	44	0.77
	CMV	50	56	54	0.96
	CA	50	58	46	0.79
	CA	200	55	50	0.91
Eel electroplax			18	3	0.17
	CMV	50	20	5	0.25
	CMV	400	29	10	0.34
	CMV	1000	32	20	0.63
	CA	50	20	4	0.20
	CA	1000	32	9	0.28
Walking leg nerve of lobster			925	337	0.36
	CMV	100	900	442	0.49
	CMV	1000	886	698	0.79
	CA	1000	900	475	0.53
Frog sartorius muscle			32	13	0.41
	CMV	1000	32	27	0.84
Rabbit cerebral cortex			260	138	0.53
	CMV	1000	285	152	0.53
	CA	1000	256	156	0.61

[a] The permeability constant (PC) is the ratio of AChE activity of intact and homogenized tissue. CMV = *Agkistrodon piscivorus* venom; CA = *Crotalus adamanteus* venom. All AChE activities are expressed as μM ACh hyd/g/hr except for the electroplax results which are presented as μM ACh hyd/cell/hr (average cell weight is 40 mg) (Rosenberg and Dettbarn, 1967, 1964).

in increasing permeability of CMV as compared to rattlesnake (*Crotalus adamanteus*) venom agrees with previous findings in other systems that rattlesnake venom is less effective in its ability to disrupt membranes. Since the venoms used have no AChE activity themselves (Rosenberg and Dettbarn, 1964; Zeller, 1949), their effects must be attributed to making AChE more accessible than in the control preparation. The increased permeability caused by the venoms in lobster nerves agrees with the findings that CMV decreases the concentration of ACh required to affect electrical activity (Dettbarn, 1963).

Because, as discussed above, substrates such as ACh do not penetrate to all of the AChE, it is difficult to determine the total enzyme activity in intact nerve fibers. Several procedures have been tried, but none has been completely satisfactory (Dettbarn and Rosenberg, 1962; Dettbarn and Hoskin, 1962; Rosenberg, 1960). Our results indicate that venoms may be useful in future studies where it is essential to obtain an indication of the total AChE activity in the intact preparation.

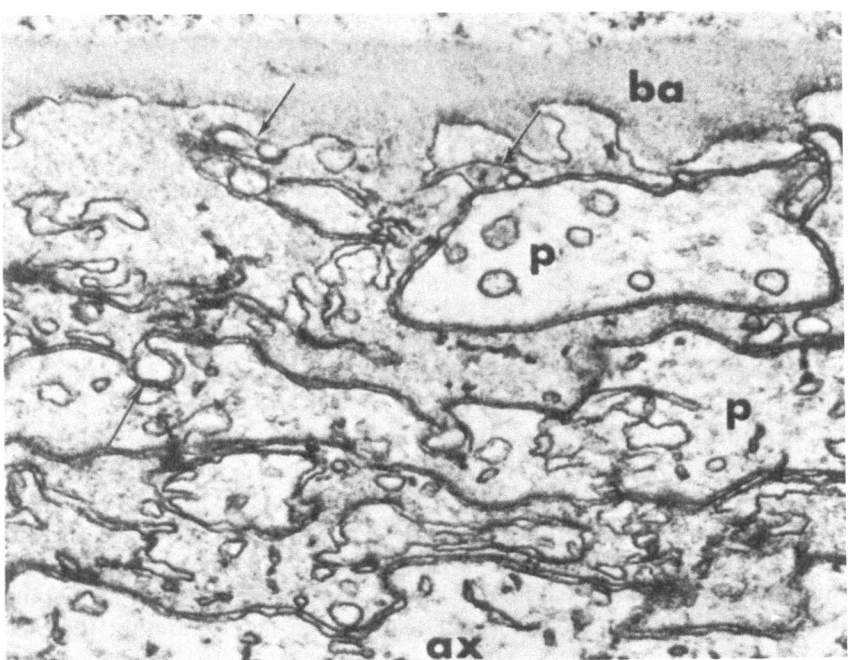

Fig. 5. Schwann sheath of a control giant axon (*ax*) fixed in permanganate immediately after dissection. The sheath is formed by several processes (*p*) and surrounded by a prominent basement membrane (*ba*). At the arrows, there are either transversely cut fingerlike extensions or globular postmortem artifacts. × 42,500. (Martin and Rosenberg, 1968).

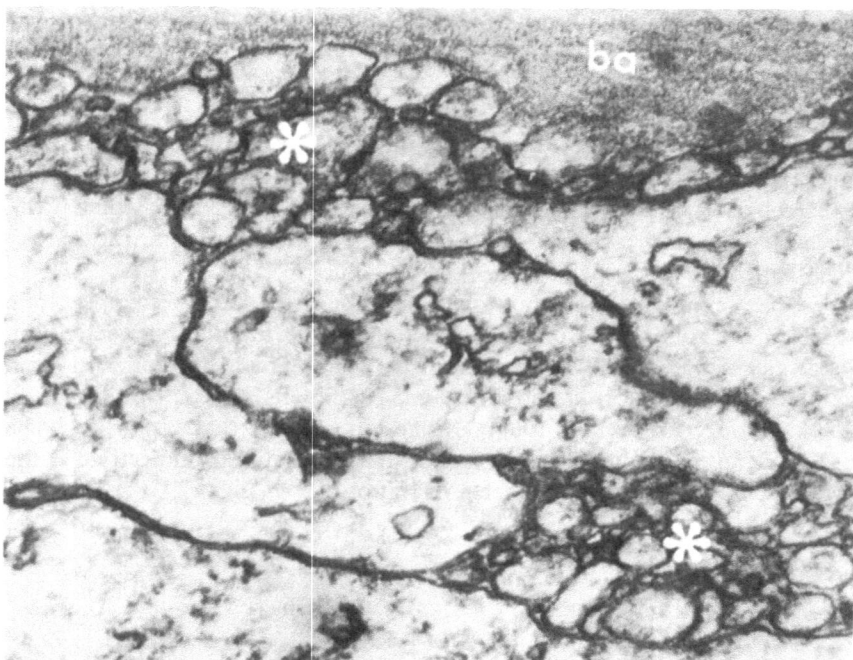

Fig. 6. Effect of 100 μg/ml of CMV on the structure of the sheath of a giant axon fixed in permanganate. At (*) there are nests of cytoplasmic globules produced by the treatment. × 50,000. (Martin and Rosenberg, 1968).

B. Structural Alterations Associated with Increased Permeability

Electron microscopic studies have been undertaken to determine whether structural modifications may be observed in venom-treated squid nerves (Martin and Rosenberg, 1968). The venoms of cottonmouth, ringhals, and cobra all caused a marked breakdown in the structure of the Schwann sheath (*cf* Figs. 5 and 6). Rattlesnake venom, the direct lytic factor obtained from ringhals venom, and hyaluronidase caused few observable changes in structure. This correlates with their inability to increase permeability. Since high amounts of venom had no noticeable effect on the basement membrane or connective tissue, it would appear that these structures are not the sites of the permeability barriers. Villegas and Villegas (1960) have shown that Schwann cells are traversed by relatively large channels, yet their tortuous nature may still make penetration difficult. The venom results indicate that the Schwann cell may be the major permeability barrier in the squid giant axon.

VI. PHOSPHOLIPID FUNCTION IN NERVE

A. Component of Venom Responsible for Effects on Axon

Besides nonenzymic components, venoms contain many enzymes including PhA, hyaluronidase, proteolytic enzymes, *l*-amino acid oxidase, phosphodiesterase, etc. (Bücherl *et al.*, 1968; Russell, 1967; Braganca and Aravindakshan, 1962; Buckley and Porges, 1956). In addition, colubrid venoms contain AChE (Zeller, 1949). It is obviously of great interest to determine the component of venom responsible for increasing permeability, since we might then have a clue as to those components of the membrane which are responsible for maintaining its permeability properties. Phosphodiesterase, *l*-amino acid oxidase, proteolytic enzymes, hyaluronidase, a direct lytic factor from ringhals venom, and a neurotoxic fraction from cobra venom were all unable to render squid axons sensitive to curare (Condrea and Rosenberg, 1968; Rosenberg and Ng, 1963; Rosenberg and Podleski, 1962; Rosenberg and Ehrenpreis, 1961). In lobster axons, it was found that neither proteases nor hyaluronidase had any significant effect on the action or resting potentials (Narahashi and Tobias, 1964; Tobias, 1958; 1955).

The first indication we had that PhA was the component of venom responsible for increasing axonal permeability was the observation that alkaline-heated solutions of CMV and *Naja naja* venom did not render axons sensitive to curare, while acid-heated solutions were effective (Rosenberg and Podleski, 1962). PhA is known to be resistant to boiling at acid pH, but it is destroyed by boiling at an alkaline pH (Rosenberg and Ng, 1963; Magee and Thompson, 1960; Braganca and Quastel, 1953; Hughes, 1935). An acid-heated solution of cobra venom has been found to decrease membrane potential, threshold potential, action potential, and membrane resistance in giant axons of lobster (Narahashi and Tobias, 1964; Tobias, 1955). A partially purified preparation of PhA was isolated from ringhals (*Hemachatus hemachatus*) venom by electrophoresis (Condrea and Rosenberg, 1968; Condrea *et al.*, 1967). This isolated fraction increased permeability, sensitized axons to curare and ACh, and in higher concentrations blocked conduction of axons from the walking leg nerve of lobster (Condrea *et al.*, 1967). PhA also reproduced the venom effects which were observed on the squid axon: 10 μg/ml renders the axon sensitive to ACh and curare and 50 μg/ml blocks conduction. The direct effects of PhA on conduction are shown in Fig. 7. PhA produced vesiculations of the Schwann cell similar to those reported for whole venoms (Martin and Rosenberg, 1968), and almost completely destroyed the permeability barrier to the penetration of radioactive ACh (Condrea and Rosenberg, 1968). Other

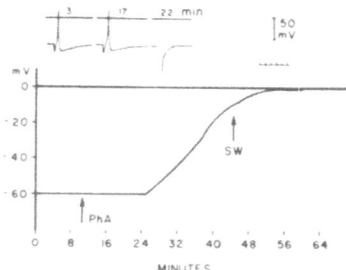

Fig. 7. Effects of PhA on the resting and action potentials of the squid giant axon. Intracellularly recorded action potentials are shown at top of figure, and time course change in resting potential is shown below. PhA (50 μg/ml) applied at 10 min, blocked conduction at 22 min and subsequently depolarized the membrane. SW=sea water. Time signal calibration in msec is shown beneath the calibration for mV. Squid giant axons with fibers were used (Condrea and Rosenberg, 1968).

preparations may differ from the squid giant axons, since Tobias has reported that block of conduction in lobster giant axon by acid-heated *Naja naja* venom is not associated with observable structural changes (Tobias, 1958).

B. Mechanism of Phospholipase A Effects on Conduction and Permeability

The effects of PhA could be due to a direct disruption of the PL or due to the production of lysophosphotides (Chap. 4, Sec. II). For example, lysolecithin, a compound with detergent properties, is formed by PhA by hydrolysis of the fatty acid ester at the β position of lecithin. (Fig. 8). Indirect hemolysis of red blood cells by venoms is due to the action of evolved lysophosphatides (Roy, 1945; Delezenne and Ledebt, 1912; 1911). Block of conduction in lobster nerves by heated venom solutions may also be due to the formation of lysophosphatides (Tobias, 1955). A cationic detergent,

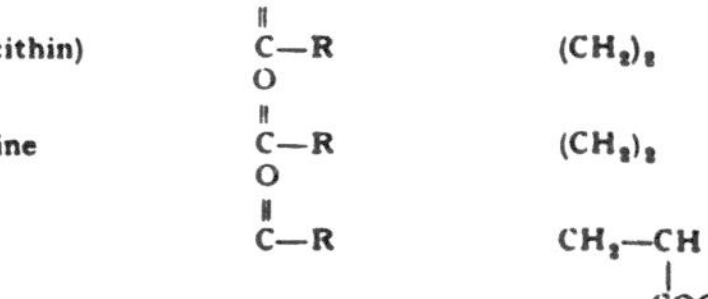

	X_1	X_2	X_3
Phosphatidylcholine (lecithin)	$\overset{O}{\underset{\parallel}{C}}$—R	$(CH_2)_2$	$(CH_3)_3$
Phosphatidylethanolamine	$\overset{O}{\underset{\parallel}{C}}$—R	$(CH_2)_2$	H_3
Phosphatidylserine	$\overset{O}{\underset{\parallel}{C}}$—R	CH_2—CH $\underset{COO^{(-)}}{\mid}$	H_3
Phosphatidalcholine (choline plasmalogen)	$CH=CH$—R	$(CH_2)_2$	$(CH_3)_3$

Fig. 8. Structure of several glycerophosphatides. A, C, and D indicate the points of hydrolysis by phospholipase A, C, and D, respectively. R=hydrocarbon chain (Rosenberg and Ng, 1963).

cetyltrimethyl ammonium, has effects on axons similar to that of venoms and PhA (Martin and Rosenberg, 1968; Walsh and Webb, 1963; Rosenberg and Ehrenpreis, 1961; Walsh and Deal, 1959).

In most of our studies we used for convenience giant axons containing adhering small nerve fibers. The observation was later made that CMV is inert on giant axons dissected free of adhering small nerve fibers, neither increasing permeability nor rendering axons sensitive to curare and ACh (Martin and Rosenberg, 1968; Rosenberg and Hoskin, 1965; Rosenberg and Podleski, 1962). A partially purified sample of PhA was also inactive on finely dissected axons (Condrea and Rosenberg, 1968). A likely explanation for these findings is that in the closely dissected axon there is less substrate on which PhA can act and therefore less lysophosphatide is formed. To check this possibility, ringhals venom was incubated with giant axons containing adhering small nerve fibers, and a lipid extract of this incubate was diluted in sea water and applied to finely dissected axons. This lysophosphatide mixture blocked conduction, rendered axons sensitive to ACh, and increased the penetration of ACh (Rosenberg and Condrea, 1968). A synthetic sample of lysolecithin had similar effects. We concluded that the enzymatic formation of lysophosphatides within the membrane is responsible for the increased permeability of the squid giant axon produced by venoms. In all studies using PhA it is necessary to dissociate the effects of PL splitting *per se* from the secondary effects of evolved toxic products.

C. Maintenance of Conduction and Permeability in Presence of Phospholipid Splitting

Various venoms and isolated PhA resulted in approximately identical percentages of splitting of PL in giant axons with or without adhering small nerve fibers, although blocking conduction only in those preparations containing small nerve fibers (Table IV; Condrea and Rosenberg, 1968). The percentage of splitting of PL by concentrations of PhA and venom which blocked conduction was greater than that produced by lower concentrations which rendered axons sensitive to curare. A correlation between PL hydrolysis and block of axonal conduction was also confirmed in axons from the walking leg nerves of lobster (Condrea *et al.*, 1967). CMV and ringhals venoms blocked conduction and split PL, whereas palestinae viper and eastern diamondback rattlesnake venoms were inactive on the intact axons although they split PL in homogenized preparations. PhA from various sources differs in its ability to hydrolyze PL in biological material, as also found previously on red cells, brain slices and other tissues (Condrea *et al.*, 1965; 1964; Kirshmann *et al.*, 1964; Klibansky *et al.*, 1964).

We tested PhC, which hydrolyzes PL, yielding nontoxic diglycerides and phosphorylated bases (Fig. 8). PhC occurs in the toxin of *Clostridium*

Table IV.
Effects of Phospholipases on Phospholipids in Squid Axons[a]

Phospholipase	Concentration (mg/ml)	Preparation	% Splitting			
			L	PE	PS	SM
Ends of axons tied						
A	0.05	GAF	48	37	10	0
	0.05	GA	26±12	39±9	10	0
	0.05	Axoplasm	36±5	50±3		
C	2.0	GAF	55±1	29±2	13±0	52±4
	20.0	GAF	84	50	3	84
	20.0	GA	56	27	7	100
	20.0	Axoplasm	54	21		
	2.0[b]	GAF	95	86	30	69
End of axons open						
C	2.0	GAF	69±4	48±1	17±9	74±3
	2.0	GAF	64	57	33	100

[a] All incubations at pH 7.6 to 8.0. GA=giant axon free of nerve fibers; GAF=
giant axon surrounded by small nerve fibers; L=lecithin; PE=phosphatidyl
ethanolamine; PS=phosphatidyl serine; SM=sphingomyelin. (Rosenberg and
Condrea, 1968.)

[b] Axon was homogenized in the presence of phospholipase C.

welchii (Long and Maguire, 1954; Macfarlane and Knight, 1941) and the
venom of *Bothrops alternatus* (Vidal Breard and Elias, 1950). In concentrations as high as 20 mg/ml, it had no effect on the height of the conducted
action potential, did not render the axons sensitive to curare nor increase the
penetration of ACh (Rosenberg and Condrea, 1968), although it induced
extensive splitting of PL in giant axons with or without adhering nerve
fibers (Table IV). Most of the diglyceride formed as a result of PhC action
remains tightly bound to the membrane, whereas most of the phosphorylated
bases leave the membrane and appear in the aqueous external media (Rosenberg, 1970).

These findings are of special interest in regard to the essentiality of PL
for the maintenance of structural and bioelectrogenic properties of membranes. Goldman (1964) has proposed that phosphate groups in the
membrane act as exchange sites through which ions pass and may be
intimately involved in the genesis of bioelectricity. Tobias concluded that
in the lobster axon the chemical associated with membrane resistance and
capacitance is more likely to be PL than protein (Narahashi and Tobias,
1964; Tobias, 1960). It has also been suggested that PL are involved in active
transport (Hokin and Hokin, 1963), and in interaction with local anesthetics
(Feinstein, 1964). In the squid giant axon, however, conduction and mem-

brane permeability can be maintained in the presence of extensive PL splitting (Table IV). Any conclusions are somewhat speculative since we cannot distinguish between the extent of hydrolysis in the excitable membrane proper and that occurring in the Schwann cell or connective tissue. However, considerable splitting of axoplasmic lecithin and phosphatidyl ethanolamine occurred, thus indicating that hydrolysis of PL in the axolemma might have occurred.

The Davson–Danielli–Robertson type model of the membranes has a PL bilayer with the polar heads oriented outward and bound to surrounding protein by electrostatic forces (Robertson, 1963). Another possible structure (Lenard and Singer, 1966; Wallach and Zahler, 1966) is with the polar heads of the PL and the charged groups of the proteins at the surfaces of the membrane, while the interior of the membrane contains the rest of the protein bound by hydrophobic interactions to the hydrophobic tails of the PL. Our results with PhC appear in support of the latter model, since the phosphoester bonds in the intact membrane are exposed to the enzyme molecule and hydrolysis of the polar heads does not alter conduction or permeability of the membrane, which one might expect to be altered if electrostatic binding were of major importance. Lenard and Singer (1968) have similarly observed that release of about 70% of the total red cell membrane phosphorus with PhC does not alter membrane integrity or average protein conformation.

Caution must be advised in generalizing to other membranes, such as red blood cells, muscles, or spinal cord, where hemolysis, changes in permeability, and demyelination are produced by PhC (Habermann and Krusche, 1962; Habermann, 1960; Morrison and Zamecnik, 1950). PhC is also able to block conduction of axons from the walking legs and nerve cord of lobster, as well as Ranvier nodes from the frog sciatic nerve (Nelson, 1958; Tobias, 1955; Rosenberg and Condrea, unpublished observations).

VII. NEURONAL METABOLISM

A. Function and Structure of Mitochondria

Venoms, PhA, and PhC have been extensively used to study the role of PL in mitochondrial respiration (Fleischer et al., 1966; Elliott et al., 1966; Vidal et al., 1966; Petrushka et al., 1959; Edwards and Boll, 1954; Nygaard et al., 1954; Nygaard and Sumner, 1953; Braganca and Quastel, 1953). Since the properties of the nervous system are ultimately dependent on a supply of metabolic energy, we will consider how the use of venoms has aided our understanding of metabolism.

Heated snake venoms produced an initial stimulation, followed by a rapid decline in rate of respiration in brain mitochondria (Petrushka *et al.*, 1959). PL protected against this inhibitory effect on respiration. The effects on respiration of PhC were similar to those of PhA, but PL had no protective effect against PhC action. In addition to uncoupling oxidative phosphorylation, venoms also caused mitochondria to be inhibited by adenosine 5'-diphosphate (reverse acceptor control) (Elliott *et al.*, 1966; Ziegler *et al.*, 1965). A fall in respiratory activity has been observed in spinal cord slices incubated with heated cobra venom (Hudson *et al.*, 1960). There is reduced turnover of ^{32}P and reduced incorporation in the adenosine triphosphosphate-adenosine diphosphate fractions in the presence of venom.

Lysophosphatides might be implicated in the suppression of enzyme activities brought about by PhA. Lysolecithin, for example, has been reported to uncouple oxidative phosphorylation and alter mitochondrial structure (Witter *et al.*, 1957; Witter and Cottone, 1956; Nygaard *et al.*, 1954). That there are differences in the actions of lysolecithin and PhA is emphasized by the findings that the former increases the activity of cytochrome oxidase while the latter, as well as whole cobra venom, inhibits cytochrome oxidase (Witter *et al.*, 1957; Braganca and Quastel, 1953; Chatterjee, 1949). That disruption of PL *per se* can affect tissue respiration, independent of the formation of lysolecithin, is shown by the findings that PhC, whose action does not give rise to lysolecithin, inhibits cytochrome oxidase and the aerobic oxidation of succinate (Macfarlane, 1950; Wooldridge and Higginbottom, 1938). Due mainly to studies of Green and Fleischer (1963), it is possible to believe mitochondrial PL essential by providing a medium of low dielectric constant in which reactions abetted by such a medium can proceed. In general, those metabolic enzyme systems inhibited by venom or acid-heated venom solutions (as a source of PhA) are those which are associated with mitochondria and which require specific membrane structure for their activities (Braganca and Quastel, 1953). In contrast, those enzyme systems not attacked by venom are soluble and active in aqueous tissue extracts.

Both PhA from venoms and lysophosphatides have been reported to produce a characteristic disruption of mitochondrial membranes (Nygaard *et al.*, 1954). Because of this property of venom PhA, Fleischer *et al.*, (1966) were able to determine the specific PL requirement of a particular mitochondrial enzyme. They released β-hydroxybutyrate dehydrogenase from mitochondria by treatment with heated *Naja naja* venom solutions, which inactivated this mitochondrial enzyme. They then systematically added back various PL, of which only lecithin was effective in restoring activity. Since lecithin has no net charge it is inferred that the enzyme may require a hydrophobic region for its activity.

B. Acetylcholine—Synthesis, Storage, Release, and Hydrolysis

Nerves metabolize compounds which have specific functions either along the entire axon or at the axon terminal. It should be noted that ACh, as well as the enzymes which synthesize (choline acetylase) and hydrolyze (AChE) this ester, are found all along the nervous system and not solely at junctional regions (Nachmansohn, 1969; 1959; Dettbarn and Rosenberg, 1966; Brzin et al., 1966).

Heated cobra venom (source of PhA) appears initially to increase the rate of synthesis of ACh by brain homogenates, either by accelerating the formation of free ACh from bound ACh or by changing the permeability of mitochondria for ATP (Braganca and Quastel, 1952). A decrease in ACh synthesis ultimately occurs when respiratory activity and formation of ATP is markedly depressed. Cobra venom and lysolecithin were both found to release "bound" ACh from guinea pig brain homogenates (Gautrelet and Corteggiani, 1939; 1938). With the use of cobra venom (as well as other treatments) it was possible to demonstrate two types of bound ACh in nerve endings from the central nervous system (Whittaker, 1961). Cobra venom appeared to release that portion of the ACh present within particles in simple solution, while more drastic treatment was required to release that portion bound more firmly to the matrix of particles.

Cobra venom and cardiotoxin isolated from cobra venom appear to decrease the release of ACh from nerve endings (Lee and Chang, 1966). Bungarus multicinctus venom and β-bungarotoxin isolated from this venom act presynaptically to reduce the ACh output from the rat phrenic nerve (Lee and Chang, 1966; Chang, 1960). In contrast, it was observed in axons from the walking legs of lobster that CMV increased the efflux of ACh, probably by directly increasing membrane permeability (Dettbarn and Rosenberg, unpublished observations).

Venoms may be useful in studying the transport mechanisms for neurohumors and other physiological compounds. Both PhA (Purified from Naja nigricollis venom) and PhC decrease the active uptake of atropine and ACh in brain cortex slices of mice (Heilbronn, 1969), suggesting the participation of PL in some stage of active transport (Hokin and Hokin, 1963). The possible involvement of PL in explanation of the data of Heilbronn (1969) is difficult to relate to the findings of Klibansky et al. (1964) that while Naja naja venom and its isolated PhA split PL of cat brain homogenates, they have no effect on the PL in brain slices. Neither did CMV have any effect on the permeability of rabbit brain slices (Rosenberg and Dettbarn, 1964).

The ability of venoms to decrease permeability barriers in the squid axon and expose AChE to ACh (Fig. 4; Table III) opened up the possibility of designing experiments to test for the essentiality of AChE in nerve conduction. Organophosphates, such as diisopropyl-fluorophosphate (DFP) or diethyl-*p*-nitrophenyl phosphate (Paraoxon), phosphorylate and thereby irreversibly inhibit AChE and block electrical activity (Nachmansohn, 1969; 1959). It is possible to reactivate the phosphorylated enzyme with certain nucleophilic compounds, among which pyridine aldoxime methiodide (PAM) is extremely potent and specific (Wilson and Ginsburg, 1955). Attempts to restore conduction with PAM after blockage by organophosphates are extremely difficult to carry out, because PAM, like ACh and curare, cannot penetrate the conducting membranes of nerve or muscle. In the lobster axon, where the permeability barriers are decreased, (Dettbarn, 1963; Dettbarn and Davis, 1963), it was possible to overcome conduction block by Paraoxon with PAM (Dettbarn *et al.*, 1964). We therefore tested on the venom-treated squid axon (where the permeability barriers are reduced and the active sites of AChE exposed) whether PAM could restore electrical activity which had been blocked by DFP or Paraoxon.

In axons not venom-pretreated the block of conduction by Paraoxon was reversible, whereas in axons treated with 25 μg/ml CMV, the block was irreversible (Rosenberg and Dettbarn, 1967). Paraoxon may be reacting with some component of the membrane other than AChE, possibly with the active site of the receptor, to cause reversible block. The irreversible conduction block by Paraoxon after venom may be either because of the greater exposure of AChE to Paraoxon or because venom pretreatment inactivates the enzyme which hydrolyzes organophosphates. It was found that the squid axon has considerable amounts of this enzymatic activity, both in the envelope and in the axoplasm (Hoskin *et al.*, 1966). Conduction in 14 out of 16 venom-treated axons was irreversibly blocked by Paraoxon, whereas in axons exposed to PAM following Paraoxon the block of conduction by Paraoxon was irreversible in only 6 of 17 axons (Rosenberg and Dettbarn, 1967). PAM also restored electrical activity which had been blocked by DFP. These experiments indicate an association between electrical and ChE activity.

While these studies indicate a relationship between electrical and AChE activity, we were interested in determining the critical level of enzyme activity required for axonal conduction more directly. Consequently, we measured the permeability, detoxication, and effects on conduction and AChE activity of several organophosphates including 217 AO [$(C_2H_5O)_2P(O)SCH_2CH_2N(CH_3)_2$] and selenophos [$C_2H_5O)$ (C_2H_5) P (O) $SeCH_2CH_2N(C_2H_5)_2$] (Hoskin *et al.*, 1969; Hoskin and Rosenberg, 1967; Kremzner and Rosenberg, unpublished observations). These compounds are potent *in vitro* AChE inhibitors, are not detoxified by biological tissue, and can penetrate rapidly into the axoplasm of the squid giant axon. They have only weak effects on conduction. These findings appear in contradiction to the earlier findings with PAM. Nevertheless, it was possible that the inhibitors penetrated through sites in the membrane without inhibiting all of the membranal AChE. Unfortunately, the unequivocal measurement of AChE activity after exposure of nerves to inhibitors is subject to many difficulties, including release of entrapped inhibitor upon homogenization or failure of the substrate to reach all of the enzyme if intact tissue is used (Hoskin and Rosenberg, 1967; Dettbarn and Rosenberg, 1962). There appeared to be another way to test the hypothesis that some membranal AChE had not been reached by the inhibitors, and this was to pretreat the axons with CMV. Following such pretreatment, the organophosphate compounds had much more potent effects on conduction, perhaps indicating a greater access to membranal AChE (Hoskin et al., 1969; Hoskin and Rosenberg, 1967). Those enzyme assays which have been performed do not demonstrate any direct and simply quantifiable relationship between electrical and AChE activity, although, as indicated above, these assays are subject to certain difficulties.

VIII. CONCLUSIONS

I have attempted to show how snake venoms can be used as pharmacological tools in studying nerve activity. This use of venoms can be added to their well-known applications in the analysis of hematological processes and enzyme mechanisms. To be sure, we are using venoms, whose composition and mechanism of action we do not completely understand, to unravel biological processes which have in the past been even more resistant to solution. At first consideration, this task may appear hopeless, but I think the tremendous potential of this tool has already been demonstrated. While I have emphasized those studies most directly related to my personal research interests, I have also mentioned other studies remote from my field of competence. It has been my intention to reveal that almost the entire life cycle of nerve has been studied with the aid of venoms or venom components.

NOTE

Abbreviations used in this chapter: acetylcholine, ACh; acetylcholinesterase, AChE; cottonmouth moccasin venom, CMV; diisopropylfluorophosphate, DFP; 3,4 dihydroxyphenylalanine, DOPA; γ-amino butyric acid, GABA; nerve growth factor, NGF; phospholipids, PL; phospholipase A, PhA; phospholipase C, PhC; pyridine aldoxime methiodide, PAM; d-tubocurarine, curare; tertiary analogue of phospholine, TP; triorthocresyl phosphate, TOCP.

IX. REFERENCES

Adams, R. D. and E. P. Richardson (1961), The demyelinating diseases of the human nervous system, *in* "Chemical Pathology of the Nervous System" (J. Folch-Pi, ed.) Pergamon Press, New York, pp. 162–194.

Angeletti, P. U., P. Calissano, J. S. Chen, and R. Levi-Montalcini (1967), *Biochim. Biophys. Acta*, **147**:180.

Beiler, J. M., R. Brendel, and G. J. Martin (1956), *J. Pharmacol. Exp. Therap.*, **118**:415.

Birkmayer, W. and E. Neumayer (1957), *Deut. Z. Nervenheilk*, **177**:117.

Boquet, P. (1964), *Toxicon*, **2**:5.

Braganca, B. M. and I. Aravindakshan (1962), Neurochemical effects of snake venoms, *in* "Neurochemistry" (A. C. Elliott, I. H. Page, and J. H. Quastel, eds.), Charles C. Thomas, Springfield, Ill., pp. 840–850.

Braganca, B. M. and J. H. Quastel (1952), *Nature*, **169**:695.

Braganca, B. M. and J. H. Quastel (1953), *Biochem. J.*, **53**:88.

Brzin, M., W.-D. Dettbarn, and P. Rosenberg (1965a), *Biochem. Pharmacol.*, **14**:919.

Brzin, M., W.-D. Dettbarn, P. Rosenberg, and D. Nachmansohn (1965b), *J. Cell Biol.*, **26**:353.

Brzin, M., V. M. Tennyson, and P. E. Duffy (1966), *J. Cell Biol.*, **31**:215.

Bücherl, W., E. E. Buckley, and V. Deulofeu (eds.) (1968), "Venomous Animals and Their Venoms," vol. 1, Academic Press, New York.

Buckley, E. E. and N. Porges (eds.), 1956, "Venoms," American Association for the Advancement of Science, Washington, D.C.

Bullock, T. H., D. Nachmansohn, and M. A. Rothenberg (1946), *J. Neurophysiol.*, **9**:9.

Chang, C. C. (1960), *J. Formosan Med. Ass.*, **59**:315.

Chatterjee, A. K. (1949), *Indian J. Med. Res.*, **37**:241.

Cohen, S. (1958), A nerve growth promoting protein, *in* "Chemical Basis of Development," Johns Hopkins Press, Baltimore, pp. 665–667.

Cohen, S. (1959), *J. Biol. Chem.*, **234**:1129.

Cohen, S. and R. Levi-Montalcini (1956), *Proc. Nat. Acad. Sci.*, **42**:571.

Condrea, E. and A. de Vries, *Toxicon*, **2**:261.

Condrea, E. and P. Rosenberg (1968), *Biochim. Acta*, **150**:271.

Condrea, E., A. de Vries, and J. Mager (1962), *Biochim. Biophys. Acta*, **58**:389.

Condrea, E., A. de Vries, and J. Mager (1964), *Biochim. Biophys. Acta*, **84**:60.

Condrea, E., Y. Avi-Dor, and J. Mager (1965), *Biochim. Biophys. Acta*, **110**:337.

Condrea, E., P. Rosenberg, and W.-D. Dettbarn (1967), *Biochim. Biophys. Acta*, **135**:669.

Delezenne, C. and S. Ledebt (1911), *C. R. Acad. Sci. (Paris)*, **152**:790.

Delezenne, C. and S. Ledebt (1912), *C. R. Acad. Sci. (Paris)*, **155**:1101.

Dettbarn, W.-D. (1963), *Life Sciences*, **12**:910.

Dettbarn, W.-D. and F. A. Davis (1963), *Biochim. Biophys. Acta*, **66**:397.

Dettbarn, W.-D. and F. C. G. Hoskin (1962), *Biochim. Biophys. Acta*, **62**:566.

Dettbarn, W.-D. and P. Rosenberg (1962), *Biochem. Pharmacol.*, **11**:1025.

Dettbarn, W.-D. and P. Rosenberg (1966), *J. Gen. Physiol.*, **50**:447.

Dettbarn, W.-D., P. Rosenberg, and D. Nachmansohn (1964), *Life Sciences*, **3**:55.

Devi, A. (1968), The protein and nonprotein constituents of snake venoms, *in* "Venomous Animals and Their Venoms" (W. Bücherl, E. E. Buckley, and V. Deulofeu, eds.), Academic Press, New York, pp. 119–165.

Eccles, J. C. (1964), "The Physiology of Synapses," Academic Press, New York.

Edwards, S. W. and E. G. Ball (1954), *J. Biol. Chem.*, **209**:619.

Elliott, W. B., J. M. Augustyn, and C. Gans (1966), *Mem. Inst. Butantan Simp. Intern.*, **33**:411.

Feinstein, M. B. (1964), *J. Gen. Physiol.*, **48**:357.

Fleischer, B., A. Casu, and S. Fleischer (1966), *Biochem. Biophys. Res. Comm.*, **24**:189.

Gautrelet, J. and E. Corteggiani (1938), *C. R. Acad. Sci.*, **207**:465.

Gautrelet, J. and E. Corteggiani (1939), *C. R. Soc. Biol.*, **131**:951.

Goldman, D. E. (1964), *Biophys. J.*, 4:167.
Green, D. E. and S. Fleischer (1963), *Biochim. Biophys. Acta*, 70:554.
Habermann, E. (1960), *Arch. Exp. Pathol. Pharmak.*, 238:502.
Habermann, E. and B. Krusche (1962), *Biochem. Pharmacol.*, 11:400.
Hadidian, Z. (1956), Proteolytic activity and physiologic and pharmacologic actions of *Agkistrodon piscivorus* venom, *in* "Venoms" (E. E. Buckley and N. Porges, eds.) American Association for the Advancement of Science, Washington, D.C., pp. 205–215.
Heilbronn, E. (1969), *J. Neurochem.*, 16:627.
Hodgkin, A. L. (1964), "The Conduction of the Nerve Impulse," C. C. Thomas, Springfield, Ill.
Hokin, L. E. and M. R. Hokin (1963), The role of phosphatides in active transport with particular reference to sodium transport, *in* "Proc. First Int. Pharmacol. Meeting," vol. 4, "Drugs and Membranes" (C. A. M. Hogben, ed.) The Macmillan Co., New York, pp. 23–40.
Hoskin, F. C. G. and P. Rosenberg (1964), *J. Gen. Physiol.*, 47:1117.
Hoskin, F. C. G. and P. Rosenberg (1965), *J. Gen. Physiol.*, 49:47.
Hoskin, F. C. G. and P. Rosenberg (1967), *Science*, 156:966.
Hoskin, F. C. G., P. Rosenberg, and M. Brzin (1966), *Proc. Nat. Acad. Sci.*, 55:1231.
Hoskin, F. C. G., L. T. Kremzner, and P. Rosenberg (1969), *Biochem. Pharmacol.*, 18:1727.
Hudson, A. J., J. H. Quastel, and P. G. Scholefield (1960), *J. Neurochem.*, 5:177.
Hughes, A. (1935), *Biochem. J.*, 29:437.
Hunter, W. K. (1909), *Proc. R. Soc. Med.*, 3:105.
Ibraham, S. A., H. Saunders, and R. H. S. Thompson (1964), *Biochem. J.*, 93:588.
Jiménez-Porras, J. M. (1968), *Annual Review of Pharmacology*, 8:299.
Katz, B. (1966), "Nerve, Muscle and Synapse," McGraw-Hill Book Co., New York.
Kellaway, C. H. and H. F. Holden (1932), *Aust. J. Exp. Biol. Med. Sci.*, 10:167.
Kirshmann, Ch., E. Condrea, N. Moav, S. Aloof, and A. de Vries (1964), *Arch. Int. Pharmacodyn.*, 150:372.
Klibansky, C., J. Shiloah, and A. de Vries (1964), *Biochem. Pharmacol.*, 13:1107.
Lamb, G. and W. K. Hunter (1904), *Lancet*, 1:20.
Lee, C. Y. and C. C. Chang (1966), *Mem. Inst. Butantan Simp. Int.*, 33:555.
Lenard, J. and S. J. Singer (1966), *Proc. Nat. Acad. Sci.*, 56:1828.
Lenard, J. and S. J. Singer (1968), *Science*, 159:738.
Levi-Montalcini, R. (1958), Chemical stimulation of nerve growth, *in* "Chemical Basis of Development" (W. D. McElroy and B. Glass, eds.), Johns Hopkins Press, Baltimore, pp. 646–664.
Levi-Montalcini, R. and P. U. Angeletti (1961), Biological properties of a nerve growth promoting protein and its antiserum, *in* "Regional Neurochemistry" (S. S. Kety and J. Elkes, eds.), Pergamon Press, New York, pp. 362–376.
Levi-Montalcini, R. and P. U. Angeletti (1968a), *Physiol. Rev.*, 48:534.
Levi-Montalcini, R. and P. U. Angeletti (1968b), Biological aspects of the nerve growth factor, *in* "Ciba Found. Symp. Growth of the Nervous System" (G. E. W. Wolstenholme and M. O'Connor, eds.), Churchill, London, pp. 126–147.
Levi-Montalcini, R. and B. Booker (1960a), *Proc. Nat. Acad. Sci.*, 42:373.
Levi-Montalcini, R. and B. Booker (1960b), *Proc. Nat. Acad. Sci.*, 42:384.
Levi-Montalcini, R. and S. Cohen (1956), *Proc. Nat. Sci.*, 42:695.
Long, C. and M. F. Maguire (1954), *Biochem. J.*, 57:223.
Macfarlane, M. G. (1950), *Biochem. J.*, 47:267.
Macfarlane, M. G. and B. C. J. G. Knight (1941), *Biochem. J.*, 35:884.
Magee, W. L. and R. H. S. Thompson (1960), *Biochem. J.*, 77:526.
Martin, R. and P. Rosenberg (1968), *J. Cell Biol.*, 36:341.
Meldrum, B. S. (1965), *Pharmacol. Rev.*, 17:393.
Minton, S. A. (1956), Some properties of North American pit viper venoms and their correlation with phylogeny, *in* "Venoms" (E. E. Buckley and N. Porges, eds.),

American Association for the Advancement of Science, Washington, D.C., pp. 145–151.

Morazain, R. and P. Rosenberg (1970), Lipid changes in triorthocreasyl phosphate-induced neuropathy, *Toxicol. Applied Pharmacol.*, **16,** 461.

Morrison, L. R. and P. C. Zamecnik (1950), *Arch. Neurol. Psychiat.*, **63**:367.

Nachmansohn, D. (1959), "Chemical and Molecular Basis of Nerve Activity," Academic Press, New York.

Nachmansohn, D. (1969), *J. Gen. Physiol.*, **54**:187s.

Narahashi, T. and J. M. Tobias (1964), *Amer. J. Physiol.*, **207**:1441.

Nelson, P. G. (1958), *J. Cell. Comp. Physiol.*, **52**:127.

Nygaard, A. P. and J. B. Sumner (1953), *J. Biol. Chem.*, **200**:723.

Nygaard, A. P., M. V. Dianzani, and G. F. Bahr (1954), *Exp. Cell. Res.*, **6**:453.

Okonogi, T., S. Hoshi, M. Honma, M. Mitsuhashi, S. Maeno, and Y. Sawai (1960), *Jap. J. Microbiol.*, **4**:297.

Petrushka, E., J. H. Quastel, and P. G. Scholefield (1959), *Canad. J. Biochem. Physiol.*, **37**:975.

Robertson, J. D. (1963), Unit membranes: a review with recent new studies of experimental alterations and a new subunit structure in synaptic membranes, *in* "Cellular Membranes in Development" (M. Locke, ed.) Academic Press, New York, p.1.

Rosenberg, P. (1960), *Biochem. Pharmacol.*, **3**:212.

Rosenberg, P. (1965), *Toxicon*, **3**:125.

Rosenberg, P. (1966), *Mem. Inst. Butantan Simp. Int.*, **33**:477.

Rosenberg, P. (1970), *Toxicon*, in press.

Rosenberg, P. and E. Bartels (1967), *J. Pharmacol. Exp. Therap.*, **155**:532.

Rosenberg, P. and E. Condrea (1968), *Biochem. Pharmacol.*, **17**:2033.

Rosenberg, P. and W.-D. Dettbarn (1963), *Biochim. Biophys. Acta*, **69**:103.

Rosenberg, P. and W.-D. Dettbarn (1964), *Biochem. Pharmacol.*, **13**:1157.

Rosenberg, P. and W.-D. Dettbarn (1967), Use of venoms in testing for essentiality of cholinesterase in conduction, *in* "Animal Toxins" (F. E. Russell and P. R. Saunders, eds.), Pergamon Press, New York, pp. 379–388.

Rosenberg, P. and S. Ehrenpreis (1961), *Biochem. Pharmacol.*, **8**:192.

Rosenberg, P. and H. Higman (1960), *Biochim. Biophys. Acta*, **45**:348.

Rosenberg, P. and F. C. G. Hoskin (1963), *J. Gen. Physiol.*, **46**:1065.

Rosenberg, P. and F. C. G. Hoskin (1965), *Biochem. Pharmacol.*, **14**:1765.

Rosenberg, P. and H. G. Mautner (1967), *Science*, **155**:1569.

Rosenberg, P. and K. Y. Ng (1963), *Biochim. Biophys. Acta*, **75**:116.

Rosenberg, P. and T. R. Podleski (1962), *J. Pharmacol. Exp. Therap.*, **137**:249.

Rosenberg, P. and T. R. Podleski (1963), *Biochim. Biophys. Acta*, **75**:104.

Rosenberg, P., H. Higman, and D. Nachmansohn (1960), *Biochim. Biophys. Acta*, **44**:151.

Rosenberg, P., H. G. Mautner, and D. Nachmansohn (1966), *Proc. Nat. Acad. Sci.*, **55**:835.

Rossiter, R. J. (1961), The chemistry of wallerian degeneration, *in* "Chemical Pathology of the Nervous System" (J. Folch-Pi, ed.), Pergamon Press, New York, pp. 207–230.

Rothenberg, M. A., D. B. Sprinson, and D. Nachmansohn (1948), *J. Neurophysiol.* **11**:111.

Roy, A. C. (1945), *Nature*, **155**:696.

Russell, F. E. (1967), *Clin. Pharmacol. Therap.*, **8**:849.

Russell, R. E. and T. E. Long (1961), Effects of venoms on neuromuscular transmission, *in* "Second International Symp. on Myasthenia gravis," vol. III (H. R. Viets, ed.), Charles C. Thomas, Springfield, Ill., pp. 101–116.

Russell, F. E. and P. R. Saunders (eds.) (1967), "Animal Toxins," Pergamon Press, New York.

Russell, F. E. and R. S. Scharffenberg (1964), "Bibliography of Snake Venoms and Venomous Snakes," Bibliographic Associates, Inc., West Covina, Calif.

Sabatini, M. T., A. P. deIraldi, and E. deRobertis (1965), *J. Exp. Neurol.*, **12**:370.

Sarkar, N. K. and A. Devi (1968), Enzymes in snake venoms, *in* "Venomous Animals and Their Venoms" (Bücherl, W., Buckley, E. E., and Deulofeu, V., eds.), vol. 1, Academic Press, New York, pp. 167–216.

Sjöstrand, F. X. (1963), The structure and formation of the myelin sheath, *in* "Mechanisms of Demyelination" (A. S. Rose and C. M. Pearson, eds.), McGraw-Hill, New York, pp. 1–43.

Swank, R. L. (1961), "A Biochemical Basis of Multiple Sclerosis," Charles C. Thomas, Springfield, Ill.

Tasaki, I. (1968), "Nerve Excitation. A Macromolecular Approach," Charles C. Thomas, Springfield, Ill.

Thompson, R. H. S. (1964), Lipolytic enzymes and demyelination, *in* "Metabolism and Physiological Significance of Lipids" (R. M. C. Dawson and E. N. Rhodes, eds.), Wiley & Sons, New York, pp. 541–551.

Tobias, J. M. (1955), *J. Cell. Comp. Physiol.*, **46**:183.

Tobias, J. M (1958), *J. Cell. Comp. Physiol.*, **52**:89.

Tobias, J. M. (1960), *J. Gen. Physiol.*, **43**:57.

Toman, J. E. P. (1949), *Electroenceph. Clin. Neurophysiol.*, **1**:33.

Vidal, J. C., B. N. Badano, A. O. M. Stoppani and A. Bovens (1966), *Mem. Inst. Butantan Simp. Int.*, **33**:913.

Vidal Breard, J. J. and V. E. Elias (1950), *Arch. Farm. Bioquim. Tucman*, **5**:77.

Villegas, G. M. and R. Villegas (1960), *J. Ulstrastruct. Res.*, **3**:362.

Wallach, D. F. H. and P. H. Zahler (1966), *Proc. Nat. Acad. Sci.*, **56**:1552.

Walsh, R. R. and S. E. Deal (1959), *Amer. J. Physiol.*, **197**:547.

Walsh, R. R. and G. D. Webb (1963), *Biochem. Pharmacol.*, **12**:451.

Webb, G. D. and H. G. Mautner (1966), *Biochem. Pharmacol.*, **15**:2105.

Whittaker, V. P. (1961), *Biochem. Pharmacol.*, **5**:392.

Wilson, I. B. and S. Ginsburg (1955), *Biochim. Biophys. Acta*, **18**:168.

Witter, R. F. and M. A. Cottone (1956), *Biochim. Biophys. Acta*, **22**:364.

Witter, R. F., A. Morrison, and G. R. Shepardson (1957), *Biochim. Biophys. Acta*, **26**:120.

Wooldridge, W. R. and C. Higginbottom (1938), *Biochem. J.*, **32**:1718.

Zeller, E. A. (1949), *Helv. Chim. Acta*, **32**:94.

Zeller, E. A. (1951), Enzymes as essential components of bacterial and animal toxins, *in* "The Enzymes," vol. 1, pt. 2 (J. B. Sumner and K. Myrback, eds.), Academic Press, New York, pp. 986–1013.

Zeller, E. A. (1966), *Mem. Inst. Butantan Simp. Intern.*, **33**:349.

Ziegler, F. D., L. Vázquez-Colón, W. B. Elliott, A. Taub, and C. Gans (1965), *Biochemistry*, **4**:555.

Chapter 6

Fugu (Puffer-Fish) Poisoning and the Pharmacology of Crystalline Tetrodotoxin in Poisoning

Yasumi Ogura

Department of Pharmacology
Faculty of Dentistry, Tohoku University
Sendai, Japan

I. INTRODUCTION

Fugu (puffer-fish) is one of many poisonous fishes. It produces a potent, toxic substance that is found in various of its organs, for example, the ovaries, liver, intestine, skin, and spawn. Although fugu is dangerous to eat, it is very interesting that there are special restaurants for cooking fugu in Japan. Such restaurants are obligated by the Japanese government to prepare the fish in such a way that fugu intoxication will not be a hazard to diners. One will naturally raise the question—what reasons have Japanese for this dangerous custom. This point-blank question is fired at us by many foreigners. Dangerous, but interesting, eating habits have been rooted among Japanese for a long time; in fact, such habits are localized to Japan. However, the white meat of fugu can please the Japanese palate without causing danger, because a very good technique was developed by our ancestors for treating organs contaminated with its toxic substance. This is a rather unique example of food–life history.

Fugu meat is well-appreciated by the Japanese as well as by the Chinese. However, there is a difference in fugu species between Japan and China. In China, fugu live in fresh water, and the species is *Fugu ocellatus obscurus*

(Ogura, 1965a). This species migrates up various rivers during spawning season. On the contrary, in Japan, almost all species of fugu are marine, the present number of known species being 28.

The first reference to fugu in Japan appeared in the first Japanese pharmacopeia Honzo-Wamyo (本草和名, *The Book of Medicine or Herbs*) published in the Heian era (794–1192). In this book, fugu was referred to by the Japanese term fuku (布久). The name referred to the ability of the fish to distend its abdomen, and it can be translated reasonably as blowfish, globefish, swellfish, or porcupine fish, popular terms now in common use in English. In the late eighteenth century in Japan, there were books describing fugu intoxication. From the archaeological point of view, we can assume that in the neolithic era in Japan our ancestors used fugu for food, because the characteristic bone of fugu is frequently found among other fish bones dug up from shell-heaps. In Egypt, the puffer has been identified in hieroglyph on the tomb of the Egyptian pharaoh Ti of about 3100 B.C. (Halstead, 1958). An expression of "dissatisfaction" seems evident because the fugu is characterized with a distended abdomen.

Remy was the first to study the intoxication of fugu as a scientific endeavour. He was particularly awed by the fact that Japanese take pleasure in eating a poisonous fish, so he investigated the action of the toxin with the intention of sending a warning about intoxication to Japan. His first report was published in 1883. After that, studies on the toxin of fugu were centered on extraction of a true, effective substance, and Japanese researchers were most active in this work. Tawara, in 1902, extracted a purified toxin from the ovaries of fugu and named it tetrodotoxin (see Ogura, 1965a). Fukuda and his collaborators delved into studies of Tawara's toxin in the light of pharmacological and physiological knowledge available at their time, and their results have acquired a distinct historical value to studies on the toxin (*see* Ogura, 1965, 1958a, 1969b).

On the other hand, chemical studies on the toxin also proceeded, but the progress was difficult. In 1950, Tsuda *et al.*, were the first to masscrystallize tetrodotoxin. At the IUPAC Symposium on the Chemistry of Natural products in Kyoto, Japan, April 1964, studies on the structure of tetrodotoxin were reported by Tsuda, Hirata, Woodward, and Mosher. The structure of tetrodotoxin as presented by Tsuda's group was finally recognized during this congress. It has a very unusual structure for a natural product; three possible hemilactal rings in its structure are regarded as a kind of "bird cage" as represented in adamantanlike compounds. We should be aware that 60 years intervened between the naming of tetrodotoxin and the determination of its unique structure. After the crystallization of tetrodotoxin, two great currents in pharmacological as well as physiological research ensued: (1) Studies on the release of a chemical transmitter in the synapse and ganglion and (2) studies on the sodium-carrying system in excitable membranes. It is the purpose of this paper to relate problems of clinical toxicology to molecular pharmacology, paying close attention to the actual conditions of fugu intoxication.

II. ACTUAL CONDITIONS AND STATISTICAL SURVEY OF FUGU POISONING

A. Varieties of Fugu

It is known that throughout the world there are about 30 species of puffer. The fish are distributed widely in the Japanese Sea, Pacific Ocean, Chinese Sea, Indian Ocean, and Mediterranean Sea. It is very intriguing that 28 species are found in the sea around Japan. Table I shows a list of the Latin names and the Japanese names of these fish. Among them, *Fugu rubripes*, *Fugu vermicularis porphyreus*, *Fugu vermicularis vermicularis* are very frequently used as food. These fugu are known to contain higher concentrations of tetrodotoxin in their tissues (ovaries, liver, intestine, skin, etc.) than the others. The meat from poisonous fugu is much more appetizing than that from the nonpoisonous fugu. This is one factor in production of fugu poisoning.

B. Localization

Tetrodotoxin is localized mainly in the ovaries, muscle, and liver, but not in blood or testicles. These fundamental facts had been established by the extensive study of Tani (1945) (*see* Table I). In some species of fugu, toxin in detectable concentrations is also found in the intestine and skin.

C. Influence of Season

Tetrodotoxin does not disappear with change of seasons. However, the concentration of tetrodotoxin in fish organs begins to increase in the winter and reaches the highest values just prior to the spawning period, May to July (Tani, 1945; Ogura, 1958b). On the other hand, the incidence of human poisoning in Japan is highest in the winter months, November, December, January, and February, somewhat lower during March, April, May, September, and October, and lowest in the summer months (Ogura, 1958b). Therefore, it seems that the incidence of human poisoning is directly related to tetrodotoxin content of fish organs.

D. Statistical Survey

Statistical data on fugu poisoning, compiled from authentic sources, has accumulated over a long period of time in Japan. The incidence of

Table I.

Species of Fugu and Toxicity of the Organs. (cf Tani, 1945)

Species	Japanese name	Ovaries	Testicles	Liver	Skin	Intestine	Muscle	Blood
Fugu niphobles	Kusa-fugu	3+	1+	3+	2+	3+	1+	
[a]*Fugu poecilonotus*	Komon-fugu	3+	2+	3+	2+	2+	1+	
[a]*Fugu pardalis*	Higan-fugu	3+	1+	3+	2+	2+	—	—
[a]*Fugu vermicularis*	Shosai-fugu	3+	—	3+	2+	2+	1+	
[a]*Fugu verm. porphyreus*	Ma-fugu	3+	—	3+	2+	2+	—	
Fugu ocellatus	Me-fugu	3+	—	2+	2+	2+	—	—
Fugu basilewskianus		2+	—	2+	1+	2+	—	
[a]*Fugu chrysops*	Akame-fugu	2+	—	1+	1+	1+	—	
Fugu pseudommus		2+	—	1+	1+	1+	—	
[a]*Fugu rubripes*	Tora-fugu	2+	—	2+	—	1+	—	
[a]*Fugu xanthopterus*	Shima-fugu	2+	—	2+	—	1+	—	
Fugu stictonotus	Goma-fugu	2+	—	2+	1+	—	—	
Lagocephalus laevigatus inermis	Kana-fugu	—	—	2+	—	—	—	
[a]*Lagocephalus eunaris*	Saba-fugu	—	—	—	—	—	—	
Fugu cutaneus	Kawa-fugu	—	—	—	—	—	—	
Canthigaster rivulatus	Kitamakura	—	—	1+	2+	1+	—	
Diodon holacanthus	Harisenbon	—	—	—	—	1+	—	
Chilonycterus affinis	Ishigaki-fugu	—	—	—	—	1+	—	
Ostracion tuberculatus	Hako-fugu	1+	—	—	—	1+	—	
Lactoria diaphana	Umisuzume	—	—	—	—	1+	—	
Kentrocapros	Itomaki-fugu	—	—	—	—	1+	—	

[a]   Fugu generally used for cooking.
+   Relative toxicity.
—   Nontoxic.

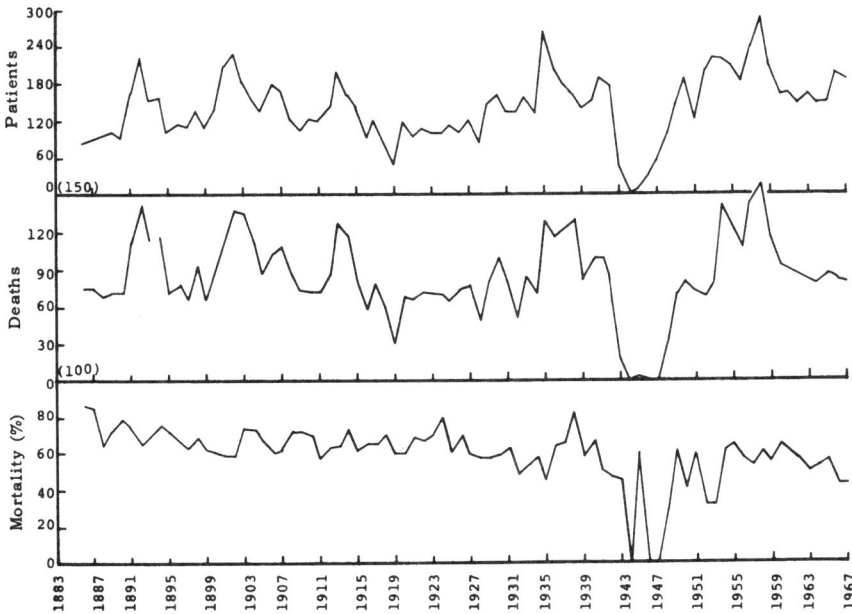

Fig. 1. Statistical survey of fugu-poisoning in Japan (1886–1967).

human poisoning due to fugu is quite important, because mortality due to this intoxication holds a high rank among all forms of fatal food poisoning, although the gross number of patients afflicted by this poisoning is comparatively low. Figure 1 represents the available statistics on fugu poisoning (number of patients, deaths, and mortality) in Japan between 1886 and 1967 (Ogura, 1958b; 1963b; 1965a; 1967). A mortality of 50–60% is obtained throughout the 81 years. However, the mortality during the recent decade (1957–1967) has declined to 40–50%. There is no explanation for this decrease, but the author (1969b) speculates that it is the result of the licensing of fugu cooks. Factors in cooking fugu appropriately arouse public attention to the possibilities of poisoning.

E. Difference between Fugu Poisoning and Ciguatera

The disease known as "ciguatera," or tropical fish poisoning, is not uncommon in the tropical Indo-Pacific area and Caribbean. The toxic signs produced by ciguatera are very similar to those of fugu poisoning. Ciguatoxin, which refers to a possibly pure toxin extracted from ciguatera fishes, is chemically different from tetrodotoxin. Furthermore, if ciguatera fish are kept in sea unpolluted by ciguatera, the toxin content declines and may reach zero. Such a fact is not recognized in the case of fugu (Banner, 1967; Ogura *et al.*, 1968; Scheuer *et al.*, 1967; Banner and Helfrich, 1964).

III. CLINICAL SYMPTOMS AND TREATMENT OF FUGU INTOXICATION

In the case of fugu intoxication, toxic signs generally appear within 30–60 min after ingesting the fish. Dr. T. Fukuda, Professor Emeritus of the University of Kyushu, has proposed that the toxic signs may be conveniently divided into the following four categories.

First degree: Numbness of the lips, of tongue, and often of fingers is present. Nausea, vomiting, and anxiety are seen frequently.

Second degree: Numbness of the above-described areas becomes progressively more marked. Muscular paralysis of extremities occurs without loss of tendon reflexes.

Third degree: Ataxia and motor incoordination become progressively more severe and paralysis develops. Consciousness is present at this time. Voice production is very difficult because of paralysis of the vocal chords.

Fourth degree: Consciousness may progressively deteriorate, and respiratory paralysis may cause death.

Prognosis is generally unfavorable in the following conditions: (1) rapid appearance of toxic signs, (2) existence of intensive vomiting, (3) development of symptoms of the third or fourth degree. In nonfatal cases, no special symptoms remain. Furthermore, no immunity to tetrodotoxin develops. Therefore, one who ingests fugu must have uppermost in his mind that he is constantly exposing himself to the danger of the intoxication.

No antagonists (antidotes) for tetrodotoxin exist at present. During intoxication, anticurare agents and antibarbiturates are of no practical use. Although tetrodotoxin is quickly decomposed under alkaline conditions *in vitro*, it is not possible to divert this chemical observation to the treatment of intoxication directly. The following measures, however, are used as practical treatments.

a. Gastric Lavage. In the begining stage of intoxication, the stomach is washed out by 2–5% sodium bicarbonate, and frequently with animal charcoal powders. If more than 30 min intervene between ingestion and treatment, it is necessary to lave the intestine with sodium chloride solution of 2–5%. The lavage produces satisfactory results for alleviation of symptoms.

b. Emetic Agents. These agents are of no particular therapeutic efficacy. Vomiting produced by the toxin itself is useful for the purpose of removing the toxin. Anti-emetics do not affect vomiting, as will be explained in a later section.

   c. Cathartics. Magnesium sulfate and castor oil are used on occasion with gastric lavage, but these must be used very carefully in the advanced stage, because this treatment may increase the cardiac load.

   d. Respiration. Artificial respiration must be initiated as quickly as possible by any available artificial respiration apparatus, and the treatment must be powerfully and continuously practiced to prevent respiratory arrest. If respiration is supported for 8–9 hr after ingestion, many patients, seemingly near death, can be revived. Therefore, artificial respiration must be employed even in advanced cases. At the same time, it is possible to use central stimulants: lobeline, coramine, morpholamine, aminocordine, ephedrine, caffeine, amphetamine, vitacamphor, methylamphetamine, etc. However, one must avoid depending on drugs only.

   e. Cardiotonics. The maintenance of cardiac movement and respiration is a chief point in the treatment of intoxication. Adrenaline, noradrenaline, neosynephrine, ephedrine, amphetamine, neosynesine, morpholamine, etc. are generally used. The infusion of Ringer's solution or 5% glucose solution may also be used to reduce cardiac load. An antitoxic serum does not exist in the case of tetrodotoxin. Further, it is doubtful that blood-exchange transfusion is effective in intoxication.

   f. Diuretics. Tetrodotoxin is quickly accumulated in the kidneys and produces inhibition of urine secretion. Diuretics with central stimulatory action may be advised.

   g. Liver-activating drugs. Tetrodotoxin does not produce dysfunction of liver. Use of liver-activating drugs is not valuable.

IV. PHARMACOLOGICAL ACTIONS UNDERLYING CLINICAL SYMPTOMS

A. Emetic Action

   Vomiting normally appears as the first sign of intoxication induced by tetrodotoxin. This response is always observed in cats and dogs, and very frequently in humans. However, in very high concentrations, tetrodotoxin will produce respiratory failure without producing any sign of emetic reaction. When tetrodotoxin (1 μg/kg) was subcutaneously injected in dog, vomiting, but no other objective sign, occurred. Hayama and Ogura (1958, 1963) designated this dose as the standard minimum emetic dose. The latent period before vomiting is very short after intravenous injection, but more than 30 min after oral administration. The latent period of the latter resembles that of human intoxication. This suggests that tetrodotoxin is poorly absorbed from the digestive apparatus.

The emetic action of tetrodotoxin has been investigated in detail in dogs (Hayama and Ogura, 1963) and in cats (Borison et al., 1963). The agent imperfectly induces vomiting in animals having ablations in the area postrema. Even a fivefold increase in the standard minimum emetic dose may be inactive. Therefore, it appears that tetrodotoxin induces the emetic reaction through stimulation of emetic chemoreceptive trigger zone (CTZ) in the area postrema. The emetic reaction is experimentally inhibited by tetra-ethylammonium (Hayama and Ogura, 1963), but not by phenothiazine derivatives. The fact indicates that there are differences in the mode of emetic actions between tetrodotoxin and apomorphine. Borison et al. (1963) observed that even when tetrodotoxin in very small doses was intracerebroventricularly or intracisternally injected in cats, vomiting was not induced.

B.   Circulation

The next remarkable pharmacological reaction to tetrodotoxin is a significant and sustained fall in arterial blood pressure. This is seen in all vertebrate animals. The hypotension is in general produced by a dose of 0.5 μg/kg intravenously. When the toxin is used in the dose of 1 μg/kg or more, blood pressure tends not to return to normal levels without artificial respiration particularly in experiments of repeated application of the toxin. In the case of the latter, artifical respiration is imperative.

During hypotension, heart rate decreases corresponding to toxin doses. The altered heart rate has been observed in dog, rabbit, guinea pig, rat, mouse (Ogura et al., 1960; Tsukada, 1957), and cat (Ogura, 1962). However, cats are more resistant to bradycardia than other animals (Ogura, 1962). Depressed heart rate was theorized on the basis of electrocardiograms to be sinoauricular bradycardia (Tsukada, 1957). This bradycardia is not prevented by vagotomy or atropinization. With large doses, cardiac slowing and irregularities occur.

The basis of hypotension produced by tetrodotoxin is not clear. However, from the results obtained by pharmacological analysis, three mechanisms may be summarized as follows: (1) depression of the peripheral vascular system, (2) ganglionic blocking action, and (3) paralyzing action of the vasomotor center. Kao et al. (1967) indicated in cross-perfusion experiments on cats and dogs that the medullary vasomotor center is relatively unimportant for producing hypotension by tetrodotoxin, and that the hypotension is due to paralysis of peripheral vascular structures. Lipsius et al. (1967) were of the similar opinion that the depression is caused by a direct action on the blood vessels with a decrease of peripheral vascular resistance. Ogura *et al.* (1966a) observed that tetrodotoxin, in large doses, inhibited the physostigmine-induced hypertension in rats, but produced no influence on the electroencephalogram activated by physostigmine. Thus, it may be said that there is as yet no convincing evidence pointing to any preferential action of tetrodotoxin on the vasomotor center, in spite of some reports that the toxin has a central action (Watanabe *et al.*, 1967; Murtha and Stabile, 1957).

On the other hand, hypertensive reactions produced by nicotine, serotonin, sodium cyanide, carotid arterial occlusion, or acetylcholine with the pretreatment of atropine, and hypotensive reactions produced by electric stimulation of the vagus, are suppressed by tetrodotoxin. Blood pressure reaction to adrenaline, noradrenaline, histamine, anal acetylcholine is not influenced (Ogura *et al.*, 1960; Tsukada, 1960). Response of the nictitating membrane to electrical stimulation of the cervical sympathetic nerve in dogs (Tsukada, 1960), rabbits (Ogura, 1967), and cats (Ozawa and Sugawara, 1967) was depressed by the toxin. From this and other results, Ogura (1967) suggested that tetrodotoxin-induced hypotension may be explained in part by a ganglionic blocking action.

Finally, it is necessary to consider cardiac function to understand the mechanism of hypotension induced by tetrodotoxin. Ogura (1962) investigated the effect of tetrodotoxin on the cardiac contractile force in urethane-anesthetized rabbits and chloralose-anesthetized cats, and the obtained results show that toxin produces a decrease in cardiac contractile force, and that this action is potentiated by repeated administration of the toxin. Cats have a lower sensitivity than rabbits to this reaction.

It is known that some hypotensive drugs have a histaminelike or histamine-releasing action. However, tetrodotoxin itself has no irritant action (Ogura and Mori, 1968), and no influence on the permeability of capillary blood vessels (Ogura and Nara, 1963; Ogura, 1959). In the past, for commercial stocks of tetrodotoxin, benzylalcohol had been used as solvent. Now the commercially available tetrodotoxin preparation (Sankyo) contains 500 μg of sodium citrate for each 100 μg tetrodotoxin. This fact may have led investigators to the incorrect belief that tetrodotoxin releases histamine from tissue materials.

C. Respiration

Death in fugu intoxication is due to respiratory failure. The mechanism of respiratory depression is not yet clear, but a number of results presented by different investigators may by divided broadly into two categories: one is depression of the respiratory center, and the other is paralysis of the respiratory nerves and muscles. The evidence in support of the former is: (1) during tetrodotoxin depression, increased respiratory responses induced by electric stimulation of afferent nerves is not provoked, but the reaction of the phrenic nerve as produced by electric stimulation is sustained (Takahashi and Inoko, 1890; Iwamoto, 1955; Kimura, 1927); at death, the diaphragm is still responsive (Iwamoto, 1955); (2) central analeptics have no effect on the remarkable depression of respiration (Takahashi and Inoko, 1890); and (3) very small doses of tetrodotoxin applied by intracerebroventricular or intracisternal routes produced more respiratory and cardiovascular failure, when compared to the use of intravenous routes (Elmqvist and Feldman, 1965; Nomiyama, 1942). On the other hand, evidences of peripheral effects are: (1) a marked increase in the threshold of phrenic nerve to electric stimulation occurs after tetrodotoxin administration (Cheymol and Bourillet, 1966; Ishihara, 1918); (2) paralysis of respiratory nerve and muscle is induced as the main action of tetrodotoxin, from the cross-perfusion experiments in dogs (Kao et al., 1967; Wang et al., 1968); and (3) with slow intravenous infusion, action potentials in the diaphragm disappeared before they did in the phrenic nerve. Nikethamide could provoke a response from the phrenic nerve without causing a corresponding contraction of diaphragm (Sakai et al., 1961).

D. Excitable Cells

In the two chapters which follow, molecular mechanisms of tetrodotoxin are discussed in detail. For the purpose of the present discourse, a short resumé will suffice.

1. Nerve

The resting membrane potential is not influenced by tetrodotoxin, even when the agent is present at rather high concentrations. On the other hand, tetrodotoxin does block the normal rising phase of the action potential. Two explanations have been offered for the blocking phenomenon. Nakamura et al. (1965a,b), Narahashi et al. (1964), Goldman (1965), and Takata et al. (1966) concluded that tetrodotoxin selectively depresses inward membrane permeability to sodium ions. Watanabe et al. (1967) indicated that cation exchange at macromolecular sites on nerve membrane is the primary physicochemical event leading to excitation, and that strong binding of tetrodotoxin to charged sites can hinder the necessary exchange of small cations.

2. Neuromuscular Junction

Neither the spontaneous release of acetylcholine, as manifested by spontaneous miniature endplate potentials, nor the sensitivity of endplate receptors is markedly altered by tetrodotoxin. This has been demonstrated in frog muscle (Ogura and Nara, 1964; Miledi, 1967; Katz and Miledi, 1967a, b), crayfish abdominal ganglion (Ogura et al., 1964), rat phrenic nerve–

diaphragm (Elmqvist and Feldman, 1965), and squid stellate ganglion (Miledi, 1967; Katz and Miledi, 1967a,b). Nevertheless, release of acetylcholine after nerve stimulation is depressed in both nerve–diaphragms (Cheymol et al., 1962a,b) and transmurally stimulated guinea pig ileum (Ogura et al., 1966b). Apparently the toxin has a selective effect on the excitable phenomenon produced by electrical stimulation.

3. Muscle

As described for the nerve, the conception that tetrodotoxin inhibits selectively the passage of sodium across excited membranes has been advanced (Narahashi et al., 1960; Nakajima et al., 1962). Tetrodotoxin has no effect on either the excitation–contraction coupling system or on contraction itself (Ogura and Nara, 1964; Ogura, 1965b).

4. Smooth Muscle

Tetrodotoxin does not produce either contraction or relaxation in isolated smooth muscle preparations. Although it seems evident that tetrodotoxin can block ganglia that impinge upon smooth muscle (Ogura, 1958a, 1967), there is no convincing evidence that the muscle itself is labile to poisoning.

5. Cardiac Muscle

Several preparations have been studied including sheep Purkinje fibers (Trautwein et al., 1967), frog ventricle (Hagiwara et al., 1965; Bianchi and Cedrine, 1967), perfused guinea pig heart (Coraboeuf et al., 1967), and rabbit auricle (Yamagishi and Sato, 1966). The data may be summarized as follows. Tetrodotoxin produces a disappearance of sodium current in excited cardiac muscle membrane, but inhibits pacemaker potentials only at high concentrations. At levels of 10^{-6} g/ml, the toxin has a significant, negative inotropic action and a slight, negative chronotropic action. These actions are presumably due to the decreased excitability of cardiac muscle (Ogura and Mizukami, 1966a,b, 1967a,b).

E. Nonexcitable Cells

In this section, various cells other than nerve and muscle are considered.

1. Sensory Receptor Cells

Lowenstein et al. (1963), Ozeki and Sato (1965), and Nishi and Sato (1966) have investigated Pacinian corpuscles. The results obtained in these studies indicate that tetrodotoxin is without influence on production of receptor potentials, these being regarded as generator potentials, but inhibits spike components. According to Katsuki et al. (1966), and Konishi and

Kelsey (1968), cochlear microphonics show almost no change, while the action potentials diminish gradually to less than 50% of their original amplitude by 30 min after tetrodotoxin application. They regarded the cochlear microphonic responses as receptor potentials.

Ogura and Kobayashi (1965) observed that an air-blowing-induced wave in rabbit olfactory brain, and slow potentials produced by chemical stimulation of toad olfactory bulb were not affected by tetrodotoxin, but the superimposed spike components completely disappeared. Tucker and Shibuya (1965) reported the same results on the electro-olfactogram in turtles.

A graded sensory response in the eye of *Limulus* (Benolken and Russell, 1967; Dowling, 1968), the slowly adapting stretch receptor neuron of lobster (Albuquerque and Grampp, 1968), and the isolated muscle spindle of frog (Albuquerque *et al.*, 1968) have led to the same conclusions as the above-mentioned experiments.

2. Red Cells

Tetrodotoxin has no hemolytic action, nor methemoglobin-forming property, like procaine (Ogura, 1969b). Procaine, xylocaine, and chlorpromazine have a stabilizing action on the red cell membrane, but tetrodotoxin has no such action. This may be explained by the fact that red cell membrane stabilization is controlled by a higher K-ion dependency. Nakazawa and Ogura (1960) showed that tetrodotoxin, even in high concentrations, had no influence on the activity of carbonic anhydrase and ATPase in red cell. Therefore, it appears that both active and passive permeabilities of red cell membrane are unaffected by tetrodotoxin, a basic difference from the excitable membrane of muscle and nerve.

3. Renal Tubular Cells

Uptake and release of *p*-aminohyppuric acid (PHA) in kidney slice are not affected by tetrodotoxin, but uptake of PHA is increased by citrate and acetate in the presence of tetrodotoxin (Yohida and Ogura, 1968). An explanation for these data is not available. An inhibitory action of tetrodotoxin on urine secretion in animals was observed by Ogura (1960), but this does not appear to be due to an interaction with antidiuretic hormone. Pullman *et al.* (1968) observed that when tetrodotoxin was directly perfused through the renal artery into the kidney, a significantly increased excretion of sodium was induced.

4. Other Cells

Na- and K-flux in the toad bladder (Marumo *et al.*, 1967), and short circuit current in the frog skin (Kao and Fuhrman, 1963) are not affected by tetrodotoxin. The lifetime of HeLa cells (Cheymol *et al.*, 1965) and of bacteria (Ogura and Nara, unpublished data) is impervious to tetrodotoxin.

F. Biochemical Aspects

At present, a chemical determination method for tetrodotoxin is not established, and therefore it is very difficult to investigate the *in vivo* metabolism of the substance. The function of respiratory enzyme systems in various organs of rats, of oxygen consumption by frog nerves, and of Pasteur's effect in rat brain are not affected by tetrodotoxin (Nakazawa and Ogura, 1969; Kao and Fuhrman, 1963). Aldolase efflux from muscle cells of diaphragm immersed in media containing 5 mM or 67 nM K^+ was unaffected by the toxin (Ogura and Fujimoto, 1963). Oxidation of pyruvate and glutamate in homogenates of brain and liver, plus cytochrome oxidase, were unaffected (Nakazawa and Ogura, 1960). Tetrodotoxin has no effect on the activity of cholinesterase (Ogura, 1958a). Increased oxygen consumption of rat brain slice by current stimulation or by removal of Na-influx was inhibited by tetrodotoxin (Chan and Quastel, 1967). On the other hand, incorporation of amino acids and phosphate into brain is not altered by tetrodotoxin. This differs from the action of ouabain (Swanson, 1968).

G. Relationship Between Chemical Structure and Pharmacological Action

Seven compounds related to tetrodotoxin are known, and these are illustrated in Chap. 8. These related compounds are made by chemical

Table II.

Comparative Effect Between Local Anesthetic Activities and Lethal Dose of Tetrodotoxin Derivatives (Ogura and Mori, 1968)

Compounds	Crayfish test[a] (μM)	Guinea pig test[b] (mM)	LD$_{50}$[c] (mg/kg)
Tetrodotoxin	3×10^{-7}	7.5×10^{-5}	0.011
Deoxytetrodotoxin	3×10^{-2}	7.5×10^{-4}	0.054
Methoxytetrodotoxin	3×10^{-1}	3.0×10^{-2}	0.322
Tetrodoaminotoxin	1.5	3.2×10^{-2}	0.477
Anhydrotetrodotoxin	2.5	3.9×10^{-3}	0.986
Monoformylanhydrotetrodotoxin	2.5	6.0×10^{-3}	1.2
Diacetylanhydrotetrodotoxin	10	7.8×10^{-1}	94.4
Tetrodonic acid	2.5×10^2	1.8	64.8
Dibucaine	1.0×10^3	7.8×10^{-1}	3.8
Procaine	2.0×10^4	30	58.2

[a] Conduction-blocking test in the desheathed crayfish abdominal nerve fibers.
[b] Test of the intradermal wheals in guinea pigs.
[c] Mouse, intravenously.

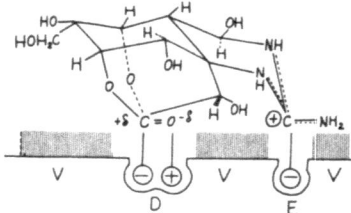

Fig. 2. Model of binding of tetrodotoxin molecule to the surface at the receptor site by: V, van der Waals; D, dipole–dipole interaction; E, electrostatic force.

treatment of tetrodotoxin, and are classified into three groups depending on their structure. The first group is represented by tetrodotoxin, the second by anhydrotetrodotoxin, and the third by tetrodonic acid. Local anesthetic activities generally are in the following decreasing order: first group>second group>third group. Among these compounds, tetrodotoxin has the highest activity and tetrodonic acid has the lowest. The same results hold true for toxicity and other pharmacological actions (Table II) (Ogura and Mori, 1968).

Each group possesses a positively-charged guanidyl group, a hydroxy-methyl group at carbon atom C_6, and a quinazoline ring. Quinazoline and its derivates are inactive as local anesthetics (Ogura, 1969c). The introduction of some substituents at C_6 does little to influence the local anesthetic activity. Therefore, it seems that the guanidyl group, coupled with negatively-charged oxygen at carbon atom C_{10}, plays an important role in combining with the nerve receptor. Furthermore, the presence of the hemilactal ring is useful for potentiating local anesthetic activities.

It is believed that at equilibrium, tetrodotoxin in water solution can exist as two different cations or as a zwitterion (*see* Chap. 8). In experiments on desheathed frog sciatic nerve (Camougis *et al.*, 1967), and desheathed cray-fish abdominal nerve cord (Ogura and Mori, 1968), the pH of a physiological solution containing tetrodotoxin was altered over a reasonable range such as 7–9. This was done to determine whether the zwitterion is more or less potent in blocking excitation than the cationic forms. This in turn might tell us something about a possible mechanism for interaction of tetrodotoxin with a receptor site. As an outcome, it was found that the cations represent the active form. In studies in which the external nerve sheath was not re-moved, tetrodotoxin was found to be more effective in alkaline solutions. Therefore, the toxin apparently crosses the sheath in the uncharged form. Once inside the sheath, the uncharged molecule enters a relatively neutral environment controlled by the buffer action of tissue. A large proportion of the uncharged molecule is then converted back to the cationic form, which in turn reacts with the receptor to block conduction.

Büchi and Perlia (1960) stated that common local anesthetics are bound to the receptor by three types of physicochemical forces, namely, van der Waals forces, dipole–dipole interactions, and electrostatic binding. On the basis of this hypothesis and in the light of a theoretical electron analysis by Löfgren (1948), a model of binding of tetrodotoxin to its receptor was presented by Ogura and Mori (1968), as illustrated in Fig. 2. With the highly reactive carbonyl group at carbon atom C_{10}, the electron cloud at the oxygen is sufficiently dense to act as an electron donor capable of forming hydrogen bonds. A greater negativity associated with the oxygen atom of the carbonyl group is important in producing local anesthetic action. It is highly unlikely that van der Waals forces will contribute to receptor binding of the polar components of the hemilactal ring and the free hydroxyl group at atom C_9. It seems much more probable that hydrophobic and hydrogen binding will be involved. The lack of an hemilactal ring form and the formation of an ether linkage between carbon atoms C_9 and C_4, as seen in the case of tetrodonic acid, induces the lowering of local anesthetic activity.

H. Absorption, Distribution, and Excretion

As shown in Table III, toxicity of tetrodotoxin varies with the route of administration. The order of toxicity is as follows: per os $<$ subcutaneous $<$

Table III.
Toxicity of Crystalline Tetrodotoxin in Various Animals (Ogura, 1963b)

Experimental animal	Injection routes	LD50 (μg/kg)
Mouse	s.c.	14
	i.p.	11
	i.v.	10 (8^a)
	p.o.	180
	i.c.	0.3^c
Rat	s.c.	14
	i.p.	12
	i.v.	10
	p.o.	147
Rabbit	s.c.	10
	i.v.	2
	p.o.	200^c
Cat	i.v.	2^c
Dog	s.c.	15^c
	$s.c.^b$	0.7
	$i.v.^b$	0.3
	$p.o.^b$	70

[a] Presented by Cheymol and Bourillet (1966).
[b] Minimum emetic dose.
[c] Minimum lethal dose.

intramuscular < intraperitoneal < intravenous < intracerebroventricular.   In mice, the oral LD_{50} is 10–20 times more than the intravenous LD_{50}. In the case of the emetic action of tetrodotoxin in dogs, the difference is 200-fold. The potency of tetrodotoxin according to route of administration does not vary among experimental animals.

Ishihara (1918) reported that application of large doses of tetrodotoxin to the rabbit cornea did not cause death of the animal. However, Ogura and Mori (1968) reported toxic signs caused by crystalline tetrodotoxin using the same application as that of Ishihara.

There is relatively little knowledge concerning the distribution of tetrodotoxin in the body. The lack of a good microassay for tetrodotoxin lies at the center of the problem. Thus, estimation of toxin depends on a biological assay. In our laboratory (Ogura, 1958a), it has been found that after a single subcutaneous injection of the toxin, detectable amounts are present in the kidneys, heart, liver, lungs, intestine, brain, and blood. The peak concentration in these tissues was reached in 20 min. The concentrations are highest in the kidneys and lowest in the brain and blood. Tetrodotoxin is not found in the blood, brain, intestine, and lung after 2 hr. In the heart, tetrodotoxin appears and disappears relatively quickly. The relatively rapid appearance of high concentrations of tetrodotoxin in the kidneys and liver, plus the slow disappearance from these organs, may indicate that an appreciable amount of tetrodotoxin is excreted in the urine in an unchanged form. Little is known about the fate of the toxin in the body. Tetrodotoxin has a relatively significant antidiuretic action (Ogura, 1960). This action may delay recovery from fugu intoxication. In pathological and histological studies, no particular abnormalities were present, although congestive changes were found in the kidneys and lungs (Hori, 1957, 1958).

V. LEGISLATIVE CONTROL FOR PREVENTING FUGU POISONING IN JAPAN

Only in Japan is fugu poisoning a public health problem, but it cannot be considered a public health hazard. Legislative control has been exercised for preventing fugu poisoning. The effectiveness of such legislation is undeniable. Most poisoning results from cooking managed by amateurs, and poisoning due to cooking by restaurants with special licenses is almost nonexistent (Ogura, 1958b). A license is granted by the Ministry of Health and Welfare only when the common cuisinier is judged knowledgeable on the species and seasonal variations in toxicity, is capable of eviscerating toxic organs from fish without cutting the liver, ovaries, or intestine, and is capable of preventing toxic substances from contaminating meat.

Table IV.
Clinical Use of Crystalline Tetrodotoxin in Various Cases

	Number of cases	Effec-tive	Ineffec-tive	Percent-age
Breast pain	4	4	0	100
Vascular pain (Raynaud's disease)	6(2)	6	0	100
Shoulder stiffness	15	15	0	100
Articular pain	27	19	8	70
Neuralgia	22	15	7	68
Muscular pain	9	6	3	67
Feeling of cold	12	8	4	66
Dorsal pain	13	8	5	61
Neuralgia	25	15	10	60
Carcinomatosal pain	14	8	6	57
Contusive pain	15	8	7	53
Low back pain	58	30	28	52
Asthma	6	2	4	33
Hypertension	23	6	17	26
Parkinson's disease	12	2	10	17
Erythema	2	0	2	0
Postoperative pain	8	0	8	0
Arrythmia	2	0	2	0
Gallbladder disease	4	0	4	0

VI.   TESTED CLINICAL USE OF CRYSTALLINE TETRODOTOXIN

In the past, purified tetrodotoxin (injection solution contained 0.5%
phenol) was sold and used clinically in diseases such as neuralgia, in particular leprotic neuralgia, pruritus, asthma, gastralgia, tetanic convulsion,
enuresis, nocturia, etc. Since mass production of tetrodotoxin in the crystalline form is now performed by the chemical industry, clinical application has
been reinvestigated using the crystalline material. Many clinicians have
participated in these studies, dating from 1959 to 1963. Table IV illustrates
the results recaluculated by the author on the basis of clinical reports obtained during the past 4 years. These results suggest that tetrodotoxin is
effective against the symptoms of breast pain, pain due to vascular diseases,
and stiffness of the shoulders. The fact that tetrodotoxin showed good results
in two cases of Raynaud's disease is very interesting, especially in light of
the mode of action of tetrodotoxin [vasodilatation and autonomic ganglionic blocking action (Ogura, 1967)]. Other diseases with pain were judged
similarly whether crystalline or purified tetrodotoxin was used. During
therapeutic treatment with tetrodotoxin, many have complained of a sense

of warmth. Therefore, tetrodotoxin was given to patients who felt cold, and recognized to be 60% effective (unpublished data). However, it remains as a problem that the number of cases is small. Hypertension, cardiac disease with arrythmia, and gastric hypersecretion are not effectively treated with tetrodotoxin because of attendant toxicity.

Tetrodotoxin does have value in the area of experimental pharmacology (Ogura and Hori, 1961; Ogura and Mizukami, 1966b, 1967a; Ogura, 1967, 1969b; Tsukada, 1960). Its use in experimental pharmacology, as well as its (limited) medical efficacy, lead me to hope that tetrodotoxin can be a useful agent in a peaceful world.

ACKNOWLEDGMENTS

In the preparation of this article, I have enjoyed the friendly help and advice of many people at Chiba University. Foremost among these are Drs. T. Hayama, T, Nakazawa, M, Hori, J, Hamada, O. Tsukada, Y. Watanabe, and T. Sato, and Mr. K. Mizukami, Mr. S. Yoshida, Mr. N. Irie, Mrs. K. Fujimoto, Mrs. Y. Mori, Mrs. J. Tamura, Mrs. K. Moroi, Miss J. Nara, Miss S. Takahashi, Miss K. Sano, and Miss J. Shoji. I am also indebted to Dr. K. Tsuda of Tokyo University, and to Dr. M. Matsui, Dr. G. Sunagawa, and Dr. F. Koishi of Sankyo Co. Ltd. for generous supplies of crystalline tetrodotoxin.

VII.   REFERENCES

Albuquerque, E. X. and W. Grampp (1968), *J. Physiol.*, **195**:141.
Albuquerque, E. X., S. H. Chung, and D. Ottoson (1968), *Fed. Proc.*, **27**:407.
Banner, A. H. (1967), Marine toxin from the pacific. I, Advances in the investigation of fish toxins, *in* "Animal toxins," Pergamon Press, New York, pp. 157–165.
Banner, A. H. and P. Helfrich (1964), *Hawaii Mar. Lab. Tech. Rept.*, **3**:48.
Benolken, R. M. and C. J. Russell (1967), *Science*, **155**:1576.
Bianchi, D. and L. Cedrini (1967), *Bull. Soc. Ital. Biol.*, **43**:1581.
Borison, H. L., L. E. McCarty, W. G. Clark, and N. Radhakrishnan (1963), *Toxic. Appl. Pharmac.*, **5**:350.
Büchi, J. and X. Perlia (1960), *Arzneim-forsch.*, **10**:1.
Camougis, G., B. H. Takman, and J. R. P. Tasse (1967), *Science*, **156**:1625.
Chan, S. L. and J. H. Quastel (1967), *Science*, **156**:1752.
Cheymol, J. and F. Bourillet (1966), *Actual. Pharmacol.*, **19**:1.
Cheymol, J., F. Bourillet, and Y. Ogura (1962a), *Med. Exp.*, **6**:79.
Cheymol, J. F. Bourillet, and Y. Ogura (1962b), *Arch. Intern. Pharmacodyn.*, **139**:187.
Coraboeuf, E. and G. Vassort (1967), *C. R. Acad. Sci.*, **D264**:1072.
Dowling, J. E. (1968), *Nature*, **217**:28.
Elmqvist, D. and D. S. Feldman (1965), *Acta Phys. Scand.*, **64**:475.
Goldman, D. E. (1965), Contributions of electropharmacology to the analysis of membrane structure, *Abstracts 23rd Int. Cong. Physiol. Sci.*, p. 59.
Hagiwara, S. and S. Nakajima (1965), *Science*, **149**:1254.
Halstead, B. W. (1958), *Public Health Rept. U.S.*, **73**:302.

Hayama, T. and Y. Ogura (1958), *Ann. Rept. Inst. Food Microbiol. (Chiba Univ.)*, **11**:77.
Hayama, T. and Y. Ogura (1963), *J. Pharmac.*, **139**:94.
Hayashi, H. and K. Muto (1902), *Arch. Exp. Pathol. Pharmak.*, **47**:209.
Hori, H., 1957, *Ann. Rept. Inst. Food Microbiol. (Chiba Univ.)*, **10**:70.
Hori, H. (1958), *Ann. Rept. Inst. Food Microbiol. (Chiba Univ.)*, **11**:71.
Ishihara, F. (1918), *Mitteil. Med. Fal. Tokio Univ.*, **20**:375.
Iwamoto, M. (1955), *Igaku Kenkyu*, **25**:832.
Kao, C. Y. (1966), *Pharmac. Rev.*, **18**:997.
Kao, C. Y. and F. A. Fuhrman (1963), *J. Pharmac.*, **140**:31.
Kao, C. Y., T. Suzuki, A. L. Kleinhaus, and M. J. Siegman (1967), *Arch. Intern. Pharma-
        codyn.*, **165**:438.
Katsuki, Y., K. Yanagisawa, and J. Kanzaki (1966), *Science*, **151**:1544.
Katz, B. and R. Miledi (1967a), *J. Physiol.*, **192**:407.
Katz, B. and R. Miledi (1967b), *Proc. Roy. Soc. B.*, **167**:8.
Keatinge, W. R. (1968), *J. Physiol.*, **194**:169.
Kimura, S. (1927), *Tohoku J. Exp. Med.*, **9**:41.
Konishi, T. and E. Kelsey (1968), *J. Acoust. Soc. Amer.*, **43**:471.
Lipsius, M., M. J. Siegman, and C. Y. Kao (1967), *Fed. Proc.*, **26**:736.
Löfgren, N. (1948), "Studies on local anesthetics xylocaine, a new synthetic drug," Ivar
        Haeggstrom, Stockholm, p. 52.
Lowenstein, W. R., C. A. Terzuolo, and Y. Washizu (1963), *Science*, **142**:1180.
Marumo, F., Y. Asano, T. Sasaoka, and S. Koshikawa (1967), *Proc. Jap. Acad.*, **43**:404.
Miledi, R. (1967), *J. Physiol.*, **192**:379.
Nakamura, Y., S. Nakajima, and H. Grundfest (1965a), *J. Gen. Physiol.*, **48**:985.
Nakamura, Y., S. Nakajima, and H. Grundfest (1965b), *J. Gen. Physiol.*, **49**:321.
Nakazawa, T. and Y. Ogura (1960), *Ann. Rept. Inst. Food Microbiol., (Chiba Univ.)*,
        13:59.
Narahashi, T., T. Deguchi, N. Urakawa, and Y. Ohkubo (1960), *Amer. J. Physiol.*,
        198:934.
Narahashi, T., J. W. Moore, and W. Scott (1964), *J. Gen. Physiol.*, **47**:965.
Nishi, K. and M. Sato (1966), *J. Physiol.*, **184**:376.
Nomiyama, S. (1942), *Folia Pharmacol. Jap.*, **35**:458.
Ogura, Y. (1958a), *Seitai-no-kagaku*, **9**:281.
Ogura, Y. (1958b), *Ann. Rept. Inst. Food Microbiol. (Chiba Univ.)*, **11**:79.
Ogura, Y. (1959), *Ann. Rept. Inst. Food Microbiol. (Chiba Univ.)*, **12**:105.
Ogura, Y. (1960), *Folia Pharmacol. Jap.*, **56**:142.
Ogura, Y. (1962), Contribution á l'étude du mécanisme d'action de la tétrodotoxine au
        niveau de la jonction neuromusculaire, thèse de l'université de Paris (France).
Ogura, Y. (1963b), Fugu-poisoning, *in* "Food Hygiene (Shokuhin Eiseigaku)," Asakura
        Shoten, Tokyo, pp. 186–199.
Ogura, Y. (1965a), *Popular medicine (Karada-no-kagaku)*, **6**:100.
Ogura, Y. (1965b), *Ann. Rept. Inst. Food Microbiol. (Chiba Univ.)*, **18**:99.
Ogura, Y. (1967), *Sogo-Rynsho*, **16**:749.
Ogura, Y. (1969a), *Igaku-no-Ayumi*, **68**:243.
Ogura, Y. (1969b), *Ann. Rept. Inst. Food Microbiol. (Chiba Univ.)*, **21**:1.
Ogura, Y. (1969c), *Med. Biol.*, **79**:201.
Ogura, Y. and K. Fujimoto (1963), *Ann. Rept. Inst. Food Microbiol. (Chiba Univ.)*, **16**:57.
Ogura, Y. and Hori H. (1961), *Folia Pharmacol. Jap.*, **57**:274.
Ogura, Y. and T. Kobayashi (1965), *Folia Pharmacol. Jap.*, **61**:8.
Ogura, Y. and K. Mizukami (1966a), *Med. Biol.*, **73**:262.
Ogura, T. and K. Mizukami (1966b), *Med. Biol.*, **73**:305.
Ogura, Y. and K. Mizukami (1967a), *Med. Biol.*, **74**:19.
Ogura, Y. and K. Mizukami (1967b), *Med. Biol.*, **74**:55.
Ogura, Y. and Y. Mori (1968), *European J. Pharmac.*, **3**:58.
Ogura, Y. and J. Nara (1963), *Ann. Rept. Inst. Food Microbiol. (Chiba Univ.)*, **16**:61.
Ogura, Y. and J. Nara (1964), *Ann. Rept. Inst. Food Microbiol. (Chiba Univ.)*, **17**:53.

Ogura, Y. and S. Yoshida (1968), *Folia Pharmacol. Jap.*, **64**:169.

Ogura, Y., J. Hamada, and O. Tsukada (1960), *Folia Pharmacol. Jap.*, **56**:35.

Ogura, Y., K. Mizukami, and T. Kobayashi (1966a), *Folia Pharmacol. Jap.*, **62**:91.

Ogura, Y., Y. Mori, and Y. Watanabe (1966b), *J. Pharmac. Exp. Ther.*, **154**:456.

Ogura, Y., J. Nara, and T. Yoshida (1968), *Toxicon*, **5**:131.

Ogura, Y., Y. Watanabe, and Y. Mori (1964), *Ann. Rept. Inst. Food Microbiol. (Chiba Univ.)*, **17**:61.

Ogura, Y., Y. Watanabe, and Y. Mori (1966c), *Jap. J. Pharmacol.*, **16**:173.

Ozawa, H. and K. Sugawara (1967), *Jap. J. Pharmacol.*, **17**:287.

Ozeki, M. and M. Sato (1965), *J. Physiol.*, **180**:186.

Pullman, T. N., A. R. Lavender, and I. Aho (1968), *Proc. Nat. Acad. Sci.*, **60**:822.

Remy, C. (1883a), *Mem. Soc. Biol.*, **35**:1.

Remy, C. (1883b), *C. R. Soc. Biol.*, **35**:263.

Sakai, F., A. Sato, and K. Uraguchi (1961), *Arch. Exp. Pathol. Pharmak.*, **240**:313.

Scheuer, P. J., W. Takahashi, J. Tsutsumi, and T. Yoshida (1967), *Science*, **155**:1267.

Swanson, P. D. (1968), *Biochem. Pharmacol.*, **17**:129.

Takahashi, D. and Y. Inoko (1890), *Arch. Exp. Pathol. Pharmac.*, **26**:401.

Takata, M., J. W. Moore, C. Y. Kao, and F. A. Fuhrman (1966), *J. Gen. Physiol.*, **49**:977.

Tani, I. (1945), "Toxicological studies in Japanese puffers," Teikoku Tosho, Tokyo, p. 103.

Tsukada, O. (1957), *Ann. Rept. Inst. Food Microbiol. (Chiba Univ.)*, **10**:78.

Tsukada, O. (1960), *Chiba Med. J.*, **36**:1369.

Tucker, D. and T. Shibuya (1965), *Cold Spring Harbor Symp. Quant. Biol.*, **30**:207.

Watanabe, A., I. Tasaki, I. Singer, and L. Lerman (1967), *Science*, **155**:95.

Wang, H. H., T. F. Huang, N. Kahn, and S. C. Wang (1968), *Fed. Proc.*, **27**:651.

Chapter 7

Paralytic Shellfish Poisoning and Saxitoxin

Edward J. Schantz

Biological Sciences Laboratories
Fort Detrick
Frederick, Maryland, U.S.A.

I. OCCURRENCE AND DISTRIBUTION OF PARALYTIC SHELL-FISH POISONING

During the past 200 years or more, medical records from various parts of the world have reported sporadic outbreaks of poisoning in humans following the ingestion of shellfish. This type of poisoning, termed shellfish or mussel poisoning, results in death or a temporary incapacitating illness that lasts a day or two. The symptoms begin with a numbness in the lips, tongue, and fingertips, and they may be apparent within a few minutes after eating poisoned shellfish. This is followed by a feeling of numbness in the legs, arms, and neck, with general muscular incoordination. A feeling of lightness, as though floating on air, is often described by the afflicted persons. Other associated symptoms may be listed as dizziness, weakness, drowsiness, incoherence, headache, and the like. The mental symptoms vary, but most patients appear calm and remain conscious during the illness. As the illness progresses, respiratory distress and muscular paralysis become more and more severe, and death results from respiratory paralysis within 2–12 hr, depending upon the magnitude of the dose. If one survives 24 hr the prognosis is good, and there appears to be no lasting effect from the ordeal.

There is no effective antidote for shellfish poisoning. In cases where humans have had the misfortune to collect and eat toxic shellfish, emesis should be induced immediately after symptoms begin to appear. If respiratory difficulties appear, artificial respiration should be applied and continued for several hours. Meyer (1953) believed that artificial respiration may have saved persons who obtained a marginal dose of the poison, but larger doses usually caused death, regardless of the treatments given. The clinical picture of symptoms and therapy of shellfish poisoning is quite similar to that of fugu poisoning (*see* Chap. 6).

Shellfish poisoning is unique in that the poison is produced by a dinoflagellate and reaches man through the food chain. This is in contrast to such food poisoning as that caused by the organisms *Clostridium botulinum* or *Staphylococcus aureus*; these produce toxins directly in food. Because of this fact and the lack of knowledge regarding poisonous dinoflagellates, the origin of the brief and sporadic occurrence of the paralytic poison in shellfish remained unknown until about 1937. Halstead (1965) has presented a thorough review of marine toxins and Schantz (1960) has reviewed the developments in shellfish poisoning. The problem was complicated by the fact that shellfish, in areas where they had been collected and eaten for many years, would suddenly become extremely poisonous, causing much sickness and many deaths among persons who had eaten them. Other persons, unaware of what had happened, would consume shellfish from this same area a week or two later and experience no difficulties whatsoever, indicating that no poison was present in the shellfish at the later date. This was the story of events in many places throughout the world, particularly in certain areas along the coasts of western Europe and the North Sea, the North Atlantic coast of North America, the Pacific coasts of North America from central California through Alaska, and the Asian coast throughout Japan. Other areas that have experienced considerable difficulties with shellfish poisoning are along the coasts of southern Africa and New Zealand. All of these areas are 30° or more north or south latitude.

The expeditions of Captain Cook and Captain Vancouver along the Pacific coast of North America during the latter part of the eighteenth century at times experienced heavy losses from eating shellfish that happened to be poisonous at that particular time. Also, the Russian expeditions in Alaska and to the south along the Pacific coast to California experienced similar difficulties.

In 1885 an unusually large outbreak of poisonings occurred near Wilhelmshaven, Germany, killing many people who had eaten mussels picked from this area. This outbreak stimulated many investigations on the cause and nature of the poison occurring in mussels. Little success was attained, however, because of the rapid disappearance of the poison in the mussels after these unexpected occurrences. The investigators (Brieger, 1889; Salkowski, 1885; Wolff, 1885) found that the poison was located in the dark gland or hepatopancreas of the mussels and could be extracted readily with slightly acid water. Brieger claimed to have isolated the poisonous principle in the pure state, but later work showed that the isolate was an organic compound contaminated with some of the poison. No solution to the question regarding the cause of the poison was achieved at that time, but several theories were proposed to explain the phenomenon, such as infections of the shellfish with bacteria causing putrefraction or the concentration of certain metallic salts in the shellfish.

The solution to this problem came about 50 years later during several serious outbreaks of poisoning that occurred along the central California coast during the period 1928–1948. During this period several investigators from the University of California (Sommer and Meyer, 1937; Sommer *et al.*, 1937) observed that the presence of poison in California sea mussels occurred only when a particular marine dinoflagellate was blooming in the water around the mussel beds. This dinoflagellate was identified as *Gonyaulax catenella* Wedon Kofoid. Sommer collected the organisms from the ocean and found that extracts of these organisms killed mice with symptoms identical to those from extracts of the mussels. He also placed nonpoisonous mussels in tanks of sea water in which this dinoflagellate was growing and found that the mussels became poisonous, thus proving unequivocally that the poison in the mussels resulted from feeding on the poisonous organisms. When poisonous mussels were placed in tanks containing nonpoisonous organisms, the poison in the mussels disappeared within 1–2 weeks. The poison from the organisms was bound in the dark gland of the shellfish and caused no apparent change in its appearance or physiological function.

The discovery of the relationship of *Gonyaulax catenella* to mussel poisoning by California investigators was soon followed by discoveries of other organisms that caused shellfish to become poisonous. Koch (1939) found that *Pyrimidium phoenus* was responsible for the poison in Belgian mussels. Needler (1949) and Prakash (1963, 1967) found that *Gonyaulax tamarensis* was responsible for the toxicity of clams and mussels and scallops along the North Atlantic coast, and Prakash and Taylor (1966) found *Gonyaulax acatenella* to be responsible for the poison in clams along the coast of British Columbia. Blooms producing a red tide of these poisonous dinoflagellates, as well as species of nonpoisonous organisms, become apparent when the number of organisms reaches 20,000–30,000 or more/ml. However, mussels may become too poisonous for human consumption when the number of poisonous organisms reaches 200–500/ml. When the count gets into the thousands, mussels become poisonous very quickly because they are taking up the poison at a much faster rate than they are destroying or excreting it. When such a bloom, which may last 2–3 weeks, recedes to a sufficiently low level, the poison in the mussels soon disappears and the mussels are again safe for human consumption.

II. SHELLFISH POISONING AS A PUBLIC HEALTH PROBLEM

On the basis of the number of deaths and cases of poisoning, shellfish poisoning is not a general world public health problem. Medical records show only about 1000 cases with about 200 deaths actually recorded. However, these are limited to small areas and in these areas shellfish poisoning is an important public health problem. In cases of shellfish poisoning, the persons involved are the local people and picnickers who collect mussels and clams occasionally for food. Another and much broader public health problem is the control that must be placed on international and intranational shipments of shellfish for commercial markets to make certain that harmful amounts of poison are not contained in the shellfish for human consumption. In this respect, the U.S. Food and Drug Administration has set a tolerance level for fresh, frozen, or canned clams of no more than 400 mouse units, or about 80 μg/100 g of clam meat. The mouse unit (MU) and its equivalent weight of poison will be defined in Sec. III of this chapter.

The amount of poison required to cause sickness or death in humans varies considerably. In an attempt to determine these figures, Sommer and Meyer counted empty mussel shells left by persons who became sick or died from eating mussels. After determining the number of mussels consumed, they assayed the remaining mussels to determine the amount of poison consumed. From these data it was estimated that sickness may result from about 1000 to about 20,000 MU, and the minimum amount to cause death is about 20,000 MU or more (Meyer, 1953). Using similar techniques, Canadian workers Bond and Medcof (1958) found lower values for sickness and death. In many cases sickness occurred at about 600 MU and death at 3000–5,000 MU. The lower figures were explained on the basis that these persons had not consumed shellfish regularly and had not acquired any tolerance to the poison by consuming small doses.

Many government agencies carry out assays from May to October, to check for poison in areas where shellfish are collected for food; if the shellfish are dangerously poisonous they post signs of warning. In spite of these warnings some persons will collect shellfish for food because they were perfectly good a week or so ago. In fact, it has been the experience of this author that those of us collecting poisonous mussels along the California coast for isolation of the poison, on occasions encountered persons collecting them for food. Education of the public by public health agencies regarding the dangers of the sporadic occurrence of the poison and its cause is very important, especially in the areas where shellfish poisoning is common, and is no doubt responsible for the rarity of occurrences of poisoning in recent years. Regulations on the commercial collection and processing of shellfish are described by the U.S. Public Health Service (1959).

The poison in the Alaska butter clam, and to some extent in other species, presents a somewhat complicated problem in that the bulk of the poison in the clam is retained in the siphon for long periods of time, precluding human consumption. The butter clam is one of the most palatable of the species of clams and is an important food item in the economy of Alaska. Another difficulty in handling the problems of poison in clams and other shellfish is that the poison is quite stable to heating. Canned clams processed at 240°F in the normal manner may still retain 50% or more of the poison in the raw clams. Attempts to destroy the poison in the clams by increasing the pH during processing were successful only when the pH was high enough to destroy the palatability of the clams (Magnusson and Carlson, 1951). Removing the siphons (which contain 60–80% of the poison) from the clams will sometimes reduce the poison sufficiently to pass the maximum tolerance limit, but the process is expensive. Transplanting poisonous clams to beds where the clams are not poisonous required a year or more to show any appreciable decrease in the poison content (Schantz and Magnusson, 1964). The source of the poison in the Alaska butter clam is not known definitely, but it is believed to be in the dinoflagellate, *Gonyaulax catenella*, or a closely related species (Schantz and Magnusson, 1964; Prakash and Taylor, 1966).

III. DETECTION OF SHELLFISH POISON

The proper control and protection of the public against shellfish poisoning necessitates an effective method of assay for the poison. A very good method and the only practical one at present was devised by Sommer and Meyer (1937). These investigators defined a mouse unit (MU) of poison as the amount that will kill a 20-gram white mouse in 15 minutes when one ml of the poison solution is injected intraperitoneally. Higher concentrations of poison will kill in less time. The curve relating time from challenge to death and the amount of poison per ml may be constructed as follows: times of 3, 4, 6, 8, and 15 min are equivalent to 3.7, 2.5, 1.6, 1.25, and 1.0 MU. If the logarithm of the dose is plotted against the reciprocal of the time, a straight line is obtained. The dose may be calculated directly from the equation

$$\log \text{dose} = (145/t) - 0.2$$

where t is the time to death in seconds. Although the mouse unit was defined as the amount that will kill a mouse in 15 min, the most accurate determination in all cases is made when the time to death is between 240 and 480 sec (Schantz, 1958). The pH of the assay solutions should be between 3 and 4.

The assay was modified when the paralytic shellfish poison was isolated in pure form (see Sec. IV). This allows inclusion of the *pure material* as a standard, and puts the assay on the basis of the actual amount of poison in a sample of shellfish (Schantz, 1958). The mouse unit is a variable quantity depending upon the strain, weight, and many environmental conditions. As a result, assays between laboratories could vary as much as 60–70% and in certain cases much more. By measuring the response of the mice to a definite weight of poison, more consistent assays between laboratories have been obtained (McFarren, 1959). The assay procedure with this modification has been designated an official method by the Association of Official Agricultural Chemists (1959).*

An alternative procedure applicable in some cases for the assay of shellfish poison is based on the reaction of the purified poison (Schantz *et al.*, 1957; Mold *et al.*, 1957) with certain nitrophenols to give a color almost identical to that obtained with creatine in the Jaffe test. This test correlated closely with the mouse assay and suggested a possible chemical test for the poison. Studies on use of the test for the quantitative determination of the poison in shellfish meat indicated that traces of substances in shellfish altered the reaction with the poison to some degree and made the method somewhat unreliable for a practical test in this respect (McFarren *et al.*, 1958). The test is very reliable for studies on the purified poison.

IV. ISOLATION AND CHARACTERIZATION OF SHELLFISH POISONS

The outbreak of shellfish poisoning along the central California coast gave Sommer and his associates an opportunity to study the poison from California sea mussels (*Mytilus californiasus*). Muller (1939), working with Sommer, and Bendien and Sommer (1941) investigated various methods of purification and demonstrated the stability of the poison to oxidation in acid solution and its lability in alkaline solution. Later, cooperative studies with Sommer were carried on at Northwestern University and at Fort Detrick. One of the most difficult problems in this study was to obtain the poisonous mussels at the proper time. The sporadic occurrence of the poisonous dinoflagellate and resulting poisonous mussels made it necessary to carry on a continual assay program along the California coast. When areas of poisonous mussels were located, they were collected at low tide and the dark gland was removed and preserved in acidified aqueous ethanol

---

* Samples of the shellfish poison standard for bioassay purposes may be obtained free of charge from the Shellfish Sanitation Section, Department of Health, Education, and Welfare, Washington, D.C.

(15%) at pH about 2 until isolation procedures could be carried out. Because of the basic nature of the poison, Sommer *et al.*, (1948a, 1948b) and Riegel *et al.*, (1949a, 1949b) investigated several cation exchangers and chromatography on carbon for purification and obtained a preparation with a potency of 1,600 MU/mg.

In an attempt to increase the supply of poison for study, poisonous Alaska butter clams (*Saxidomas giganteus*) were collected in southeastern Alaska with the cooperation of the Fishery Products Research Laboratory, United States Department of the Interior, and the Alaska Experimental Commission, Ketchikan, Alaska. Poisonous scallops (*Pecten grandis*) were also obtained through the assistance of the Canadian Defence Research Council, Ottawa, Ontario. Siphons from the butter clams were frozen and held for processing, and the dark glands of the scallops were preserved like those of the mussels. The poison was extracted from the ground dark glands and siphons by mixing them with a filter aid (Celite 545) and percolating acidified water at pH 2 through the mixture. Working in cooperation with Sommer and Riegel, Fort Detrick scientists employed chromatography on carboxylic acid exchange resins followed by chromatography on alumina to purify the poison from mussels and clams. They obtained a preparation with a potency of 5500 MU/mg (Mold *et al.*, 1957; Schantz *et al.*, 1957). However, the poison from the scallops, which has its origin in *Gonyaulax tamarensis*, could not be purified directly by this procedure, which indicates the chemical structure of the poison produced by this organism may be slightly different than that from *Gonyaulax catenella*. Further chromatography or subjection to countercurrent distribution studies on the preparations from the mussels and clams did not increase the potency or change any of the chemical and physical properties. The poisons, therefore, were considered to be in a highly purified state.

The purified poisons are white hygrosopic solids, very soluble in water and methanol and to some extent in ethanol, but insoluble in all lipid solvents. The specific toxicity as determined by a number of laboratories is 5500 ± 500 MU/mg (Schantz *et al.*, 1958). The poisons have a specific optical rotation of $128 \pm 5°$, have no absorption in the visible or ultraviolet above 220 mμ, and absorb strongly in the infrared at 3, 6, and 9 μ. They have two basic titrable groups, pK_a at 8.2 and about 11.5. The molecular formula is $C_{10}H_{17}O_4N_7 \cdot 2HCl$. The poisons react with certain aromatic nitrocompounds to form colored complexes in much the same way as creatinine reacts with dinitrophenol in the Jaffe test and with dinitrobenzoic acid in the Benedict–Behre test. When the poisons are reduced with hydrogen at a pressure of one atmosphere in the presence of platinum black, a dihydroderivative is formed that is nonpoisonous and no longer reacts in the

Jaffe test or the Benedict–Behre test (Mold *et al.*, 1957; Schantz *et al.*, 1961).

The purified clam poison was studied by Rapoport *et al.* (1964) at the University of California in Berkeley. They proposed an unusually substituted tetrahydropurine structure and named the poison "saxitoxin." The complete chemical structure has not been determined at this time.

After the poison had been purified from toxic mussels and clams, studies were initiated to culture *Gonyaulax catenella* and isolate the poison from this organism to compare it with the poison from clams and mussels. An axenic culture of *Gonyaulax catenella* was obtained through the courtesy of Luigi Provasoli, Haskins Laboratory, New York, and used for these studies. This organism was cultured in sterile sea water in 2-liter Fernbach flasks and supplemented with small amounts of salts. After 17 days at 13°C, the cell count was about 30,000/ml. The cells were filtered from the medium and lysed with dilute HCl at pH 2–3. This extract was processed through the carboxylic acid ion exchange resins and acid-washed alumina, exactly as were the extracts of poisonous mussels and clams. The final product from this process was equal in its toxicity to mice and identical in all of its chemical and physical properties to those of the mussel aud clam poisons. The elemental analysis and molecular weight determination showed that the poison from *Gonyaulax catenella* has the same molecular formula, $C_{10}H_{17}O_7N_4$ ·2HCl. Details on the culturing, purification, and characterization of this poison were reported by Schantz *et al.* (1966). Degradation studies by Rapoport have shown that the chemical structures of the poison from mussels, clams, and the dinoflagellate *Gonyaulax catenella* are identical.

The biological characteristics of the poison from these sources place it among the most potent known to man. In terms of the purified poison, one mouse unit, as defined previously, is equal to 0.18 μg. The intravenous dose for a rabbit weighing 1 kg is 3–4 μg. If it is assumed that 3000 MU is a lethal oral dose for man, then the minimum weight of poison to cause death in man would be about 0.5 mg.

One of the main remaining problems is the search for an effective antidote to be used in localities where shellfish poisoning is a public health problem. The Klamath Indians chewed the gum from the sugar pine tree to overcome the poisonous effects after eating mussels collected along the coast of northern California (Thompson, 1916). However, studies with extracts of these gums have not proven that anything in them is really an effective antidote (Schantz, 1968). Certain salts such as sodium chloride, and alcohols such as ethanol, reduce the effects of the poison to some degree in mice but not sufficiently to be used as an antidote. In addition to clinical problems, the purified poison has been found important for studies on the transmission of impulses in nerve and muscle cells. These studies are described in Chapter 9.

V. REFERENCES

Bendien, W. H. and H. Sommer (1941), *Proc. Soc. Exp. Biol. Med.*, **48**:715-717.

Bond, R. M. and J. C. Medcoff (1958), *Canad. Med. Assoc. J.*, **79**:19-24.

Brieger, L. (1889), *Pathol. Anal. U. Physiol.*, **112**:549.

Halstead, B. W. (1965), Poisonous and venomous marine animals of the world, vol. 1, Invertebrates, pp. 1-278. U.S. Govt. Printing Office, Washington, D.C.

Koch, H. J. (1939), La cause des empoisonnements paralytiques provoque par les moules. *Assoc. Franc. Avan. Sci. Paris*, 63rd Session, p. 654-655.

Magnusson, H. W. and C. J. Carlson (1951), Technological studies on the Alaska butter clam—review of problem of occurrence of a toxin. *Tech. Rept.* No. 2, Fisheries Expt. Comm. Alaska, Fishery Products Lab., Ketchikan, Alaska.

McFarren, E. F., E. J. Schantz, J. E. Campbell, and K. H. Lewis (1958), *J. Assoc. Office Agr. Chem.*, **42**:399.

McFarren, E. J. (1959), *J. Assoc. Office Agr. Chem.*, **42**:263-271.

Meyer, K. F. (1953), *New Engl. J. Med.*, **249**-848-852.

Mold, J. D., J. P. Bowden, D. W. Stanger, J. E. Maurer, J. M. Lynch, R. S. Wyler, E. J. Schantz, and B. Riegel (1957), *J. Amer. Chem. Soc.*, **79**:5235-5238.

Muller, H. (1939), *J. Pharmacol. Exp. Therapy*, **53**:67.

Needler, A. B. (1949), *J. Fish. Res. Bd. Canada*, **7**:490-498.

Prakash, A. (1963), *Fish. Res. Bd. Canada*, **20**:983-996.

Prakash, A. (1967), *Fish. Res. Bd. Canada*, **24**:1589-1606.

Prakash, A. and F. J. R. Taylor (1966), *J. Fish. Res. Bd. Canada*, **23**:1265-1270.

Rapoport, H., M. S. Brown, R. Oesterlin, W. Schuett (1964), Saxitoxin, *147th National Meeting*, *Amer. Chem. Soc.*, Philadelphia, Penna.

Riegel, B., D. W. Stanger, D. M. Wikholm, J. D. Mold, and H. Sommer (1949a), *J. Biol. Chem.*, **177**:7-11.

Riegel, B., D. W. Stanger, D. M. Wikholm, J. D. Mold, and H. Sommer (1949b), *J. Biol. Chem.*, **177**:1-6.

Russel, F. E. (1967), *Fed. Proc.*, **26**:1206-1224.

Salkowski, E. (1885), *Virchows Arch.-Pathol. Anal. Physiol.*, **102**:578.

Schantz, E. J., J. D. Mold, D. W. Stanger, J. Shavel, F. J. Riel, J. P. Bowden, J. M. Lynch, R. S. Wyler, B. Riegel, and H. Sommer (1957), *J. Amer. Chem. Soc.*, **79**: 5230-5235.

Schantz, E. J., McFarren, E. F., Schafer, M. L., and Lewis, K. H. (1958), *J. Office Agr. Chem.*, **41**:160-177.

Schantz, E. J. (1960), *Anal. N.Y. Acad. Sci.*, **90**:843-855.

Schantz, E. J., J. D. Mold, W. L. Howard, J. P. Bowden, D. W. Stanger, J. M. Lynch, O. P. Wintersteiner, J. D. Dutcher, D. R. Walters, and B. Riegel (1961), *Can. J. Chem.*, **39**:2117-2123.

Schantz, E. J. and H. W. Magnusson (1964), *J. Protozol.*, **11**:239-242.

Schantz, E. J., J. M. Lynch, G. Vayvada, K. Matsumoto, and H. Rapoport (1966), *Biochem.*, **5**:1191-1195.

Schantz, E. J. (1968), *Agr. Food Chem.*, **17**:413-416.

Sommer, H., W. F. Whedon, C. A. Kofoid, and R. Strohler (1937), *A. M. A. Arch. Pathol.*, **24**:537-559.

Sommer, H. and K. F. Meyer (1937), *A. M. A. Arch. Pathol.*, **24**:560-570.

Sommer, H., R. P. Monnier, B. Riegel, D. W. Stanger, J. D. Mold, D. M. Wikholm, and E. S. Kiralis (1948a), *J. Amer. Chem. Soc.*, **70**:1015-1018.

Sommer, H., B. Riegel, D. W. Stanger, J. D. Mold, D. M. Wikholm, and M. B. McCaughey (1948b), *J. Amer. Chem. Soc.*, **70**:1019-1021.

Thompson, L. (1916), "To The American Indian," Cummins Print Shop, Eureka, Calif., p. 28.

U.S. Public Health Service (1959), "Manual of recommended practice for sanitary control of the shellfish industry," Part I, Washington, D.C.
Wolff, M. (1886), *Virchows Arch. Pathol. Anal. Physiol.*, **103**:187.

Chapter 8

Mechanism of Action of Tetrodotoxin (TTX) and Saxitoxin (STX)

Wolf-Dietrich Dettbarn*

Department of Pharmacology
Vanderbilt University School of Medicine
Nashville, Tennessee, U.S.A.

I. INTRODUCTION

Marine toxins such as TTX and STX have aroused the interest of physiologists, biochemists, pharmacologists, and biological warfare people, as well as writers of spy and mystery stories. In the hands of the neuroscientist they have been turned into helpful instruments vital for the study of nerve function and excitable membranes. In this chapter on modes of action, I shall limit myself to the studies of TTX and STX on nerve and muscle. On these tissues they have been studied extensively and in some depth. Neither the historical development nor chemistry of these compounds will be discussed, because there are a number of excellent papers available covering the subject (Kao, 1966). Before discussing the mode of action of TTX and STX, one must say something about the nature of the nerve impulse.

II. THE NATURE OF THE NERVE IMPULSE

The morphological and physiological complexities of the nervous system have offered many difficulties in the study of nervous activity. During

* Supported by Health Science Advancement Award No. 5 S04 FR06067.

the last two decades, work in many laboratories, and especially the work of Hodgkin and Huxley (1952), provided good evidence for the ionic basis of conduction of the nerve impulse; however, little is known about the molecular mechanism by which the observed permeability changes are affected during excitation. Pharmacological studies have shown that by the use of certain drugs as tools, specific components of the ionic currents can be studied. The pharmacological approach has become of great interest insofar as it may help in at least a partial pharmacological dissection of the excitable membrane. Drugs that have been useful in this approach are the poisons of the puffer (*Tetradon honckenyi*) and California newt (*Taricha torosa*). The active compound is tetrodotoxin (TTX), which inhibits selectively the transient sodium current. Similar actions are attributed to saxitoxin (STX), the mussel or shellfish poison. STX is produced by a dinoflagellate (*Gonyaulax catenella*).

Nerve fibers are surrounded by a plasma membrane, the axolemma, across which is a resting potential of about 60–70 mV electrically negative on the axoplasmic side. The basis of this potential is the ionic composition of the interior and the exterior of the fiber and the selective permeability characteristics of the nerve membrane. Not unlike the muscle fiber, the interior of the nerve fiber, the axoplasm, contains a high concentration of potassium and relatively little sodium and chloride. The extracellular fluid has a high concentration of sodium and chloride and but little potassium. The general description of the membrane potential assumes the relative impermeability of the axolemma to sodium and organic anions and a high permeability to potassium under resting conditions. More recent investigations, however, have shown that all these ions can penetrate the membrane. Potassium and chloride penetrate with equal ease, while the penetration of sodium is reduced by a factor of 50. The organic anions are assumed to be nonpermeating. The membrane potential can be described as a potassium concentration potential and follows within limits changes in the outside potassium concentration. However, isotope studies have shown that in addition to potassium and chloride, the membrane is permeable to sodium. Since the sodium concentration remains constant inside and at a much lower level than that of the outside, it follows that in addition to concentration gradients and voltage gradients, something else contributes to the control of the membrane potential. Since sodium ions tend to run down their concentration gradient, some active work must be done to transport sodium ions out again. This involves an active process called the sodium pump and requires energy produced by cellular metabolism. Thus, the membrane potential is generated by the movements of sodium and potassium ions down their concentration gradients and by the action of a sodium–potassium pump. The pump extrudes sodium and transports potassium ions inward and in this way contributes to the generation of the ionic concentration gradients. This by itself will cause no separation of charges on opposite sides of the membrane. The charges are separated by the different rates with which these ions diffuse. Potassium will diffuse 50 times faster than sodium. It is this excess of outward diffusion of potassium ions that charges the outside of the membrane in a positive direction and thus generates the transmembrane voltage.

While many cells have the properties just described, that is, a steady transmembrane potential, some cells possess the characteristic of being excitable. The characteristic of an excitable cell, such as nerve and muscle, is the ability for rapid changes in permeability to ions. A decrease in the membrane potential causes a transient increase in the membrane permeability to sodium ions. Any stimulus, whether electrical, chemical, or mechanical of a certain critical threshold strength, will cause this change in the permeability to sodium and gives rise to an action potential which is then conducted along the nerve fiber. Whereas the properties of excitable membranes in relation to conductance changes are well understood, not much is known about the underlying molecular mechanism that causes the permeability change which gives rise to the action potential. During the ascending phase of an action potential, the membrane permeability is increased to sodium ions which move to the inside of the fiber. During the descending phase of the action potential, the sodium permeability decreases and that for potassium increases. Thus potassium moves out of the fiber and repolarizes the membrane.

During the action potential, the membrane potential is not only reduced to zero but becomes positive on the inside as compared to the outside. The size of this depolarization and overshoot is dependent upon the sodium concentration. Just as the resting potential approaches a potassium equilibrium potential, the action potential approaches a sodium equilibrium potential. Once an action potential has been generated, current flows from the activated to an adjacent inactive region and thus progressively discharges the membrane. The return current flows back through the interstitial fluid to the active region and moves inward as sodium current. This current flow reduces the membrane potential at the inactive region; the inactive region then becomes active and the permeability to sodium increases rapidly. It is this local circuit of electrical flow that activates the adjacent inactive regions and propagates the action potential along the fibers. Since nerve fibers conduct impulses at high frequencies of up to 300/sec, the amount of sodium entering during the activity is about 100 times as great as that during rest. In order to maintain excitability, the inside concentration of sodium must remain low and potassium high. During the phase that follows nerve activity the sodium must, therefore, be pumped out again at a much higher rate.

III. CELLULAR ACTIONS OF TTX AND STX

While marine toxins have attracted the attention of investigators for their systemic effects (*see* Chap. 6), the variety of excitable membranes responsive to TTX and STX makes it difficult to speculate on a simple solution to their mode of action. To appreciate fully the mechanism of action, we will focus our attention on the most thoroughly studied preparation, the peripheral nerve. It is with this preparation that a beginning was made in elucidating the mechanisms by which TTX and STX exert their toxic effects.

A. Peripheral Nerve

It has been known for years that TTX and STX exert powerful effects on the excitable membrane of nerve and muscle (Kao, 1966). What made these compounds so attractive was that they were active in low concentrations and their actions were reversible. However, from early investigations it was not clear whether the block of conduction along nerve and muscle was caused by depolarization, and additional information was needed to decipher their action on the neuromuscular junction and neuronal synapses.

1. The Effect of TTX and STX on Myelinated Nerve Fibers

The earlier observations were made on nerve bundles; more recently, desheathed bundles or isolated single nerve fibers have been used. When the sciatic nerve of frog is used, the minimum concentration of TTX that causes block of conduction is 0.001 μg/ml. Higher concentrations (e.g., 0.01 μg/ml) also block conduction reversibly. All fibers within the nerve bundle are equally and simultaneously affected, and no depolarization of the membrane potential is observed. When isolated myelinated fibers of the frog sciatic nerve are used, the concentration of TTX needed to block conduction is still smaller. A concentration of 1×10^{-9} M TTX or 1×10^{-8} M STX blocks conduction within seconds (Dettbarn *et al.*, 1960; 1965). From observations of TTX on single fibers, it was concluded that the major action is on the maximum rate of rise of the action potential, which indicates a change in the sodium permeability. Little or no effect was seen on the rate of fall of an action potential. No changes in the resting potential or the resting membrane resistance were seen (Kao and Fuhrman, 1963).

More precise and conclusive data have been available since voltage clamp studies were used for the investigation of the action of TTX on single nerve fibers. In concentrations of 1×10^{-9} to 1×10^{-7} M, TTX quickly abolishes the action potential of single myelinated fibers. An analysis of the sodium currents shows that low concentrations of TTX or STX reduce the maximum sodium conductance without affecting the time course of the

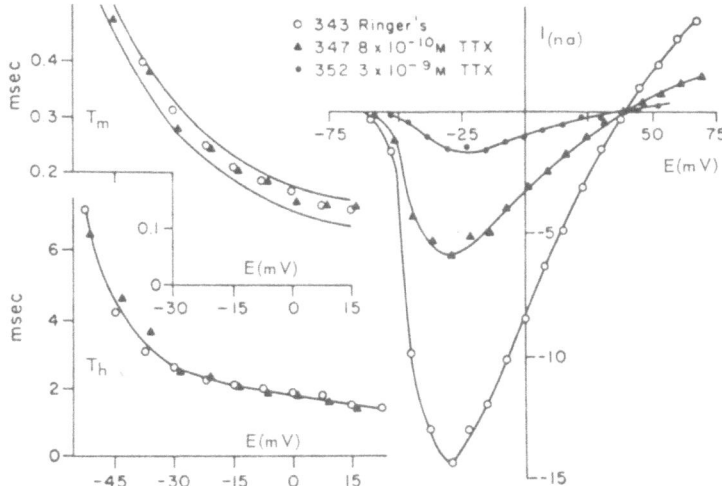

Fig. 1. Analysis of sodium currents in TTX. The time constants, T_m and T_h (left), and the peak current–voltage diagram (right) of the sodium currents of a node before and during treatment with TTX. The two lines drawn on the graph of T_m indicate the band of uncertainty in the measurement. T=2.5°C. Taken from Hille (1968).

remaining sodium current (Hille, 1968). Figure 1 shows that the time constants related to the rising and falling phases of the sodium current (sodium activation and inactivation) show a similar voltage dependence whether in normal Ringer's solution or in TTX. The magnitude of the sodium current reduction depends on the concentration of TTX or STX used. This effect of the toxins is not sodium-specific as is shown in Fig. 2 where sodium ions

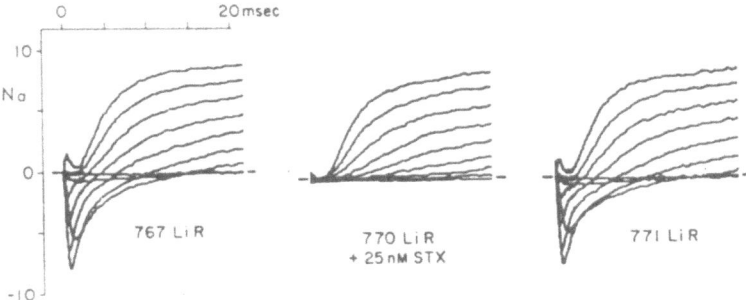

Fig. 2. Lithium currents and STX. The time courses, drawn by computer, of the voltage clamp currents minus leakage currents in sodium-free lithium Ringer's solution before, during, and after treatment with 25 nM STX. The curves are recorded at 15 mV intervals from about −60 mV to +60 mV but with a small drift of the amplifiers between the three measurements. T=6.5°C. Taken from Hille (1968).

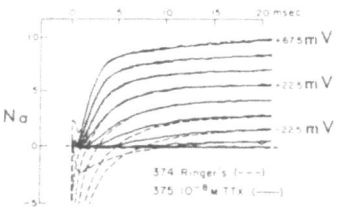

Fig. 3. Potassium currents in TTX. The superimposed voltage clamp currents minus leakage currents of a node before (dashed curves) and during (solid curves) treatment with 10 nM TTX. The maximum inward sodium current in the Ringer solution is about -17 Na, but the records are truncated at -5 Na in this figure. The maximum depolarization is to $+67.5$ mV. Taken from Hille (1968).

are replaced by lithium ions. The same is true of other ions such as guanidinium, ammonium, etc., which are used as substitutes for sodium ions in the generation of an action potential. The early inward current carried by lithium instead of sodium is quickly abolished by STX. The effect of STX is easily reversed in Ringer's solution. That the potassium currents are not affected by either TTX or STX was seen in Fig. 2 and is shown in more detail in Fig. 3. After an initial delay, the potassium currents recorded in the absence and presence of TTX are identical, thus demonstrating the absence of any action on the permeability to potassium ions. Similar results can be seen with STX.

The specificity of TTX and STX for the sodium conductance is shown in Fig. 4. When the sodium conductance is plotted against toxin concentration, the addition of tetraethylammonium, a chemical that specifically acts on potassium currents, does not change the action of STX. The dark line in Fig. 4 is a theoretical curve calculated on the assumption that each fraction of the sodium conductance is abolished by interaction of one STX molecule with one receptor. All the experimental points are close to the theoretical line. These data are taken from Hille (1968).

2. The Effect of TTX and STX on Giant Axons

The action potential is quickly abolished when concentrations of 1×10^{-9} M to 1×10^{-7} M TTX or STX are used on giant axons dissected from the circumesophageal connectives of lobster. The resting potential is not

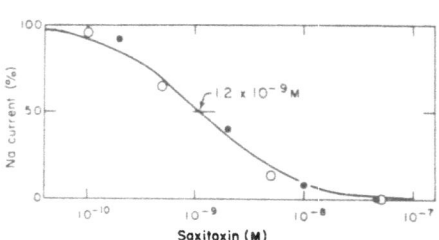

Fig. 4. Dosage–response to STX. The maximum sodium conductance at various concentrations of STX relative to that in Ringer's solution. The filled circles are from experiments in which the potassium currents have been eliminated by 5 mM TEA. All the measurements are from two nodes. The solid line is the dose–response relation of a system, in which one STX molecule binds reversibly to its receptor to produce a fraction of the inhibitory effect. $T=4°C$. Taken from Hille (1968).

affected. Lower concentrations are still effective in blocking the action potential, but the time needed to block electrical activity is increased between 4–8 min. In studies using the sucrose gap technique, TTX actions are poorly reversible. However, after the whole axon is repeatedly washed, the response to TTX is reversible (Narahashi *et al.*, 1964, 1967). Application of TTX in a concentration that blocks conduction under voltage clamp conditions causes a complete block of the sodium current while the potassium current is unchanged. These effects are partially reversible in sea water. When the conductances are measured, it is found that the sodium conductance drops to very low levels when 10^{-8} M TTX is used. In contrast to these pronounced effects on the sodium conductance, the conductance for potassium undergoes little or no change. Similar data are obtained when giant axons of the squid are used for studying TTX action on the conduction of nerve impulses and the generation of action potentials. TTX has no effect on the resting potential of the axon nor upon the membrane resistance under resting conditions. If the axon is exposed to TTX only, for periods of time less than 10 min, complete reversibility was usually observed. In all experiments when an effective dose of TTX is used, the inward current component that is carried by sodium is abolished (Nakamura *et al.*, 1965). The usually observed

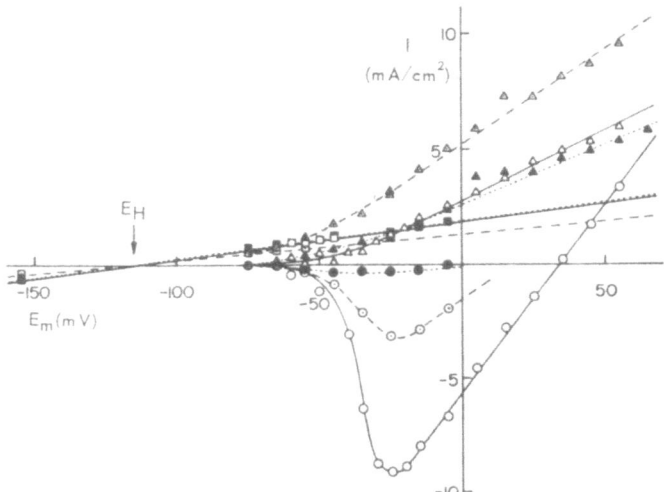

Fig. 5. Current–voltage relations before (open symbols and solid lines) and during (filled symbols and dotted lines) treatment with tetrodotoxin 3×10^{-8} g/ml, and after washing with normal sea water (open symbols with dots and broken lines). Circles refer to peak sodium current corrected for leakage current, and squares refer to leakage current. *I*, designated component of the membrane current (inward direction negative); *EM*, membrane potential; E_H, holding potential. Preparation 116-Af. Taken from Narahashi *et al.* (1960).

leakage current is unaffected by the marine toxins. The same is true for the outward current usually due to potassium activation (Fig. 5). The voltage clamp data on lobster and squid giant axons as well as those of single myelinated fibers of frog demonstrate that TTX and STX have a specific action on the mechanism which initiates the early inward current usually attributed to sodium ions. Neither the resting conductance nor the potassium activation is affected by TTX (Narahashi et al., 1964; Nakamura et al., 1965; Takata et al., 1966; Kao and Nishiyama, 1965; Takata et al., 1966; Narahashi et al., 1967).

B. Skeletal Muscle

1. The Muscle Fiber

When a muscle twitch is induced by direct or indirect stimulation, TTX at a concentration of 1×10^{-7} M quickly blocks the twitch. The effect of indirect stimulation is blocked sooner. TTX blocks the muscle fiber without causing any marked depolarization of the resting potential. Neither a graded nor propagated response can be elicited while TTX is present. This is seen even when the depolarization with cathodal current is far more than needed for the normally critical depolarization. Muscle fibers stimulated through an intracellular electrode in the presence of TTX show an increased threshold and decreased spike height. Increased concentrations abolish the conducted response totally and only graded responses are seen. From studies of the current–voltage relation, it can be concluded that TTX affects the sodium permeability only and not that of potassium or chloride (Narahashi, et al., 1960).

2. The Neuromuscular Junction

Some attempts have been made to clarify the nature of the neuro-muscular block caused by TTX and STX. The effect observed on either nerve or muscle is a block of the conducted response without depolarization. However, there is no change in the sensitivity of the endplate membrane to acetylcholine. The neuromuscular block produced by TTX or STX is quite different from that of curare or decamethonium. Neither repetitive stimulation nor physostigmine reverse the block, whereas acetylcholine applied in the presence of TTX or STX still produces depolarizations of the endplate. The endplate potential (epp) disappears prior to the spontaneously occurring miniature endplate potentials (mepp), which makes it likely that the axon proper is affected before the nerve terminal. The releasing mechanism of acetylcholine seems unaffected, since the latency or synaptic delay appears to be unchanged until complete block of conduction occurs. When STX is used, small decreases in the size of the mepp's are seen which makes it impossible to exclude completely an action of STX on the endplate membrane (Kao and Nishiyama, 1965; Katz and Miledi, 1967, 1968, 1969; Nishiyama, 1968; Bloedel et al., 1966, and Evans, 1969).

3. The Electroplax

In the electroplax, the minimum toxin concentration that will block the neurally evoked spike does not affect the directly elicited response; only higher concentrations in the range of 2×10^{-7} M are effective. Neither toxin interferes with the action of either acetylcholine or carbamyl choline. While both these compounds cause depolarization, the toxins block spikes without changing the membrane potential. Acetylcholine and carbamyl choline in concentrations of 5×10^{-6} or 2.5×10^{-5} M depolarize the membrane in the presence of TTX and STX at a concentration which blocks the directly evoked response. Neither TTX nor STX has an effect on the potassium efflux caused by the carbamyl choline induced depolarization. This is in contrast to local anesthetic action which prevents the acetylcholine or carbamyl choline depolarization (Dettbarn et al., 1965; Nakamura et al., 1964; Fleisher et al., 1961).

C. The Acetylcholine System

Action on cholinesterase as well as on choline acetylase activity have been tested. Neither enzyme is inhibited in the presence of these toxins in concentrations which affect electrical activity. Since marine toxins inhibit the sodium-activating mechanism, it was thought that they might compete with acetylcholine for the acetylcholine receptor. However, acetylcholine and other depolarizing agents retain their action in the presence of the toxins (Dettbarn et al., 1965). They also do not interfere with the release of acetylcholine. During block of conduction, cathodal depolarization will release transmitter substance. Abolition of the nerve impulse by TTX does not prevent the release of transmitter from nerve endings in the response to locally induced depolarization (Bloedel et al., 1966).

D. Action of TTX and STX on Generator Potentials

The site of generator potentials of sensory receptors as well as some postsynaptic membranes are electrically inexcitable and thus produce only graded responses. This is because there is no feedback between the change in membrane potential and the electrogenic process. Neither TTX nor STX affects electrically inexcitable responses. However, only the part of this graded response that is due to increased sodium permeability could be expected to be affected by TTX or STX. TTX blocks conduction in afferent fibers from frog muscle spindle without action on the generator potential.

Low sodium and TTX reduce the generator potential, which can subsequently be restored with sodium. The sodium current generating system
of the generator potential seems to be affected (Albuquerque *et al.*, 1969).
TTX blocks impulse initiation in the Pacinian corpuscle without affecting
the generator potential. Other experiments, however, indicate that the
generator potential is reduced by 60% (Oseki and Sato, 1965). Sodium-free
solutions reduce the receptor potential to 30% of normal. At least in part,
the TTX mechanism in these systems may be explained by its action on the
sodium activation (Nishi *et al.*, 1966).

IV. COMPARISON OF TTX AND STX

The similarity of TTX and STX in their actions at the cellular level
suggests that they may have similar action sites on some part of the cell
membrane. Since both compounds contain guanidinium as part of their
structure, it may well be that it is this part of the molecule that determines
their similarities. If one compares the systemic effects of these toxins, some
distinctions become obvious. The lowest dose of TTX which blocks conduction and indirectly blocks transmission is always accompanied by a drop
in blood pressure. The concentrations of STX which cause similar effects on
nerve and neuromuscular junction do not affect the blood pressure (Kao
and Nishiyama, 1965). Only in much higher concentrations than needed to
block conduction does STX produce a drop in blood pressure. TTX is also
a very potent emetic as well as hypothermic agent. These effects seem to be
exerted at the medullary chemoreceptor and the hypothalamus. So far, no
similar actions have been described for STX. Whether this is a difference in
their basic mechanisms or a greater specificity on the part of the STX remains to be seen (Kao, 1967).

There are some differences also on the cellular level. TTX has no effect
at all on the endplate of the neuromuscular junction. STX slightly reduces
the amplitude of the mepp after long exposure (Nishiyama, 1968). Even so,
it is not known how this is accomplished. Either STX reduces the release of
transmitter or decreases the sensitivity of the endplate membrane.

The two toxins also differ as to their degree of reversibility. The effects
of STX can always be quickly reversed on washing. In many experiments,
the effects of TTX cannot be reversed completely even after prolonged
washing (Hille, 1968; Narahashi *et al.*, 1967). On application of low concentrations of STX, an initial increase in the amplitude of the action potential can be observed (Kao and Nishiyama, 1965; Dettbarn *et al.*, 1965).

The most obvious difference is apparent when the two toxins are compared with respect to their actions on the nerves of the puffer and the taricha
newt (Mosher *et al.*, 1964). Both animals produce TTX. Their nerves are

insensitive to the action of TTX, but they are sensitive to STX, which blocks electrical activity. The action potential-generating mechanism of these nerves is sodium ion specific, which rules out the possibility that other ions, such as divalent cations, are involved. Calcium spikes are insensitive to TTX as well as to STX (Hagiwara and Nakajima, 1966). Whether resistance of these nerves to TTX is due to some peculiarities of the sodium current generating sites or to some enzymic detoxification mechanism remains to be seen (Kao and Nishiyama, 1965).

V. MECHANISM OF ACTION

A. The Active Form of TTX and STX

While the effects of TTX and STX on the electrical activity of nerve and muscle have been thoroughly investigated, not much is known about the underlying mechanism that produces the specific block of the peak transient inward current. Studies investigating possible molecular mechanisms have concentrated on TTX since its structural configuration is known. The molecule possesses several unique structural features of which the hemilactal link between C_5 and C_{10} and a guanidinium group is of interest (Mosher et al., 1964; Tsuda et al., 1964). According to the chemical structure, TTX can exist in equilibrium with two other forms (Fig. 6). One of the hemilactal forms has an electronegative charge at the oxygen, while the other has a proton added to the oxygen. An equilibrium exists between a zwitterion which is formed by the amino and the hydroxyl group and the cationic forms of the molecule. Whereas the guanidinium group has a positive charge and a pK_a of 11–12, the pK_a for the hydroxyl group is about 8.8. Studies of pH effects on the TTX action have indicated that the cationic forms are more potent than the zwitterion. This was revealed by the demonstration that the concentration of TTX required for blockade had to be increased when the

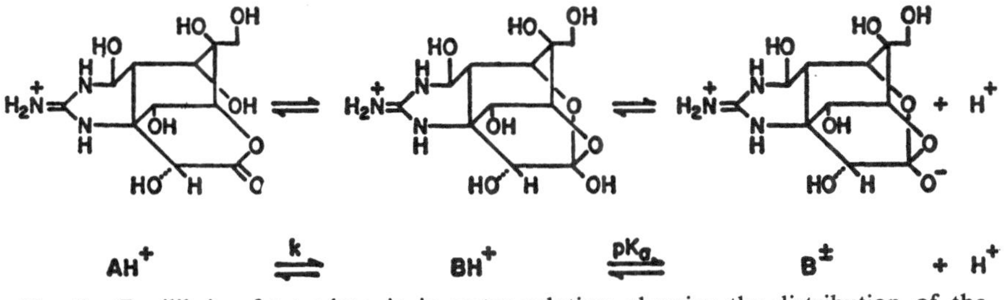

Fig. 6. Equilibria of tetrodotoxin in water solution, showing the distribution of the three molecular species. AH^+ and BH^+ are cations, while $B^{\pm}$ is a zwitterion. Taken from Camougis et al., 1967 [adapted from Woodward].

pH in the bathing solution was changed from 7 to more alkaline values (Camougis *et al.*, 1967; Narahashi *et al.*, 1969; Hille, 1968). In the pH range studied (7–9), the charge of the guanidinium would not change. This then would imply that the hemilactal-lactone part of the molecule is also of importance for the effect of TTX on the transient sodium current. Which of the two cationic forms is responsible for the action is as yet unknown. TTX does not block the action potential or the membrane sodium current when internally perfused through the giant axon, even at much higher concentrations than required to block by external application (Narahashi *et al.*, 1966). Since TTX is lipid-insoluble, it probably acts on the outer surface of the membrane only.

B. Structure–Activity Relationship

It has been suggested that the highly specific action of TTX is due to its guanidinium group, because this group can replace sodium and has approximately the same size as a sodium ion. Thus, by blocking the channels for the peak transient sodium influx, the flow of current associated with sodium ions is stopped. The electrostatic forces between the positive charge of the guanidinium group and the fixed negative charge of the sodium channel can explain only part of the effect of TTX on conduction.

In a study of several guanidinium compounds with structural features

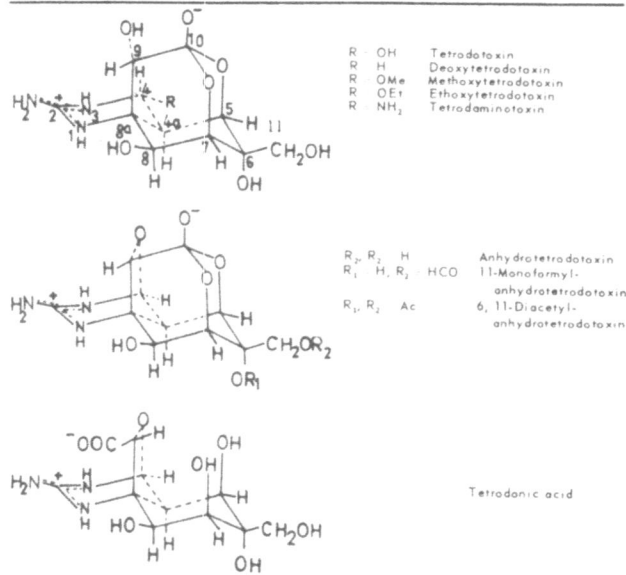

Fig. 7. Chemical structures of tetrodotoxin and its derivatives. Taken from Deguchi, 1967.

Table I.
Comparison of Tetrodotoxin and Its Derivatives[a]

Tetrodotoxin and derivatives	LD$_{50}$ for mice[b] (μg/kg)		MLD for mice (μg/kg)[c]		Blockage of frog sciatic nerve (M)	Blockage of lobster nerve (M)
	Intravenous	Oral	Intravenous	Intraperitoneal		
Tetrodotoxin	9.0	435	8.22[d]		1.6×10^{-8}	3×10^{-8}
Deoxytetrodotoxin	41.7	2,700	84.5		1.2×10^{-7}	2×10^{-7}
Methoxytetrodotoxin	341	12,700	341		4.5×10^{-7}	
Ethoxytetrodotoxin	692	25,700		692	9.6×10^{-7}	
Tetrodaminotoxin	528	26,100	841		1.7×10^{-6}	2×10^{-6}
11-Monoformylanhydrotetrodotoxin	1,380	13,600		3,000	1.8×10^{-6}	
Anhydrotetrodotoxin	1,250	16,900	4,140		2.8×10^{-6}	3×10^{-6}
6,11-Diacetylanhydrotetrodotoxin	96,700			>50,000	3.6×10^{-5}	
Tetrodonic acid	68,700		>300,000		$>5.9 \times 10^{-4}$	$>1 \times 10^{-4}$

[a] Narahashi et al., 1967. [b] After Deguchi. [c] After Tsuda et al., 1964. [d] LD$_{50}$.

common to TTX, it was shown that none of these compounds approach
TTX's toxicity. All had characteristics more common to local anesthetics
(Ranney et al., 1968). A few derivatives of TTX, deoxytetrodotoxin, meth-
oxytetrodotoxin, ethoxytetrodotoxin, tetrodoaminotoxin, monoformyl-
anhydrotetrodotoxin, anhydrotetrodotoxin, 6,11-diacetylanhydro tetrodotoxin, and tetrodonic acid are all less active than TTX. All these compounds
contain, as does TTX, the guanidinium group as part of the six-membered
ring (Fig. 7). Thus, it cannot be the guanidinium alone that determines the
specificity.

It is possible from the quantitative point of view to discuss the relation
of chemical structure and pharmacological activities and differences in
potencies among the derivatives listed here in sequence of toxicity (Table I):
(1) tetrodotoxin, deoxy-TTX, methoxy-TTX, ethoxy-TTX, and tetrodoaminotoxin, (2) monoformyl anhydro-tetrodotoxin as a carbonic acid
salt, anhydro tetrotoxin, 6,11-diacetylanhydro tetrodotoxin, and (3) tetrodonic acid. Dehydrogenation and formation of oxygen bridges between
C_4 and C_9 reduces the activity as is apparent from the comparison of the
potencies of desoxy- and anhydroderivatives. Introduction of an acetyl
group to positions 6 and 11 also decreases activity. Tetrodonic acid is substantially different from tetrodotoxin and other derivatives since its chemical
structure has no hemilactal structure and configuration at C_9. Its activity is
very low. This may indicate that the distance between the anionic and
cationic poles is important for the powerful action of TTX (Deguchi, 1967).
The guanidinium group and the hemilactal ring position seem to be important for the highly neurospecific action of TTX. However, any conclusions to be drawn from these structure–activity relationships have to be
considered with care, because contamination of the derivative with traces of
TTX can account for some of the blocking actions seen due to the extraordinarily low concentrations of TTX needed to block activity. Narahashi
et al. (1967) could show that the deoxy TTX used contained 15% TTX, and
this would account for the blocking action seen with deoxy-TTX. The even
lesser activity seen with the other active compounds could be due to still
minor contamination with TTX. Thus, the gradual diminution of the effect
with structural changes in the TTX molecule have to be considered with
caution. It is apparent that the loss of hemilactal configuration causes
reduction of activity as seen with tetrodonic acid. The same may be true for
the reduction at C_4 which results in deoxy-TTX.

C. Possible Mechanism of Interaction

TTX and STX may be bound to receptors by van der Waals' forces,
dipole–dipole interactions, and/or electrostatic bindings. With a highly

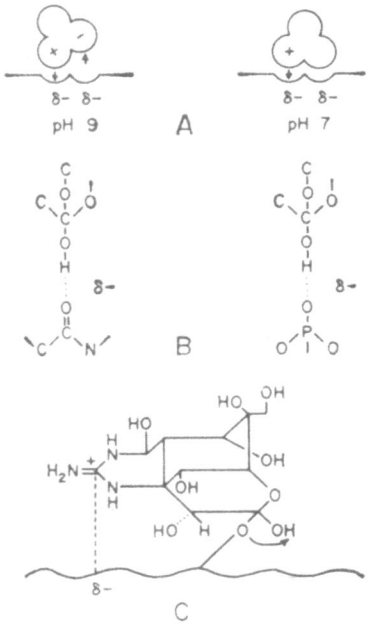

Fig. 8. A. Models of the molecular interaction of tetrodotoxin with a receptor site on the outer layer of an excitable membrane. The zwitterion is partially repelled by electronegative regions of the cell membrane. The cationic form has less repulsion, thus resulting in a higher probability of proper steric interaction with the receptor site. B. The structural formulas show possible interactions of the hemilactal part of BH^+ with an electronegative oxygen of a peptide chain, or an electronegative oxygen of a phosphate group by hydrogen bonding. C. Postulated interaction of tetrodotoxin with a receptor site by electrostatic attraction and secondary intermolecular hemilactal formation. Taken from Camougis et al., 1967.

reactive carboxyl group at C_{10}, the electron density on the oxygen may be sufficient to act as an electron donor capable of forming hydrogen bonds. The more potent a compound in the above series of analogs, the greater is the negativity associated with the oxygen of the carbonyl group. A model which entails van der Waals' forces, as well as dipole and electrostatic introductions, was illustrated in Chap. 6. However, it is unlikely that van der Waals' forces will contribute to receptor binding of the polar components of the hemilactal ring and the free hydroxy groups of TTX at C_9. It is possible that hydrophobic and hydrogen bonding are involved, since loss of the hemilactal ring and the ether linkage between C_9 and C_4 as in tetrodonic acid causes loss of the neurotoxicity. Camougis et al. (1967) suggested (Fig. 8) that the lack of electronegative charge may facilitate the binding to the membrane since this will decrease electrostatic repulsion. This would apply for either of the cationic forms. A second possibility would be that the protonic hydrogen forms a hydrogen bond between TTX and the receptor which would not be limited to proteins of the membrane but could also take place with phosphate groups. A third possibility would be that the positive charge of the guanidinium binds to a negative site of the "receptor" and an additional reaction between hydroxyl groups of the receptor with TTX could lead to a hemilactal configuration which would cause a secondary binding with another receptor site (Camougis *et al.*, 1967).

D. The Interaction of TTX and STX with Calcium

Experiments demonstrating the ability of TTX to chelate calcium have led Onishi and Ishida (1967) to the suggestion that this may be the mechanism responsible for TTX action. In their experiments, they found that TTX chelates calcium ions in a ratio of 1:2, and they suggested that the formation of a complex containing TTX, calcium, and membrane phospholipids might reduce the release of calcium ions from membrane sites. According to current theory, it is the release of calcium on stimulation that is responsible for the generation of the action potential by permitting the sodium and potassium to run down their concentration gradient. If calcium is bound tightly through the TTX action, no action potential should be generated. As attractive as this hypothesis may be, there is evidence that argues against such a mechanism of TTX action. Commercially available TTX comes as a mixture with sodium citrate (100 μg of TTX and 500 μg of sodium citrate). It is more than reasonable that the citrate may be responsible for Onishi and Tshida's observation. Hopkins and Herbst (1968) have pointed out that the binding ratio of 1:2 (TTX:calcium) corresponds to the citrate–calcium ion ratio. Furthermore, the pH effect on the calcium ion chelating mechanism is opposite to/that of the pH effect on TTX action. In the 7–9 pH range TTX is more effective in the lower ranges while the opposite is true for the citrate calcium binding. Additional evidence against the calcium binding comes from the observation that STX, which is as effective as TTX on axonal conduction, does not bind calcium ions. Another fact is that TTX is completely ineffective on preparations in which the action potential is generated by calcium ions or other divalent cations instead of sodium (Hagiwara and Nakajima, 1966).

E. Model Systems

Explanations as to the mode of action of TTX and STX are limited by our circumscribed knowledge of the nerve membrane and its functional subunits.

In recent years, model systems have been used in an attempt to explain drug action on excitable membranes through changes of some physicochemical properties of the lipid membrane which surrounds cells. Villegas and Camejo (1968) and Camejo and Villegas (1969) isolated the lipids from the squid giant axon nerve membrane and separated them into a polar fraction containing the phosphatides and into a nonpolar fraction consisting of cholesterol, fatty acids, and hydrocarbons. When TTX was tested on monolayers of both fractions, the nonpolar fraction showed an expansion on addition of TTX. On further fractionation of the nonpolar fraction, TTX expanded only the cholesterol monolayer. Tetrodonic acid, which has no effect on electrical activity, was completely ineffective when used on these monolayers. No TTX action was seen on monolayers of fatty acids or of the fatty acid hydrocarbon mixture. When cholesterol was added to these fractions the TTX effect, an expansion of volume, was observed again. Thus it is possible that cholesterol may be a critical component of that part of the membrane which controls the sodium current, and it may well be part of an active site in the interaction with TTX.

VI. CONCLUSION

While the precise mode of action of TTX and STX remains unknown, these toxins have been powerful tools in the hands of the neurophysiologist. Their ability to block the channels for the initial peak transient inward current may be explained on the basis that in their cationic form they are bound to negatively charged sites within the membrane and thus block the passage of sodium ions. The small difference of action between TTX and STX and apparent differences in their chemical structure may help in the final analysis of their mode of action. For the time being, they are useful tools in the elucidation of some aspects of excitable membranes.

VII. REFERENCES

Albuquerque, E. X., S. H. Chung, and D. Ottoson (1969), *Acta Physiol. Scand.*, **75**:301.
Bloedel, J., P. W. Gage, R. Llinas, and D. M. J. Quastel (1966), *Nature*, **212**:49.
Camejo, G. and R. Villegas (1969), *Biochim. Biophys. Acta*, **173**:351.
Camougis, G., B. H. Takman, and J. R. P. Tasse (1967), *Science*, **156**:1625.
Cheng, K. K., Y. L. Ling, and J. C. Wang (1968), *Quart. J. Exp. Physiol.*, **53**:119.
Deguchi, T. (1967), *Jap. J. Pharmacol.*, **17**:267.
Dettbarn, W-D., H. B. Higman, P. Rosenberg, and D. Nachmansohn (1960), *Science*, **132**:300.
Dettbarn, W-D., H. B. Higman, E. Bartels, and T. Podleski (1965), *Biochem. Biophy.*
    Acta, **94**:478.
Evans, M. H. (1968a), *Toxicon*, **5**:289.
Evans, M. H. (1968b), *Brit. J. Pharmacol.*, **34**:664.
Fleisher, J. H., P. J. Killos, and C. S. Harrison (1961), *J. Pharmacol.*, **133**:98.
Hagiwara, S., and S. Nakajima (1966), *J. Gen. Physiol.*, **49**:793.
Hille, B. (1968), *J. Gen. Physiol.*, **51**:199.
Hodgkin, A. L. and A. F. Huxley (1952), *J. Physiol.*, **117**:500.
Hopkins, E. W., III and E. J. Herbst (1968), *Biochem. Biophys. Res. Commun.*, **30**:528.
Kao, C. Y. (1966a), *Pharmacol. Rev.*, **18**:997.
Kao, C. Y. (1966b), Comparison of the biological actions of tetrodotoxin and saxitoxin,
    in "Animal Toxins" (F. E. Russell and P. R. Saunders, eds.) Pergamon Press Ltd.,
    Oxford, England, pp. 109–114.
Kao, C. Y. and F. A. Fuhrman (1963), *J. Pharmacol.*, **140**:31.
Kao, C. Y. and A. Nishiyama (1965), *J. Physiol.*, **180**:50.

Kao, C. Y., T. Suzuki, A. L. Kleinhaus, and M. Y. Siegman (1967), *Arch. Intern. Pharmacodyn.*, **165**:438.

Katz, B. and R. Miledi (1967), *Proc. Roy. Soc. (Biol.)*, **167**:8.

Katz, B. and R. Miledi (1968), *J. Physiol.*, **199**:729.

Katz, B. and R. Miledi (1969), *J. Physiol.*, **203**:459.

Koizumi, K., D. G. Levine, and C. McC. Brooks (1967), *Neurology*, **17**:395.

Moore, J. W., M. P. Blaustein, N. C. Anderson, and T. Narahashi (1967), *J. Gen. Physiol.*, **50**:1401.

Mosher, H. S., F. A. Fuhrman, H. D. Buchwald, and H. G. Fischer (1964), *Science*, **144**: 1100.

Nakamura, Y., S. Nakajima, and H. Grundfest (1964), *Science*, **146**:266.

Nakamura, Y., S. Nakajima, and H. Grundfest (1965), *J. Gen. Physiol.*, **48**:985.

Narahashi, T., T. Deguchi, N. Urakawa, and Y. Ohkubo (1960), *Amer. J. Physiol.* **198**:934.

Narahashi, T., J. W. Moore, and W. Scott (1964), *J. Gen. Physiol.*, **74**:965.

Narahashi, T., N. C. Anderson, and J. W. Moore (1966), *Science*, **153**:765.

Narahashi, T., J. W. Moore, and R. N. Poston (1967), *Science*, **156**:976.

Narahashi, T., H. G. Haas, and E. P. Therrjen (1967). *Science*, **157**:1441.

Narahashi, T., J. W. Moore, and D. T. Frazier (1969), *J. Pharm. Exp. Therap.*, **169**:224.

Nishi, K. and M. Sato (1966), *J. Physiol.*, **184**:376.

Nishiyama, A. (1968a), *Exp. Med.*, **95**:201.

Nishiyama, A. (1968b), *Nature*, **219**:379.

Ohnishi, T. and A. Ishida (1967), *Biochem. Biophys. Res. Commun.*, **27**:552.

Ozeki, M. and M. Sato (1965), *J. Physiol.*, **180**:186.

Ranney, B. K., F. A. Fuhrman, and J. L. Schmiegel (1968), *Arch. Intern. Pharmacodyn.*, **175**:193.

Takata, M., J. W. Moore, C. Y. Kao, and F. A. Fuhrman (1966), *J. Gen. Physiol.*, **49**:977.

Tsuda, K., R. Tachikawa, K. Sakai, C. Tamura, O. Amakasu, M. Kawamura, and S. Ikuma (1964), *Chem. Pharm. Bull.*, **12**:642.

Villegas, R. and G. Camejo (1968), *Biochim. Biophys. Acta*, **163**:421.

Chapter 9

Tetrodotoxin and Saxitoxin as Pharmacological Tools

Peter W. Gage

School of Physiology
University of New South Wales
Kensington, New South Wales, Australia

I. INTRODUCTION

A. History

Interest in the poisons tetrodotoxin and saxitoxin was initially aroused because of deaths which occurred following careless or innocent consumption of puffer-fish or shellfish. From ancient times it was well known to the Japanese and Chinese that it was hazardous to eat the ovaries and eggs of the puffer-fish (tetrodons, also known as fugu or swellfish), but rather than forsake the fish which is apparently prized by oriental gourmets, chefs were specially trained and licensed to prepare nontoxic fugu. Restaurants which were fortunate enough to have the services of such a cook could include the item in their menu (*see* Chap. 6). Natural predators were no doubt aware of puffer toxicity, and this must have been very useful in the struggle for survival of the species. One of the earliest pharmacological uses of tetrodotoxin would have been as a poison in suicide, and perhaps homicide, attempts (Kao, 1964).

Poisoning from shellfish posed a more formidable public health problem because of its sporadic nature (*see* Chap. 7). Shellfish which are nontoxic at one time of the year can suddenly, for no apparent reason, cause outbreaks of severe food poisoning, and this toxicity persists for a period of several weeks, then disappears. Some coastal tribes of Alaskan Indians who had noticed that mussels became poisonous soon after the seas became luminescent in hot weather devised an early warning system. Sentries were posted to watch for the telltale signs in the sea, and when these were seen shellfish were shunned for several weeks. Unfortunately, the only sure way of determining whether a shellfish is toxic is by bioassay.

In the early 1930s, Victor Twitty, an experimental embryologist at Stanford University, found that transplants from embryos of the salamander *Taricha torosa* caused paralysis of the embryos of another genus of salamander, *Ambystoma*, for several days. He concluded that *Taricha* embryos contained a toxic substance which selectively paralysed the nerves of *Ambystoma*. This toxin, which was originally called tarichatoxin, was extracted and purified by other biologists at Stanford. Pharmacological and chemical studies showed that tarichatoxin and tetrodotoxin were very similar, and it has recently been found that their structures are identical. The toxin from salamanders is now also called tetrodotoxin. It is extremely interesting that the toxin in the eggs of such diverse animals as puffers and newts should be the same, but why this should be so is not evident.

Tetrodotoxin occurs in the ovaries, liver, skin, and muscles of several species of the genus *Fugu* (Sphoeroides) and *Taricha torosa*. Many other tetraodontoid fish are poisonous, and all newts of the family Salamandridae which have been examined contain similar toxins, but these have not yet been identified as tetrodotoxin. Tetrodotoxin is found in very high concentration in the eggs and ovaries: the female of the species is indeed deadlier than the male. In puffers, a high concentration is found also in the liver, whereas in salamanders, the skin has a high content. The concentration of tetrodotoxin in the ovaries of puffers is highest in winter when the ova are mature but is much lower in summer. Biosynthesis of tetrodotoxin is obviously influenced by processes which control sexual maturation.

It is interesting that fish which contain tetrodotoxin are immune to its effects. Ishihara found in 1918 that of 22 species of animals tested, only the puffer itself and the Japanese newt, *Cynops pyrrogaster*, which was later found to contain tetrodotoxin, were resistant. This immunity could provide a useful method of screening new species suspected of containing tetrodotoxin.

From such beginnings has developed a powerful and finely selective pharmacological scalpel, and a gastronomic impediment has been turned into an invaluable instrument for the physiologist's kit. The historical background illustrates the type of source which may provide new and useful toxins.

B. Chemistry

1. *Tetrodotoxin*

The chemistry of the toxins is unusual, and in spite of their rather low molecular weight synthesis has not yet been achieved. Tetrodotoxin is an amino perhydroquinazoline compound ($C_{11}H_{17}N_3O_8$) with a molecular weight of 319.3. Its crystals are colorless prisms which are only sparingly soluble in water except in slightly acidic solutions, but even in such solutions the toxin is not indefinitely stable. At pHs below 3 or above 7 decomposition of tetrodotoxin occurs. In alkaline solutions the toxin is degraded into several quinazoline compounds. The purified toxin is now obtainable commercially from Sankyo Company (Tetrodotoxin, Crystalline 3X) in a mixture with a citric acid–sodium citrate buffer (pH 4.8–4.9). When using concentrations of this preparation greater than 10^{-5} g/ml, the presence of the citrate buffer may reduce the ionized calcium concentration of solutions. It is important under these conditions to ensure that the lowered calcium concentration does not affect results of experiments in which the toxin is used.

The structure of tetrodotoxin is illustrated in Chap. 8, Fig. 7. Its determination was completed only recently and proved no easy task. Chemical analysis was complicated by the sensitivity of the toxin to both acidic and basic media and by the fact that it is nonvolatile. This latter property precluded the use of mass spectrography on the pure toxin. The polar nature of the molecule and the large number of OH groups tend to make it retain water and other solvents, again making analysis more difficult. There are also some unusual structural features. The cyclic hemilactal grouping and the zwitterion structure with the guanidinium cation and hemilactal anion are unique. The normally high pK_a of the guanidine group of the toxin is masked by the acidic OH group at C_{10} which has a pK_a of about 8.5. The molecule bears no close structural relationship to any other known natural product.

2. Saxitoxin

The poison from noxious California mussels and Alaskan butter clams is called saxitoxin. It was isolated in 1954 by several groups in the United States by ion-exchange chromatography on carboxylic acid resins, followed by chromatography on acid-washed alumina in absolute alcohol. This gave a white hygroscopic product which had a potency of 5500 mouse units per milligram of solids. The structure is uncertain, but the molecule is thought to have a perhydropurine nucleus in which are incorporated two guanidinium moieties. The purified poison is a water-soluble, dibasic salt with pK_a at 8.2 and 11.5. It is stable in acidic and basic solutions and is soluble in ethanol and methanol but insoluble in all lipid solvents. Its molecular formula as a hydrochloride salt is $C_{10}H_{17}O_4N_7 \cdot 2HCl$ giving a molecular weight of 372. It has no ultraviolet absorption, gives positive Benedict–Behre and Jaffe tests, and is completely detoxified by mild catalytic reduction with the uptake of 1 mole of hydrogen per mole of poison at atmospheric pressure.

II. CELLULAR EFFECTS

Use of the toxins as pharmacological tools depends on a knowledge of their effects on cell membranes which in turn requires knowledge of current concepts of excitation phenomena in excitable membranes (cf. Hodgkin, 1964). A brief summary of excitation phenomena was given in Chap. 8. The same general material is presented here with a somewhat different perspective that should facilitate understanding the value of tetrodotoxin and saxitoxin as pharmacological tools.

A. Properties of Excitable Membranes

In excitable cells such as neurons and muscle fibers there are ionic concentration gradients across the membrane. The concentration of sodium is higher outside and the concentration of potassium higher inside the cell. There is also an electrical potential across the membrane in such a direction that the inside of the cell is negative with respect to the outside. Thus there is both an electrical and chemical force tending to drive sodium ions into the cell. However, because the membrane is only slightly permeable to sodium ions, a metabolically fueled sodium pump is able to compensate for any leakage and maintains a constant intracellular sodium ion concentration.

The inward electrical and outward chemical force on potassium ions are almost equal. However, because of the relatively greater permeability of the membrane to potassium ions, the smaller net outward force on potassium ions still results in a passive net outward flux approximately equal to the passive net influx of sodium ions. This imbalance of passive fluxes is handled by active transport of potassium ions, which is generally thought to be coupled to the active transport of sodium ions. Because the resting membrane is much more permeable to potassium than to sodium ions, the membrane potential is determined predominantly by the concentration gradient of potassium ions and values in the range -50 to -100 mV (inside of a cell with respect to the outside) have been recorded.

When an excitable membrane is depolarized, that is, the electrical potential across it is decreased, the permeability to sodium ions increases. If the depolarization is of sufficient magnitude, there occurs an explosive increase in sodium permeability which is self-terminating. The increase in the sodium permeability of the membrane is followed by an increase in permeability to potassium ions. For a short time, therefore, while sodium permeability is much higher than potassium permeability, the membrane potential reverses sign under the influence of the sodium ion concentration gradient. This reversal of membrane potential is called an action potential, which travels or propagates along a cell because of the flow of current between active and resting membrane.

Our knowledge of the permeability changes and ionic currents which occur during an action potential is derived to a large extent from the classic experiments of Hodgkin and Huxley (1952a,b,c,d). By controlling the potential across an area of membrane electronically, a technique known as "voltage clamp," it is possible when the membrane is depolarized to record two membrane resistances or conductance changes with separate time courses. For example, when the potential across the membrane of a squid nerve is "clamped" at a depolarized level, the sodium conductance starts at a very low value, rises rapidly to about 25 mmho/cm², and then declines exponentially. The potassium conductance does not change at once but rises in an S-shaped curve to a steady level. The difference in time course of the two conductance changes has led to the suggestion that sodium and potassium ions may move across excited membranes through separate conductance "channels." These channels are not completely ion-selective. For example the early transient channel allows passage of lithium, ammonium, guanidinium, and hydrazinium ions. This has prompted introduction of the terms "early transient conductance" and "late steady-state conductance" corresponding to the early transient sodium conductance and the late steady-state potassium conductance changes which occur under normal conditions. Of course a difference in time course of sodium and potassium conductance does not necessarily mean that these ions move through spatially separate channels. The differential permeability of a single channel in a membrane could change with time, giving sodium and potassium conductance changes with different time courses. Such a time-dependent change in differential permeability could reflect a sequence of changes of molecular structure in a specialized region of the membrane. However, it is convenient to talk of early transient and late steady state channels without being committed to spatially separate channels.

B. Actions of Toxins

Tetrodotoxin and saxitoxin block action potentials in a variety of cells at nanomolar (10^{-9} M, nM) concentrations. Occasionally saxitoxin, but not tetrodotoxin, causes a transient increase in the amplitude of action potentials in frog nerves. The progressive blockage of action potentials in a lobster axon following exposure to 90 nM tetrodotoxin is illustrated in Fig. 1. The numbers beside the lower four action potentials denote the time in minutes after exposure to tetrodotoxin. It can be seen that block was almost complete within 5 min at this concentration.

There are two major groups of drugs which block action potentials; those which depolarize the membrane and block presumably by causing inactivation of the sodium conductance mechanism; and those which block without causing depolarization. In the latter group are included the local

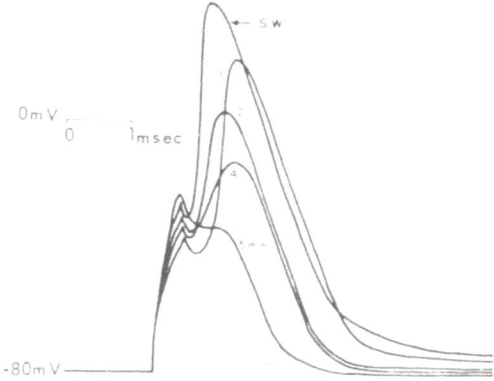

Fig. 1. Blockage of an action potential in a lobster axon over a period of a few minutes after addition of 90 nM tetrodotoxin. The time in tetrodotoxin is shown adjacent to the attenuated spikes [Takata *et al.* (1966), *J. Gen. Physiol.*, **49**:977].

anesthetics such as cocaine, which have been found to inhibit both the sodium and potassium conductance increases caused by depolarization (Shanes *et al.*, 1959; Taylor, 1959). Tetrodotoxin and saxitoxin form a new group of drugs which block only the early conductance increase leaving the late steady-state conductance completely unaffected. This can be seen in Fig. 2, which shows the result of a voltage clamp experiment in a lobster axon exposed to 90 nM tetrodotoxin. The amplitude of the early transient current, I_{Na}, and the late steady current, I_K, are plotted against the membrane potential during the clamping pulse. Inset shows the type of current record which is obtained following a depolarizing step. In the graph the

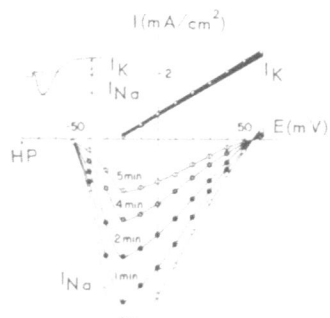

Fig. 2. Plot of the early transient sodium current (I_{Na}) and late steady potassium current (I_K) as a function of the voltage clamp potential. Only the transient sodium current is blocked by 90 nM tetrodotoxin [Takata *et al.* (1966), *J. Gen. Physiol.*, **49**:977].

downward curves show the peak sodium current which was reduced appreciably after 5 min in tetrodotoxin. The potassium current (linear superimposed lines above) was not affected by the toxin. Similar results have been obtained with saxitoxin. One difference is that saxitoxin can initially cause an increase in sodium current before the decrease (Hille, 1968), and this, no doubt, underlies the observation of a transient increase in the amplitude of action potentials in saxitoxin. Thus the increase in sodium permeability which normally follows excitation is inhibited in cells exposed to these toxins, and action potentials normally generated by such a permeability increase are inhibited.

III. PHARMACOLOGICAL USES

Sodium ions can move across resting membranes through a variety of channels or permeability processes, some of which are present in the resting state and some of which can be activated. These processes may be listed:

1. Resting Membranes
   a. Passive sodium flux. Most membranes have a small but finite permeability to sodium ions so that there is a net inward passive flux.
   b. Active sodium flux. There is normally an added movement of sodium ions against the electrochemical gradient. This flux derives energy from ATP and can be blocked by cardiac glycosides and metabolic inhibitors.
   c. Exchange diffusion. Sodium ions can cross membranes against an electrochemical gradient without utilizing ATP by exchanging for sodium ions moving in the opposite direction.

2. Activated Membranes
   a. Voltage-dependent sodium permeability. As described above, membrane depolarization causes a large transient increase in sodium permeability.
   b. Transmitter-dependent sodium permeability. Excitatory transmitters generally cause a large localized increase in sodium permeability which generates an excitatory postsynaptic potential or endplate potential.
   c. Generator potentials. Many specialized receptors (e.g., mechanoreceptors and photoreceptors) convert impinging environmental energy into an increase in sodium permeability proportional to the intensity of the stimulus. The resultant depolarization usually generates propagated action potentials.

Tetrodotoxin and saxitoxin have dramatic effects. only on the voltage-dependent early transient conductance change, and it is this specificity which makes them so extremely useful.

A. The Early Transient Channel

One of the major uses of the toxins has been in investigations of the properties of the early transient channel or conductance change.

1. Channel Specificity

It has been found that the toxins block the early transient conductance increase no matter what the ions using the channel, whether their movement is inward or outward (Tasaki and Singer, 1966; Moore et al., 1967). The late steady-state conductance increase is never affected, no matter what the ion or its direction of flow. These observations indicate that the toxins block the channel rather than impeding the movement of a specific ion. If the way in which they block the channel can be discovered, some light would be shed on the nature and specificity of some of the molecular changes which depolarization of the membrane initiates. So far, we know very little of these events.

2. Surface Specificity

There are some indications that the site of action of the toxins is very specific. In internally perfused squid axons in which 100 nM tetrodotoxin applied externally blocked the early transient channel within 1–2 min, 10 times the concentration (1000 nM) applied internally did not block the same channel (Narahashi et al., 1966). These observations indicate that tetrodotoxin blocks the early transient channel from the outside, not the inside of the membrane. It is very interesting that tetraethylammonium ions, in contrast, block the potassium conductance change in squid axons more effectively from the inside of the membrane (Armstrong and Binstock, 1965). Such observations must eventually be interpreted in terms of molecular configuration of the channels.

3. Structure Specificity

Both tetrodotoxin and saxitoxin have guanidine groups, and it has been suggested that it is this group which plugs the external gate of the early transient channel. However, minor modifications of the structure of tetrodotoxin which have left the guanidine and hemilactal groups unchanged have greatly reduced or abolished its effect on the early transient conductance change (Narahashi et al., 1966, 1967). All the compounds shown in Chap. 8, Fig. 7, were much less effective than tetrodotoxin in blocking the sodium channel. Although structure–activity relationships can only be speculative with the evidence at present available, it does seem that the unique neurotoxic properties of tetrodotoxin and saxitoxin are associated with the whole molecules and not just with the guanidine moieties or hemilactal units.

4. Channel Density

Because of its potency at very low concentrations, tetrodotoxin has been used to estimate the density of early transient (sodium) channels in an excitable membrane (Moore et al., 1967). Seven lobster nerve trunks were exposed to a small pool of solution containing 300 nM tetrodotoxin. They were then removed and the concentration of tetrodotoxin which remained in the pool after this treatment was determined by bioassay against known concentrations of toxin. The area of nerve membrane which had been exposed to the toxin and the volume of the extracellular space were estimated from light and electron micrographs of the tissues used. On the basis of these measurements, it was calculated that there were no more than 13 sodium channels per square micron of lobster axon surface. All the assumptions made in the calculations would tend to increase this estimate of channel density. This means that less than 1 part in 100,000 of the membrane surface contains an early transient channel. On the basis of these results it can be said that the area of membrane through which sodium ions flow during an action potential is only a very minute fraction of the total membrane area. Biochemical studies of the sparse locations responsible for such conductance changes will be extremely difficult.

B. Synaptic Transmission

Tetrodotoxin has proved to be a very useful agent in studies of synaptic transmission because of its selective mode of action. A prominent sign of poisoning in animals is muscular weakness, and some early investigations of the effects of the toxins at neuromuscular junctions led to the erroneous conclusion that they had a curare-like action. Before discussing synaptic effects in detail, a brief review of some aspects of synaptic transmission may be useful.

At a resting synapse, in the absence of any nerve activity there is a spontaneous, slow, random leakage of discrete, uniform "packets" or quanta of transmitter from the presynaptic terminal. The arrival of this transmitter at the postsynaptic membrane causes an increase in the conductance of the subsynaptic membrane to one or more ions (Na^+ and K^+ at many excitatory synapses; Cl^+ or K^+ or both, at many inhibitory synapses) causing "miniature" potential changes. The arrival of an action potential in presynaptic terminals causes an acceleration of the release of these quanta and hence a larger postsynaptic potential.

Use of tetrodotoxin has allowed us to examine more closely the relationship between action potentials and transmitter release. One question which had not been resolved before the advent of tetrodotoxin was whether the release of transmitter by an action potential was triggered by a conductance change, an ionic current, an ionic concentration change, or depolarization of the membrane. It had been found that the rate of release of quanta could be increased by depolarizing the presynaptic membrane, either electronically by passing current across the membrane, or chemically by increasing the extracellular potassium concentration. Liley (1956) extrapolated the relationship he obtained between the rate of release of quanta and depolari-

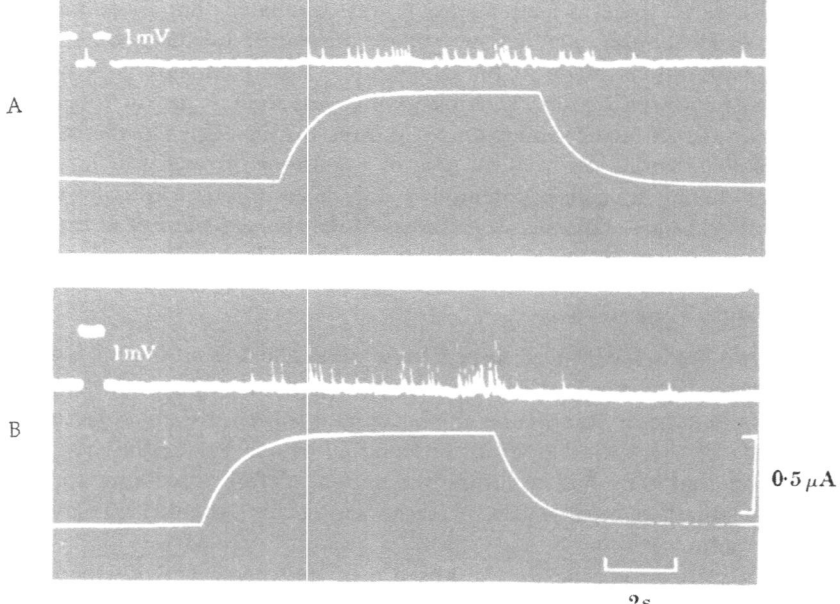

Fig. 3. Effect of electrotonic depolarization on the frequency of miniature endplate potentials. Temp. 2.5°C. The upper trace in A and B shows miniature endplate potentials recorded intracellularly; the lower trace monitors the current passed through the presynaptic terminals. The current was established slowly to avoid eliciting action potentials in the absence of tetrodotoxin. A. Normal Ringer's. B. Ringer's containing tetrodotoxin (10^{-6} g/ml). Note higher voltage amplification in upper trace in B [Katz and Miledi (1967), *Proc. Roy. Soc. B.* **167**:8].

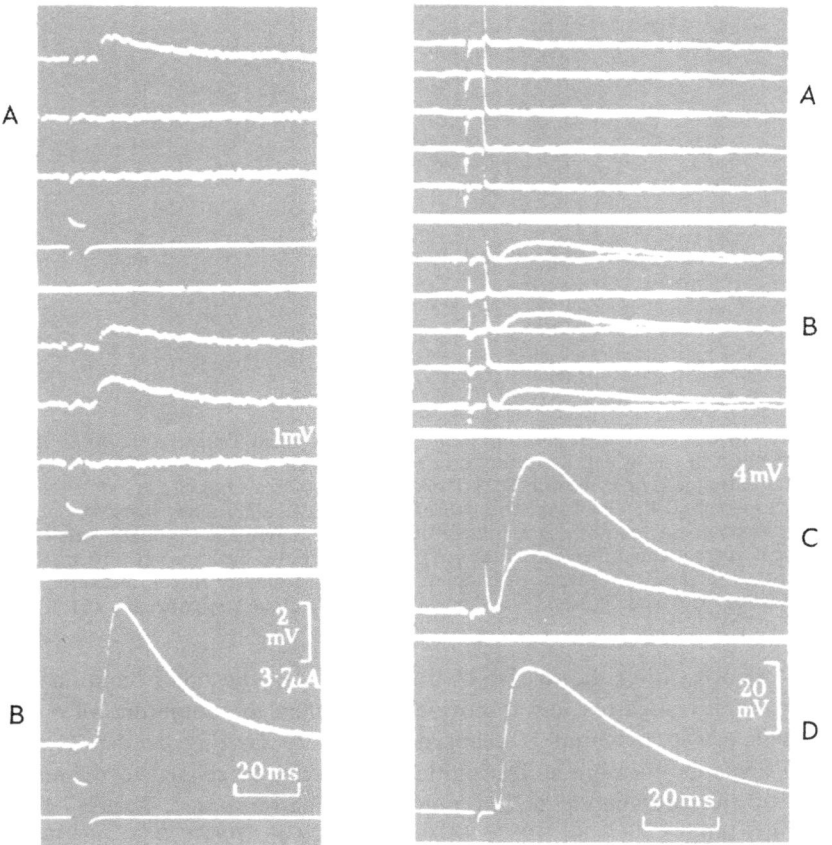

Fig. 4. Endplate potentials evoked by brief depolarizing pulses applied to nerve terminals in a preparation exposed to tetrodotoxin. The two vertical columns were recorded from different muscle fibers. Temp. 2.5°C (left); 1.5°C (right). Each block of records shows the endplate responses to brief pulses of a given strength. The pulse intensity was increased in successive blocks, from A to D. Currents are monitored in the left column only. With weak current intensities (blocks at the top), unitary endplate potentials appear in all-or-none fashion. The average size of the endplate potential greatly increases as the pulse is strengthened (lower blocks). Note the change in current amplification in the lower blocks. [Katz and Miledi (1967), *Proc. Roy. Soc. B.*, **167**:8.]

zation of the presynaptic membrane to the depolarization which occurs during an action potential and predicted that transmitter release would be increased by a factor of 10^5 by a 90 mV depolarization. This is indeed the order of magnitude of the increase which is seen following an action potential and is consistent with the hypothesis that it is membrane depolari-

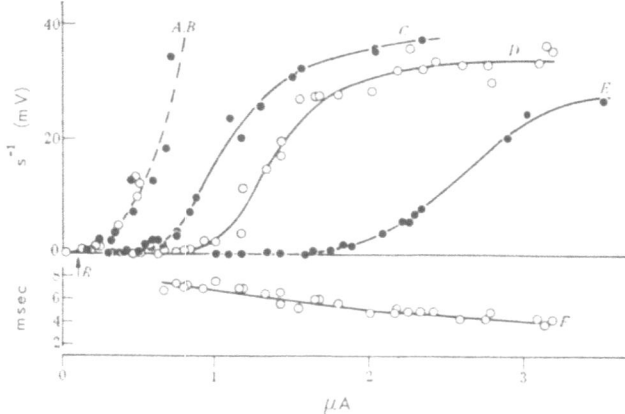

Fig. 5. Effects of strength and duration of applied current. Temperature 40°C. *A* and *B:* the effect of steady depolarization on the frequency of miniature endplate potentials. Ordinate: frequency per second (S⁻¹). Hollow circles: before; full circles: after tetrodotoxin application. *R*: 'rheobasic' strength of square pulse, determined initially. *C, D, E:* after tetrodotoxin, showing amplitudes of endplate potentials (ordinate: mV) with different current intensities (abscissa: μA), for three pulse durations (*C*, 10 msec; *D*, 5 msec; *E*, 2 msec). *F:* latency of endplate potential (ordinate: msec), measured from the start of the 5 msec pulses. [Katz and Miledi (1967), *Proc. Roy. Soc. B.*, **167**:8.]

zation which causes the release of transmitter. On the other hand, several groups of investigators had discovered that when the amplitude of a presynaptic action potential is changed by hyperpolarizing or depolarizing the presynaptic membrane, transmitter release can be related to the amplitude of the presynaptic action potential (Hagiwara and Tasaki, 1958; Takeuchi and Takeuchi, 1962; Miledi and Slater, 1966). The membrane potential at the peak of these action potentials was not significantly changed, and this led to the suggestion that there might be a relationship between current intensity during an action potential and the amount of transmitter released (Takeuchi and Takeuchi, 1962).

The question has been resolved by using preparations in which action potentials have been suppressed with tetrodotoxin, which fortunately does not change the response of the postsynaptic cell to transmitters and does not appear to interfere with the normal coupling between excitation of the presynaptic terminal and the release of transmitter (Elmqvist and Feldman, 1965; Katz and Miledi, 1967a). In Fig. 3 is shown a comparison of the effects of presynaptic depolarization on the rate of release of quanta at a neuromuscular junction in normal Ringer's (A) and in Ringer's containing 10^{-6} g/ml tetrodotoxin (B). It can be seen that tetrodotoxin does not affect appreciably the increase in the rate of release of quanta of transmitter caused by depolarization of the presynaptic membrane. To be absolutely sure that tetrodotoxin does not have any effect at all on postsynaptic conductance changes it will be necessary to do more quantitative experiments.

Katz and Miledi (1967a) applied graded depolarizing current pulses to presynaptic terminals in frog nerve–muscle preparations in which action potentials had been blocked with tetrodotoxin. They found that transmitter was released by these pulses and that the strength–response curve was very steep. Endplate potentials elicited by passing depolarizing currents through presynaptic terminals in neuromuscular junctions exposed to tetrodotoxin are shown in Fig. 4. As the intensity of current pulses was increased, the endplate potentials became larger and the relationship between current intensity and endplate potential amplitude was found to be S-shaped (Fig. 5). The release of transmitter could also be increased by lengthening the current pulse, but as there was no way of recording the transmembrane potential in these very small presynaptic terminals, it is difficult to interpret this observation.

In order to overcome this drawback, several groups of workers in the summer of 1966 poisoned squid synapses with tetrodotoxin and looked at the relationship between presynaptic depolarization and the amplitude of postsynaptic potentials (Bloedel *et al.*, 1966a,b; Katz and Miledi, 1967b; Kusano *et al.*, 1967). Depolarizations of the presynaptic terminal above the threshold caused the release of transmitter and postsynaptic potentials could be recorded. The relationship between presynaptic depolarization and postsynaptic potential amplitude appeared exponential, at least for small postsynaptic potentials, as can be seen in Fig. 6. Though it has been found consistently that the relationship between log postsynaptic

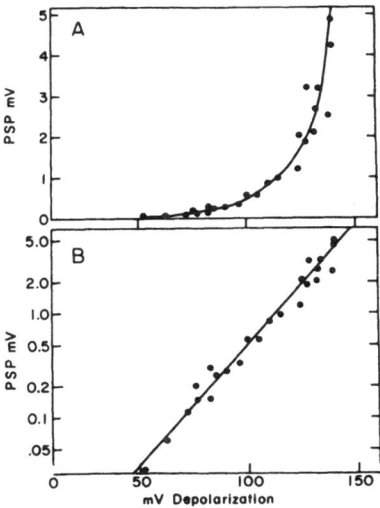

Fig. 6. Relationship between presynaptic depolarization and postsynaptic potential amplitude in the presence of tetrodotoxin (2×10^{-7} g/ml). Abscissa: presynaptic depolarization (mV). Ordinate A. Amplitude of postsynaptic potential (mV), linear scale. B. Amplitude of postsynaptic potential (mV), logarithmic scale. Temp. 8–10°C. [Gage (1967), *Fed. Proc.* **26**:1627.]

potential amplitude and presynaptic depolarization is initially linear, the relationship becomes nonlinear with a decrease in slope at more intense depolarizations. This is apparent in Fig. 7. Inset (A) shows a diagrammatic representation of the squid synapse with two electrodes (a and b) in the presynaptic terminal and one (c) in the postsynaptic axon. Current was passed through electrode (a) causing a depolarization which was recorded with electrode (b). This presynaptic depolarization is plotted against the resultant postsynaptic potential with a linear ordinate in B and C and a logarithmic ordinate in D. The decrease in slope with presynaptic depolarizations greater than 40–50 mV is very clear in D. In the experiments illustrated in Fig. 7 (Katz and Miledi, 1967b) the electrode which recorded the presynaptic membrane potential was closer to the synaptic region than in the experiment illustrated in Fig. 6, and it is probably that the curve would be even further to the left in the actual region of the membrane where transmitter is released. Consequently, the exact relationship between presynaptic depolarization and transmitter release may need to be revised when it is possible to control adequately the membrane potential over the whole of the presynaptic membrane.

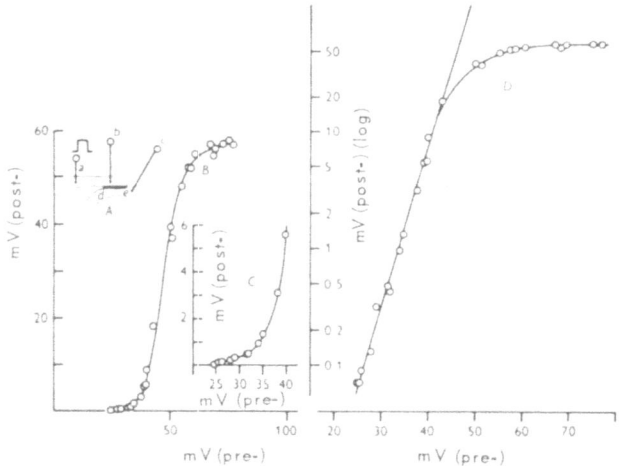

Fig. 7. Example of input/output curves. Inset A: diagram of electrode positions a and b in presynaptic axon and c in the postsynaptic. Length of synapse d–e: 0.8 mm. a: current electrode; b: prerecording electrode; c: postrecording electrode. a–d, 0.6 mm; d–b, 0.35 mm. Curve B: relation between pre- (abscissas) and post- (ordinates) potentials. 1-msec pulses. Series was taken 50 min after raising calcium concentration from 11 to 58 mM. Inset C: initial part of relation in greater detail. Curve D: semilogarithmic plot of input/output relation. Slope in D corresponds to a 10-fold change of postpotential for 7.5 mV change in prepotential. [Katz and Miledi (1967), J. Physiol., 192:407.]

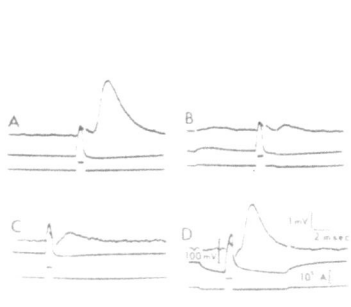

Fig. 8. Effect of background polarization on the release of transmitter in response to a standard 1-msec depolarization of the presynaptic membrane. Upper trace shows postsynaptic potentials (calibration: D, upper right), the middle trace shows presynaptic potentials (calibration: D, left), and the lower trace shows presynaptic current (calibration: D, lower right). A and B were recorded in one experiment, C and D in another. A and C show control responses produced by depolarization of the presynaptic membrane to a determined level. B, which is comparable with A, shows the postsynaptic response to the same depolarization as in A in the presence of a 10-msec background depolarization. D, which is comparable with C, shows the postsynaptic response to the same level of membrane depolarization as in C in the presence of a 10-msec background hyperpolarization. Time calibration: D, upper right. Tetrodotoxin, 2×10^{-7} g/ml. Temp. 8–10°C. [Gage (1967), *Fed. Proc.*, **26**:1627.]

When constant current pulses longer than 1 or 2 msec are injected into squid presynaptic terminals, the initial depolarization is not maintained because of an increase in potassium conductance which is not blocked by tetrodotoxin. Under these conditions, transmitter is released only by the initial peak depolarization, and this indicates that it is the membrane potential, not the current, which governs transmitter release. If this is so, why has it been found that the size of postsynaptic potentials is related to the amplitude of presynaptic action potentials modified by hyperpolarizing or depolarizing the presynaptic membrane? The results of further experiments in squid synapses exposed to tetrodotoxin (Bloedel *et al.*, 1966b; Katz and Miledi, 1967b) indicate that polarization of the presynaptic membrane directly affects excitation–secretion coupling. One of these experiments is illustrated in Fig. 8. In A, a postsynaptic potential (upper trace) was elicited by the 1-msec presynaptic depolarization shown in the middle trace. In B, a 10-msec conditioning depolarizing pulse was passed through the presynaptic membrane, and during it a 1-msec depolarizing pulse was superimposed to bring the presynaptic membrane potential to the same absolute level. It is evident that the background depolarization markedly depressed transmitter release. A similar experiment, this time using background hyperpolarization, is shown in C and D, and it can be seen that hyperpolarization increased transmitter release. In fact, hyperpolarizing pulses which were terminated up to 10-msec before a depolarizing stimulus were effective in increasing transmitter release (Bloedel *et al.*, 1966b). It seems not unlikely

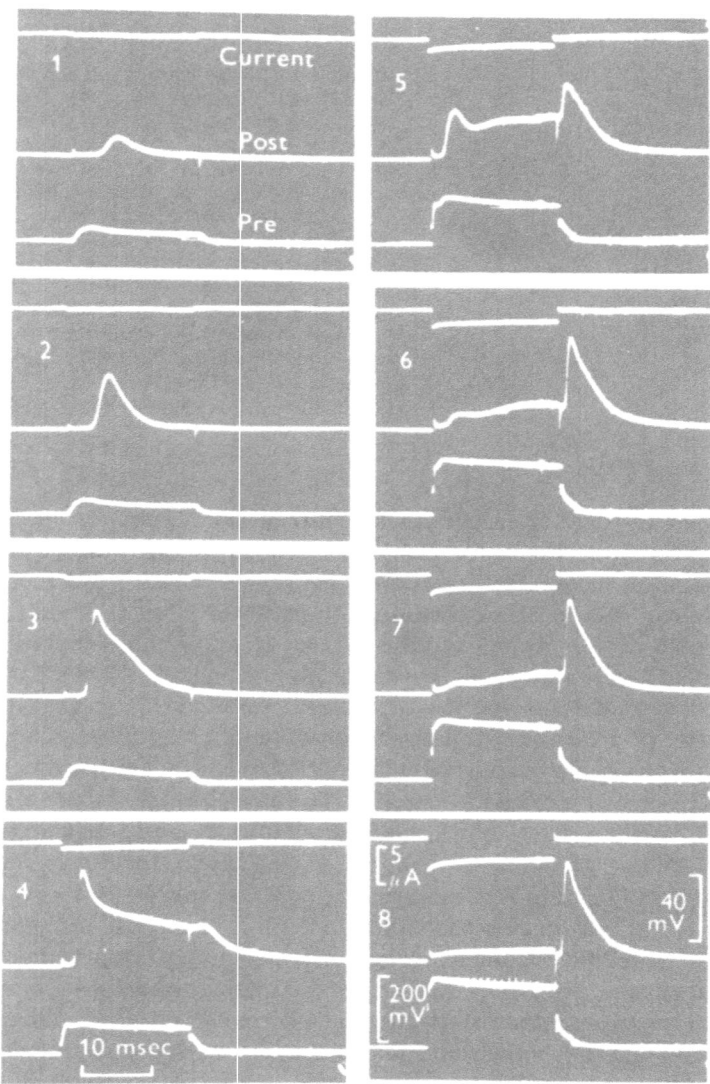

Fig. 9. Sample records of long current pulses (upper traces in each block, 1–8) and resulting pre- (lower traces) and post- (middle traces) potentials after iontophoretic loading of the terminal with tetraethylammonium. Note gradual change from ON to OFF response. [Katz and Miledi (1967), *J. Physiol.*, **192**:407.]

that imposed changes of the membrane potential of presynaptic terminals would affect in a similar way the amount of transmitter released by an action potential, and this would explain previous observations which sought to relate the amplitudes of presynaptic action potentials and postsynaptic potentials. The depression of transmitter release caused by background depolarization would also explain the depression of transmitter release which occurs in presynaptic inhibition.

In further experiments with the same preparation exposed to tetrodotoxin, Katz and Miledi (1967b) and Kusano et al., (1967) injected tetraethylammonium ions into presynaptic terminals so that potassium conductance would not increase during imposed depolarizations, which could then be prolonged. One such experiment is illustrated in Fig. 9. In each group of traces (1–8), the upper trace shows the presynaptic current injection, the middle the postsynaptic potential, and the lower trace the presynaptic potential. Transmitter release did not continue for the same length of time as the pulse. As the degree of presynaptic depolarization was increased, transmitter release during the pulse also increased at first (Fig. 9, 1–4). Then as the presynaptic membrane was depolarized even more (Fig. 9, 5–8), the postsynaptic potential became smaller during the stimulus, whereas a postsynaptic potential occurred following it. These results are consistent with the hypothesis that depolarization of presynaptic terminals causes an increase in calcium conductance. This allows an influx of calcium ions which in turn causes transmitter release. During very large depolarizations the increased internal positivity would tend to oppose inward movement of calcium ions, and hence transmitter release would tend to be inhibited. When the depolarization is terminated, it is proposed that the increased conductance of the membrane to calcium ions persists for a short time so that calcium can enter the terminal and cause transmitter release. In further such experiments, Katz and Miledi (1969) have found that depolarization of the terminals of presynaptic nerves produces a small regenerative inward current which is restricted to the presynaptic terminal and depends on the presence of calcium ions in the extracellular solution. The current increases in size and duration as the calcium concentration is increased, and it is suggested that this current represents the influx of calcium ions which causes transmitter release. By inhibiting the sodium current which normally obscures any other inward currents, tetrodotoxin has allowed the discovery of this relatively very small but important ionic flux.

It has long been known that the second of two closely spaced action potentials in a nerve terminal causes the release of more transmitter than the first, a phenomenon known as facilitation. Takeuchi and Takeuchi (1962) suggested that in the squid this was due to an increase in the amplitude of the second action potential. In tetrodotoxin-treated squid synapses it was found (Bloedel *et al.*, 1966a) that the second of two identical depolarizations caused the release of more transmitter than the first when the time interval between them was short. Thus facilitation must be due to some change in excitation–secretion coupling and is not dependent on an increase in the amplitude of a second action potential.

These experiments in which tetrodotoxin has been used as a pharmacological tool have yielded a wealth of information about the process of transmitter release. It is now clear that neither a change in sodium conductance nor an influx of sodium ions is necessary for the release of transmitter, and that the degree of activation of the release process is dependent on the level of the membrane potential of the presynaptic terminal. It is now possible to explore the relationship between presynaptic depolarization and transmitter release in these preparations free of action potentials, and further studies of the biophysics of synaptic transmission will no doubt be heavily dependent on the use of these toxins.

C. Central Nervous System

The effects of tetrodotoxin and saxitoxin on peripheral nerves have been extrapolated with some success to the central nervous system. There is need for some caution, however, since there is very little direct evidence that in all neurons in the central nervous system action potentials are sodium-dependent, or that there is an early transient channel operating as in peripheral nerve. One way of testing the effectiveness of the drugs is to record electrical activity in tissues exposed to them. In experiments where this has been done, electrical activity has indeed been abolished (Colomo and Erulkar, 1968; Blankenship, 1968). The efficacy of these drugs in blocking action potentials should of course be tested wherever they are used for this purpose.

In neurons in the central nervous system, synaptic potentials occur without stimulation of presynaptic fibers, either because of spontaneous action potentials in presynaptic terminals or because of the spontaneous release of quanta of transmitter. This constant background synaptic activity is called "synaptic noise." In cats, tetrodotoxin so reduces this noise that it was concluded that most synaptic noise is due to transmitter release evoked by spontaneous nerve impulses and can be removed by abolition of nerve impulses (Hubbard *et al.*, 1967). Blankenship (1968) and Blankenship and Kuno (1968) confirmed these observations by recording from individual motoneurons exposed to tetrodotoxin. They observed a decline of spontaneous synaptic activity and the disappearance of large potentials. On the other hand, tetrodotoxin has little effect on synaptic noise in frog neurons (Colomo and Erulkar, 1968), and it would appear that most of the spontaneous potentials are analogous to miniature endplate potentials which are not dependent on presynaptic action potentials. The observation of spontaneous hyperpolarizing potentials in the latter investigation is consistent with a quantal mechanism of transmitter release at inhibitory synapses. A possibility, which was mentioned but not excluded by Colomo and Erulkar (1968), is that some neurons with inputs to the neurons being examined may have had spontaneous action potentials which were resistant to tetrodotoxin. This is a particularly troublesome possibility since Koketsu and Nishi (1968) have found action potentials in the sympathetic ganglion of the frog are indeed resistant to tetrodotoxin.

There have been some more general investigations of the effect of tetrodotoxin on the central nervous system. Koizumi et al. (1967) injected tetrodotoxin intravenously (1–3 μg/kg) in cats and found that although neuromuscular transmission was not blocked by this dose, spinal monosynaptic and polysynaptic reflexes were depressed. Autonomic neurons were also depressed, and vasomotor reflexes were abolished before peripheral neurons were blocked. It was suggested that the hypotension produced by the toxin is due to its action on higher medullary vasomotor centers, because injections of similar quantities of toxin failed to produce significant hypotension in "spinal" animals whereas the hypotensive effect was present in decerebrate animals. It was deduced from similar evidence that respiratory depression is also due to an effect of the toxin on the central nervous system rather than on the afferent nerves or muscles of respiration. The observation that vasomotor and cortical activities were abolished at lower concentrations than were required to block peripheral axons suggests that some central nerve cells might be highly susceptible to the toxin. It would be very interesting to see the results of more direct tests of this hypothesis. However other experiments have suggested another mechanism for the hypotension. In dogs, tetrodotoxin (0.5–0.8 μg/kg) causes a fall in perfusion pressure in blood vessels of gracilis muscles isolated from the systemic circulation and perfused by a constant-volume pump (Lipsius et al., 1968). Since these doses did not block the reflex vasomotor effects on perfusion pressure caused by changes in systemic blood pressure or the effects of stimulating sympathetic nerves, the fall in perfusion pressure was attributed to a direct relaxant effect of the toxin on the vascular smooth muscle. The fall in perfusion pressure occurred even after alpha or beta adrenergic blockade. It should be possible to confirm these findings in isolated strips of vascular smooth muscle.

Tetrodotoxin appears to act on cells in the lateral geniculate body and dorsal hippocampus of cats (Hafemann et al., 1969). Injection of tetrodotoxin into the lateral geniculate reduced the amplitude of flash-evoked potentials. Crawford and Shibata (1968) injected tetrodotoxin into the lateral cerebral ventricle of rats and found that photic-evoked potentials were completely inhibited. The electroencephalogram also showed significant changes. In isolated slabs of cortex, tetrodotoxin inhibits the potentials normally evoked by electrical stimulation (Frank and Pinsky, 1966). Though these experiments demonstrate that tetrodotoxin does affect nerve cells in the central nervous system, elucidation of specific cellular or local effects will require more refined approaches.

Biochemists also have used tetrodotoxin in studies of the central nervous system. For example, Chan and Quastel (1967) have shown that electrical stimulation of slices of rat cortex usually stimulates respiration, but tetrodotoxin almost completely inhibits this effect. The increased respiration caused by stimulating the slices with potassium chloride is not affected by the toxin. The results were interpreted as indicating that it is the influx of sodium ions during action potentials which stimulates respiration in this tissue. Similar effects have been reported in slices of guinea pig neocortex by McIlwain (1966) who found that sodium entry and potassium loss in brain slices is inhibited by tetrodotoxin in stimulated but not resting preparations.

It is clear that such investigations dependent on the use of tetrodotoxin have already been fruitful, and when a more selective and quantitative approach is used, much useful information should be obtained about the central actions of the toxins at a cellular level. It would be very interesting if some areas or tracts in the brain proved to be insensitive to tetrodotoxin. This is not beyond the realm of possibility in view of the insensitivity of some cells in other species to the toxins. It may even prove feasible using electrical recording techniques to trace pathways and connections of such cells because of their persistent electrical activity in the presence of tetrodotoxin or saxitoxin.

To move to an even more speculative plane, it should prove possible to produce pharmacological lesions in the central nervous system by localized injections of the toxins. Of course some steps would have to be taken to prevent the agents which are freely diffusible from diffusing away from target areas, but such a pharmacological problem does not seem insurmountable to a physiologist.

D. Generator Potentials

Tetrodotoxin and saxitoxin can be used to eliminate action potentials in receptor organs, and investigators have not been slow to seize this opportunity. In the crustacean stretch receptor neuron, tetrodotoxin selectively inhibits action potentials but leaves generator potentials intact although the latter are sodium dependent (Lowenstein et al., 1963; Albuquerque and Grampp, 1968). The relationship between length or tension of the receptor and the size of the generator potential can be examined in these preparations without the complication of extraneous potentials caused by regenerative conductance changes in the membrane (Nakajima and Onodera, 1969a,b).

In Pacinian corpuscles, the picture is at present more complicated. Lowenstein *et al.* (1963) found that tetrodotoxin had no effect on generator potentials in these receptors, but Ozeki and Sato (1965) and Nishi and Sato (1966) observed a reduction of up to 40% in the amplitude of generator potentials after 30–60 min in the toxin. This latter observation was explained on the basis of an effect of tetrodotoxin on the sodium conductance system responsible for the generator potential. However, it is possible that tetrodotoxin does not affect directly this sodium conductance mechanism but has an indirect effect because of the inhibition of action potentials. For example, an influx of sodium during action potentials may be necessary for the maintenance of membrane integrity. Further experiments are obviously necessary to clarify this issue.

When tetrodotoxin is iontophoretically injected in the region of hair cells in the guinea pig cochlea, axonal action potentials are abolished but cochlear microphonic potentials persist (Katsuki *et al.*, 1966). This indicates that cochlear microphonics are probably not caused by sodium-dependent action potentials and probably result from a generator potential mechanism.

If the lateral eye of *Limulus* is stimulated with a flash of light, a triphasic response can be recorded from the visual cells. This response consists of a short initial pulse, a transient component and a steady-state component which persists for the duration of the stimulus. Tetrodotoxin reversibly blocks the graded transient component of this response when higher concentrations are used than required to block neural responses (Benolken and Russell, 1967). Occasionally a decline in the steady state response can be seen after prolonged exposure to higher concentrations of toxin. Before concluding that tetrodotoxin is here affecting a graded generator potential it will be necessary to demonstrate that the transient response is not in fact due to a regenerative sodium conductance increase. Indeed, it was noted (Benolken and Russell, 1967) that the transient response does exhibit regenerative properties in part of its range. It is interesting to note in this context that the receptor potential of the retinula cell of the honeybee contains a transient component which is sodium dependent and abolished by tetrodotoxin (Baumann, 1968). Transient responses with similar properties could be obtained by depolarizing the membrane. In contrast, a graded transient "spike" evoked by current or light stimulation of ventral photoreceptor cells of *Limulus* is insensitive to tetrodotoxin up to a concentration of 10^{-5} g/ml (Millecchia and Mauro, 1969).

Although there are some apparent exceptions at present, the generator or receptor potentials induced in a variety of cells by external stimuli are generally not inhibited by tetrodotoxin. This indicates some difference between the early transient voltage-dependent channel and the channels responsible for generator potentials. Tetrodotoxin should prove very useful in exploring these differences. Certainly for those who cherish unitary hypotheses, the observation that some apparent generator potentials are sensitive to tetrodotoxin should be a challenge to prove that they are not in fact generator potentials.

E. Action Potentials Not Dependent on Sodium Ions

Evidence presently available indicates that tetrodotoxin and saxitoxin block only those action potentials which are normally sodium-dependent. In some cells, the inward current during an action potential is carried by calcium ions, not sodium ions, and the calcium ions do not pass through an early transient channel sensitive to tetrodotoxin. The effect of tetrodotoxin on some of these cells will be discussed briefly.

Muscle fibers in many arthropods have these calcium-dependent action potentials which have been found to be resistant to tetrodotoxin. Action potentials in the giant muscle fibers of barnacles do not respond to tetrodotoxin but are inhibited by manganese ions, which block voltage-dependent increases in calcium conductance in many tissues (Hagiwara and Nakajima, 1966). Lobster muscles also have calcium-dependent spikes which are resistant to tetrodotoxin (Ozeki et al., 1966).

The rapid phase of the action potential in frog ventricle seems to be due to an increase in sodium conductance, while the overshoot is determined at least to some extent by an increase in calcium conductance (Orkand and Niedergerke, 1964). The rate of rise of these action potentials is markedly reduced by tetrodotoxin whereas the overshoot is little affected (Hagiwara and Nakajima, 1966). In the short Purkinje fibers of sheep, tetrodotoxin at concentrations from 10^{-5} to 10^{-8} g/ml has no effect on the rate of rise or duration of action potentials (Dudel et al., 1967). At 10^{-5} g/ml there was a progressive small depolarization, the rate of rise of action potentials was slowed and the plateau phase was shortened. However, the membrane currents recorded under voltage clamp conditions were not the same as those seen in sodium-free solutions. These results may have been affected by the presence of the citrate buffer which at these concentrations of tetrodotoxin may have lowered the calcium concentration.

In many smooth muscle fibers also, it appears that action potentials are dependent on calcium rather than sodium ions and are resistant to tetrodotoxin. The smooth muscle fibers of guinea-pig *Taenia coli* for example have action potentials which are resistant to tetrodotoxin (Kuriyama et al., 1966; Nonomura et al., 1966), but the electrical response produced by nerve elements in the same tissue is blocked by the toxin (Bulbring and Tomita, 1967). In the smooth muscle of the vas deferens of guinea pigs and mice, where it is thought that calcium ions are involved in action potentials, tetrodotoxin in concentrations up to 10^{-6} g/ml has no effect on directly elicited action potentials, though the lack of response to stimulation of afferent nerves showed that the nerves were blocked (Hashimoto *et al.*, 1967). The toxins should prove useful in studies of transmission at autonomic neuromuscular junctions since they block action potentials in presynaptic nerves but presumably do not affect the secretion or effectiveness of transmitters. Indeed, it has already been shown that tetrodotoxin does not reduce the response of smooth muscles in several tissues to nicotine, tyramine, or noradrenaline, indicating that the postsynaptic conductance changes caused by these chemicals are not impaired (Bell, 1968).

Not only muscle fibers but also some neurons have these "calcium spikes." Bullfrog sympathetic ganglion cells (Koketsu and Nishi, 1969) and molluscan nerve cells (Chamberlain and Kerkut, 1967) can produce action potentials in isotonic calcium chloride solution, and these action potentials are insensitive to tetrodotoxin.

In the giant plant cell (*Nitella*) action potentials are caused by an efflux of chloride ions, and again this sodium-independent mechanism is immune to the effects of tetrodotoxin even at high concentrations (cited by Kao, 1964).

From these examples in a variety of tissues it is clear that some cells can function quite adequately with calcium instead of sodium as the ion carrying inward current during action potentials. In many investigations the insensitivity of action potentials to tetrodotoxin has been used as evidence that they are not caused by an increase in sodium conductance. Such evidence should be complemented by the demonstration that the action potentials do not depend on the presence of sodium ions, since it is possible that some sodium-dependent action potentials may prove not to be sensitive to tetrodotoxin. This has indeed been demonstrated in nerve fibers of pufferfish and newts.

F. General

The possible influence of tetrodotoxin and saxitoxin on sodium ion movements in resting membranes will not be discussed in any detail. There have been few reports of conclusive investigations of such effects, but it has been noted that tetrodotoxin does not affect the resting membrane potential of muscle or nerve fibers (Narahashi *et al.*, 1960, 1964; Nishi and Sato, 1966; Narahashi *et al.*, 1967). If the passive fluxes of sodium were inhibited by the toxins, some membrane hyperpolarization should be seen. The most direct way of ascertaining whether the resting sodium conductance channels are blocked would be to measure unidirectional fluxes of sodium ions. At the same time exchange diffusion and active transport of sodium ions could be examined. It has been reported that tetrodotoxin at a concentration of 3.6×10^{-4} M inhibits active sodium transport and lowers oxygen consumption in toad bladder (Marumo *et al.*, 1968). This is a very high concentration of toxin and the citrate concentration was presumably high also.

In the kidney, there are large fluxes of sodium ions across the membranes of renal epithelial cells, but little is known of the permeability mechanisms responsible. When tetrodotoxin is injected into the renal arteries of dogs in concentrations of the order of 25 nM, the renal excretion of a number of inorganic ions but especially sodium is significantly increased (Pullman *et al.*, 1968). The possibility that the effect was due to the citrate ions present with the tetrodotoxin was excluded in control experiments. The observation is striking but difficult to explain. It is possible that the increased excretion of sodium is due to a vascular effect of the toxin leading to a redistribution of renal blood flow. Alternatively, tetrodotoxin may affect active sodium transport or passive sodium fluxes in these cells. It is hoped that further experiments will throw more light both on the physiology of the cells responsible and on the mode of action of tetrodotoxin in this tissue.

Tetrodotoxin is now being used regularly in experiments on muscle fibers to inhibit action potentials so that membranes can be depolarized in a graded manner without the supervention of action potentials. For example, Adrian *et al.* (1969) used tetrodotoxin so that the membrane potential of frog skeletal muscle fibers could be voltage-clamped at different levels. In these experiments an action potential from a normal muscle fiber was used as the command signal for a voltage-clamped fiber in tetrodotoxin, and it was discovered that the central myofibrils did not contract unless the imposed "action potential" was of normal size. These experiments would not have been possible without an agent like tetrodotoxin. Gage and Eisenberg (1969) used tetrodotoxin to prevent the twitches which occurred as transverse tubules were being disrupted in glycerol-treated muscle fibers and concluded that the twitches were caused by spontaneous action potentials. These could sometimes be recorded but the contractions made use of intracellular microelectrodes difficult. Tetrodotoxin stopped the twitches and allowed the electrical properties of the fibers to be investigated.

IV. CONCLUSION

It is apparent that tetrodotoxin has been used more widely than saxitoxin in physiological experiments, no doubt because tetrodotoxin is commercially available. Saxitoxin, however, would probably be more useful because its effects are more readily reversible. A wide variety of tissues has been exposed to the toxins which have now become established as useful adjuvants to the pharmacological armamentarium of physiologists. In the future, the basis of the effect of the toxins on the early transient channel may be learned, and perhaps inexpensive, equally active analogs will be synthesized. It is possible that these toxins may be the forerunners of a new family of general and local anesthetics, as well as serving as indispensable aids to physiologists in their invasion of the secrets of membranes.

V. REFERENCES

Adrian, R. H., L. L. Constantin, and L. D. Peachey (1969), *J. Physiol.*, **204**:231.
Albuquerque, E. X. and W. Gramp (1968), *J. Physiol.*, **195**:141.
Armstrong, C. M. and L. Binstock (1965), *J. Gen. Physiol.*, **48**:859.
Baumann, F. (1968), *J. Gen. Physiol.*, **52**:855.
Bell, C. (1968), *Brit. J. Pharm. Chemother*, **32**:96.
Benolken, R. M. and C. J. Russell (1967), *Science*, **155**:1576.
Blankenship, J. E. (1968), *J. Neurophysiol.*, **31**:186.
Blankenship, J. E. and M. Kuno (1968), *J. Neurophysiol.*, **31**:195.
Bloedel, J., P. W. Gage, R. Llinás, and D. M. J. Quastel (1966a), *Nature*, **212**:49.
Bloedel, J. R., P. W. Gage, R. Llinás, and D. M. J. Quastel (1966b), *J. Physiol.*, **188**:52.
Bülbring, E. and T. Tomita (1967), *J. Physiol.*, **189**:299.
Chamberlain, S. G. and G. S. Kerkut (1967), *Nature*, **216**:89.
Chan, S. L. and J. H. Quastel (1967), *Science*, **156**:1752.
Colomo, F. and S. D. Erulkar (1968), *J. Physiol.*, **199**:205.
Crawford, M. L. J. and S. Shibata (1968), *Brit. J. Pharm. Chemother.*, **32**:25.
Dudel, J., K. Peper, R. Rudel, and W. Trautwein (1967), *Nature*, **213**:296.
Elmqvist, D. and D. S. Feldman (1965), *Acta Physiol. Scand.*, **64**:475.
Frank, G. B. and C. Pinsky (1966), *Brit. J. Pharmacol.*, **26**:435.
Gage, P. W. (1967), *Fed. Proc.*, **26**:1627.
Gage, P. W. and R. S. Eisenberg (1969), *J. Gen. Physiol.*, **53**:265.
Hafemann, D. R., A. Costin, and T. J. Tarby (1969), *Brain Research*, **12**:363.
Hagiwara, S. and S. Nakajima (1966), *J. Gen. Physiol.*, **49**:793.
Hagiwara, S. and I. Tasaki (1958), *J. Physiol.*, **143**:114.
Hashimoto, Y., M. E. Holman, and A. J. McLean (1967), *Nature*, **215**:430.
Hille, B. (1968), *J. Gen. Physiol.*, **51**:199.
Hodgkin, A. L. (1964), "The conduction of the nervous impulse," Liverpool University Press, England.
Hodgkin, A. L. and A. F. Huxley (1952a), *J. Physiol.*, **116**:449.
Hodgkin, A. L. and A. F. Huxley (1952b), *J. Physiol.*, **116**:473.
Hodgkin, A. L. and A. F. Huxley (1952c), *J. Physiol.*, **116**:497.
Hodgkin, A. L. and A. F. Huxley (1952d), *J. Physiol.*, **117**:500.
Hubbard, J. I., D. Stenhouse, and R. M. Eccles (1967), *Science*, **157**:330.
Kao, C. Y. (1964), *Pharmacol. Rev.*, **18**:997.
Katsuki, Y., K. Yanagisawa, and J. Kanzaki (1966), *Science*, **151**:1544.
Katz, B. and R. Miledi (1967a), *Proc. Roy. Soc. B.*, **167**:8.
Katz, B. and R. Miledi (1967b), *J. Physiol.*, **192**:407.
Katz, B. and R. Miledi (1969), *J. Physiol.*, **203**:459.
Koizumi, K., D. G. Levine, and C. McC. Brooks (1967), *Neurology*, **17**:395.
Koketsu, K. and S. Nishi (1969), *J. Gen. Physiol.*, **53**:608.
Kuriyama, H., T. Osa, and N. Toida (1966), *Br. J. Pharmac. Chemother.*, **27**:366.
Kusano, K., D. R. Livengood, and R. Werman (1967), *J. Gen. Physiol.*, **50**:2579.
Liley, A. W. (1956), *J. Physiol.*, **134**:427.
Lipsius, M. R., M. J. Siegman, and C. Y. Kao (1968), *J. Pharm. Exp. Ther.*, **164**:60.
Lowenstein, W. R., C. A. Terzuolo, and Y. Washizu (1963), *Science*, **10**:1180.
McIlwain, H. (1967), *J. Physiol.*, **190**:39P.

212   Peter W. Gage

Marumo, F., T. Yamada, Y. Asano, T. Sasaoka, A. Yoshida, and H. Endou (1968), *Pflugers Arch.*, **303**:49.
Miledi, R. and C. R. Slater (1966), *J. Physiol.*, **184**:473.
Millecchia, R. and A. Mauro (1969), *J. Gen. Physiol.*, **54**:310.
Moore, J. W., M. P. Blaustein, N. C. Anderson, and T. Narahashi (1967), *J. Gen. Physiol.*, **50**:1401.
Moore, J. W., T. Narahashi, and T. I. Shaw (1967), *J. Physiol.*, **188**:99.
Nakajima, S. and K. Onodera (1969a), *J. Physiol.*, **200**:161.
Nakajima, S. and K. Onodera (1969b), *J. Physiol.*, **200**:187.
Narahashi, T., T. Deguchi, N. Urakawa, and U. Ohkubo (1960), *Amer. J. Physiol.*, **198**:934.
Narahashi, T., J. W. Moore, and W. Scott (1964), *J. Gen. Physiol.*, **47**:965.
Narahashi, T., N. C. Anderson, and J. W. Moore (1966), *Science*, **153**:765.
Narahashi, T., J. W. Moore, and R. N. Poston (1966), *Science*, **154**:425.
Narahashi, T., N. C. Anderson, and J. W. Moore (1967), *J. Gen. Physiol.*, **50**:1413.
Narahashi, T., J. W. Moore, and R. N. Poston (1967), *Science*, **156**:976.
Nishi, K. and M. Sato (1966), *J. Physiol.*, **184**:376.
Nonomura, Y., Y. Hotta, and H. Ohashi (1966), *Science*, **152**:97.
Orkand, R. K. and R. Niedergerke (1964), *Science*, **146**:1176.
Ozeki, M. and M. Sato (1965), *J. Physiol.*, **180**:186.
Ozeki, M., A. R. Freeman, and H. Grundfest (1966), *J. Gen. Physiol.*, **49**:1319.
Pullman, T. N., A. R. Lavender, and I. Aho (1968), *Proc. Nat. Acad. Sci.*, **60**:822.
Shanes, A. M., W. H. Freygang, H. Grundfest, and E. Amatniek (1959), *J. Gen. Physiol.*, **42**:793.
Takata, M., J. W. Moore, C. Y. Kao, and F. A. Fuhrman (1966), *J. Gen. Physiol.*, **49**:977.
Takeuchi, A. and N. Takeuchi (1962), *J. Gen. Physiol.*, **45**:1181.
Tasaki, I. and I. Singer (1966), *Ann. N. Y. Acad. Sci.*, **137**:792.
Taylor, R. E. (1959), *Amer. J. Physiol.*, **196**:1071.

Chapter 10

The Clinical Effects of Tetanus

Edward Barry Adams

Department of Medicine
University of Natal
Congella, Durban, South Africa

I. TETANUS: THE WORLD PROBLEM

At least a million people suffered from tetanus, and half of them died during the ten-year period 1951–1960, according to Bytchenko (1966) who reviewed, for the World Health Organization, available data from around the world. These stark figures establish the importance of the disease and indicate how dangerous it can be.

Asia provided the greatest number of cases, as might be anticipated from the size of its population, and although notifications were incomplete, the highest incidence appears to have been in India. Other records show 1565 people died from tetanus in Indonesia over a two-year period, 445 deaths occurred in Turkey in one year, and in Japan there were 10 times as many deaths from tetanus as from typhoid.

National totals are impressive, but a practicing physician is likely to know only one or two hospitals intimately, so some hospital statistics are quoted. One Bombay hospital had 4733 patients with tetanus over an eight-year period, almost 2% of all admissions; 2000 were admitted with this disease to a hospital in Delhi in three years; over the space of nine years 1062 children with tetanus were treated in a Djakarta hospital.

Numerous reports show how common tetanus is in Central and South America. The highest mortality rate recorded in Central America came from the Dominican Republic (63.3 deaths per 100,000). Such figures are often less impressive than actual numbers of deaths, as shown in a report from São Paulo where the mortality rate per 100,000 was 9.8, with deaths from this cause in the whole state for the period 1950–1958 amounting to 13,299.

Information from Africa is less detailed, but nevertheless indicates that tetanus is a very common cause of death in many areas. One South African hospital admits 150 cases a year (Adams *et al.*, 1966), and there is a similar prevalence in Nigeria.

As might be anticipated from the more advanced immunization programs practised, the incidence of the disease is much less in North America and in many parts of Europe. Even there however, it remains a significant cause of death. In the developed countries "factors such as industrialisation, urbanisation, mechanisation of agriculture, the widespread use of chemical fertilizers rather than animal dung and improvements in education, the standard of living, and public health services" have substantially reduced the incidence of the disease (Bytchenko, 1966).

It seems that tetanus is an important problem in most developing countries and a constant source of danger everywhere. Although the disease may occur at any age, it is the young who are most frequently affected. Tetanus neonatorum contributes significantly to the high perinatal death rate in countries with low hygienic standards and poorly developed health services; in such places the toll of deaths in children and young adults is also high. The incidence of the disease reaches a peak in the tropical countries, being favored by warm, damp climates and heavily manured soil. This distinction is clearly shown in Southern Africa where the disease is very common in the coastal belt of Natal, which is warm and humid, but rare in Lesotho, a dry, mountainous state some 200 miles away.

II. CLINICAL FEATURES

After gaining entry to the body, generally following wounding of some sort, and when anaerobic conditions develop, *Clostridium tetani* produce two toxins, tetanospasmin and tetanolysin. Only the former gives rise to significant clinical effects. Two striking manifestations are caused by this neurotoxin, and they dominate the clinical picture. These are rigidity of muscles, which occurs in every case, and reflex spasms, which are fortunately not invariably present. The cumulative effect of both of these phenomena, continued over many days, leads to one overriding danger—respiratory failure. These are the cardinal features of the disease. They are stated here in advance of a discussion of its natural history for the sake of emphasis, because the role of each must be fully appreciated if the disease is to be successfully treated.

Rigidity of muscles shows itself in various ways, several or all of which may be present at the same time. When the muscles of the jaw are stiff and the mouth cannot be fully opened, the patient is said to have trismus or "lockjaw." Stiffness of facial muscles alters the expression, particularly when the patient smiles. The peculiar sneering appearance which results from pursing of the lips and retraction of the angles of the mouth is the *risus sardonicus*, a typical feature of tetanus. Pharyngeal muscle involvement causes dysphagia, which is often an early symptom. Simultaneous neck stiffness, abdominal rigidity, splinting of the muscles of the thorax and the back, and stiffness of the arms and legs gives rise to a characteristic ram-rod appearance, and when the sardonic smile is added there can be little doubt about the diagnosis. Sometimes, however, the shortening of the long spinal muscles is excessive, the body is curved backwards and the head fully re-tracted. This is opisthotonos, a very striking manifestation of the disease.

In the case of newborn infants there are additional features. The arms and legs may be held slightly flexed, with the arms partly crossed over the abdomen and the hands clenched. Sometimes the tip of the thumb may be seen protruding between the index and middle fingers. The cry is stifled, the face wrinkling up at the same time. Pharyngeal stiffness impairs sucking. The cry and this difficulty at the breast are often the first abnormalities noticed by the mother.

A *reflex spasm* consists of a sudden exacerbation of the underlying rigidity. It may be mild in degree and last only a second or two. More commonly, however, a reflex spasm is an alarming and dramatic event. Suddenly there is simultaneous and excessive contraction of muscles and their antagonists and the posture of the patient is exaggerated for several seconds before relaxation to the previous tonic state of the muscles occurs. Such contractions cause splinting of the thoracic cage, and respiration is impeded or becomes impossible until the spasm passes off. Spasms may follow one another in rapid succession, so that pulmonary ventilation is seriously impaired and cyanosis results. Excessive secretions frequently collect in the mouth and upper air passages; breathing becomes noisy and bubbling, obviously adding to the patient's discomfort. Less obvious, perhaps, but more important, is the fact that these secretions are often inhaled into the lungs when the spasm is over and the patient is breathing deeply to make up his oxygen debt. Little areas of atelectasis follow, or if the plug is bigger, a segment of the lung collapses; since the inhaled secretions are often infected, pneumonia supervenes.

Spasm of the larynx is the most dramatic and perhaps the most dan-gerous event in tetanus. The upper respiratory passages are obstructed, gaseous exchange becomes impossible, cyanosis occurs and death may follow if the spsam does not pass off shortly, or if it is not quickly relieved by medical intervention.

Apnea may occur after repeated spasms or after laryngeal spasms, but sometimes the patient suddenly stops breathing for no obvious reason. All these events—repeated spasms impeding adequate respiration, laryngeal spasms, the inhalation of secretions, atelectasis, pneumonia, and apneic attacks—play a part in the onset of respiratory failure. This, in reality, is the central problem in the management of tetanus.

III. THE NATURAL HISTORY OF TETANUS

Initial symptoms, consisting of trismus, pain in the neck, or muscle stiffness in children and adults, usually come on a week or so after an injury of some sort; in the newborn the first manifestation—crying or refusal to suck—follow the cutting of the cord at birth without proper aseptic precautions. The *incubation period*, the time in days between the injury and the first symptom, varies considerably but is generally less than 14 days in all but the mildest cases. Short periods of 4–6 days are quite common, however, especially in neonates. Occasionally the incubation period may be only 1 or 2 days or on the other hand as long as 3 months.

As a generalization it can be said that the shortest incubation periods carry the worst prognosis. Numerous reports bear this out. In a series of 297 non-neonatal cases, the case fatality rate was over 60% when the incubation period was less than 9 days and only 25% when it was 9 days or more; the difference was even more striking in the newborn (Adams, 1968). In many cases, however, it is difficult to be sure when the contaminated wound occurred. Most cases of tetanus follow minor trauma, presumably because major wounds are more often properly dealt with; often patients with tetanus are seen to have several minor lesions or are not certain when wounding occurred. Moreover, in about 20% of cases no wound whatever can be detected. Too much reliance, therefore, should not be placed on the incubation period as a guide to prognosis.

The first spasms may occur shortly after the first symptom of the disease or many days later. The interval in hours between the first symptom and the first spasm, known as the *period of onset*, is one of the most important observations in tetanus. A short period of onset usually carries a bad prognosis, the trend being similar to that in regard to short and long incubation periods. In one large series of over 3000 cases of non-neonatal tetanus, the case fatality rate was 63% for periods of onset under 48 hr and 22% for periods longer than 48 hr (Patel *et al.*, 1965a); in the case of the newborn the difference has been shown to be just as striking (Adams, 1968).

Used as a prognostic index, the period of onset in tetanus is more valuable than the incubation period since it relies less on the patient's memory and more on medical observation, and can be applied to those cases with no history or evidence of injury.

Despite a wide range of possibilities, many cases of tetanus run a similar course. Within 48 hr of the first symptom a reflex spasm occurs, followed by another an hour or so later. The interval between spasms shortens progressively and less disturbance seems to bring them on. (It is perhaps worth noting here that tactile stimuli most readily cause spasms in this disease; noise and light are much less important. In its management, therefore, unnecessary disturbance should be avoided but conspicuous quietness and darkened rooms are not essential.) In most cases the march of events quickens over the first 3 or 4 days. Spasms occur more frequently and are feared by the patient. Secretions in the mouth and upper respiratory passages are troublesome, swallowing is difficult, and the patient suffers considerable discomfort.

The peak of the disease is usually reached within 3 days of the first sign. For the next 4 or 5 days the patient remains gravely ill. In most cases these first 8 days are all important. In those who survive, all the manifestations of tetanus wane from then on. Spasms soon abate and have generally ceased by the 12th day, but stiffness persists for several weeks. Most deaths occur in the first week. In a Spanish series, 60% of deaths were within the first 6 days (Torres Gost and Figueroa-Egea, 1965); 80% of fatalities in a large Bombay series took place the first 4 days (Vakil et al., 1965a); 90% of deaths in the Delhi study of Vaishnava et al. (1965) occurred between the 1st and the 8th day.

Spasms play a very important part in determining the outcome in tetanus. Patients with rigidity but no spasms ("mild" tetanus) usually recover, no matter how they are treated, whereas those with frequent and severe spasms often die ("severe" tetanus). Patel et al. (1965a) showed this quite clearly in their analysis of over 4000 case histories: the case fatality rate was 50% when there were spasms, but only 2% when they were absent. Even the occurrence of an occasional spasm, especially if not marked in degree ("moderate" tetanus), seems to be compatible with a good prognosis. In a series of 1472 cases (Adams, 1968) the case fatality rate was similar in mild and moderate tetanus (spasms absent or infrequent) and always less than 10%, whereas it was 51% in non-neonates and 66% in the newborn with frequently repeated spasms (severe tetanus).

These points about prognosis are made because of their importance when it comes to choosing the method of treatment, but they need some clarification. It must be admitted that the term moderate tetanus is quite arbitrary and defies precise definition; it is nevertheless useful in practice. Although most cases have declared themselves as regards severity by the end of the second day, an occasional case behaves otherwise. Although judged at first to have mild tetanus because there are no spasms, a patient may unexpectedly develop a laryngeal spasm many days later; or at a late stage frequent and severe spasms may take the place of the occasional spasms observed in the first few days. In both cases the prognosis must be regarded to have changed from good to bad. While the presence or absence of spasms and their frequency and severity are the most important factors determining the outcome, the incubation period and the period of onset must also be taken into consideration.

IV. COMPLICATIONS

The way in which respiratory complications arise has already been outlined. They are the commonest and most dangerous features of the disease. Indeed, the main problems in the management of tetanus are respiratory—excessive secretions in the mouth and upper air passages, the inhalation of such material, atelectasis, pneumonia, and laryngeal and oropharyngeal spasms.

Cardiovascular complications have recently assumed some importance. Tachycardia and sweating have long been recognized as clinical features. It was thought at one time that they were merely the result of excessive muscular activity. Since they persist after curarization, however, direct autonomic involvement by the tetanus toxin is another possible explanation. Some patients manifest wide variations in blood pressure and terminally develop hypotension and a cold periphery (Clifton, 1964; Prys-Roberts et al., 1969), but it is not known whether this state of shock is always the result of intoxication of the autonomic nervous system. Gram-negative infections are a constant danger in centers where the total paralysis regimen is practiced, and gram-negative septicemia produces the same results.

Fractures are common in tetanus, except after the total paralysis regimen of treatment. They are virtually confined to the mid-dorsal region of the spine and are often multiple. Their incidence depends on the presence and severity of spasms. Simultaneous and powerful contraction of the flexors and extensors gives rise to longitudinal compression of the spine as a whole, forcibly increasing the spinal curves. The cervical and lumbar vertebrae escape injury, apparently because their curves are supported on the inside by the neural arches. The thoracic spine, curved in the opposite direction, is forcibly flexed about a fulcrum situated in the region of the posterior part of the fifth vertebral body or its neural arch, and this compresses and fractures the anterior parts of this and adjacent vertebral bodies, which become wedge-shaped.

Despite their frequency, these fractures are not important complications. They cause no pain, lead to no neurological sequelae, and heal with little or no deformity.

V. CAUSES OF DEATH

Although morbid anatomical lesions do not explain all tetanus deaths, an examination of several large series shows that the respiratory system is incriminated in the majority of cases (Creech *et al.*, 1957). These authors attributed death to pneumonia in just under half their cases, with atelectasis, aspiration, pulmonary edema, and asphyxia bringing the respiratory causes of death up to 78%. Other large series confirm the overriding importance of these complications (Garcia-Palmieri and Ramirez, 1957; Vakil *et al.*, 1965b; Patel *et al.*, 1965b).

In a detailed study of necropsy material from neonatal cases in South Africa, Wright (1960) found distinct differences between early and late deaths. Apart from congestive changes, there was surprisingly little at necropsy to account for death in infants dying in the first 48 hr. In contrast, those dying later often showed pulmonary edema, atelectasis, aspirated milk, and especially bronchopneumonia. The results in children and adults were similar. Early deaths, it seems, are usually the result of uncontrolled spasms, apneic attacks, laryngeal spasms, and possibly brain stem intoxication; later, besides these factors, death is caused or at least hastened by pneumonia. Respiratory failure should therefore be regarded as the main cause of death in tetanus.

VI. TREATMENT

If management of this disease is to be rational one crucial fact must be recognized: the severest cases should be treated in intensive-care units equipped to manage patients with respiratory failure. Unfortunately this is a counsel of perfection, since such facilities are seldom found in places where the disease is common.

There has been controversy for some time about the therapeutic value of antitetanus serum in established tetanus. Arguments both for and against have in many instances been based on well-conducted clinical trials. The balance of probabilities, however, is in favor of the use of antitetanus serum, given in a dosage of 10,000 units after preliminary testing for sensitivity (Adams *et al.*, 1969). The intravenous route is preferred since the peak blood level may be delayed for 48–72 hr after intramuscular injection (Turner *et al.*, 1958).

A. Conservative Management

Satisfactory sedation and reduction of muscular rigidity can usually be achieved by drugs such as chlorpromazine and phenobarbitone, and in many cases the spasms can be diminished in severity and frequency. A satisfactory regimen is chlorpromazine, 50 mg, given every 4 hr with the addition when necessary of phenobarbitone sodium, 200 mg, both by intramuscular injection. Besides these anticonvulsants, a number of other drugs like paraldehyde, mephenesin, and meprobomate have proved useful, and corticosteroids and hyperbaric oxygen have been tried. Randomized trials, however, have failed to establish the superiority of any one drug over another (Laurence et al., 1958; Adams et al., 1959; Hendrickse and Sherman, 1966), but clinical experience points to the general usefulness of chlorpromazine (Adams et al., 1966).

There is little doubt that these conservative measures reduce muscular rigidity and alleviate suffering; they may also diminish the spasms. What is in considerable doubt is whether they make any difference to the death rate. Indeed it has been said that "any type of sedative or hypnotic agent when properly administered so as to avoid respiratory depression has the same effect or lack of effect upon the outcome of tetanus" (Creech et al., 1957). Nevertheless, an attempt must be made to relieve the patient's symptoms. For this purpose in mild and moderate cases of tetanus, conservative management by means of these anticonvulsant drugs is probably the treatment of choice, since the case fatality rate is always under 10% and the intermittent positive-pressure regimen (described below) carries inherent risks of at least this order. These drugs must also be used for severe cases where facilities for the management of respiratory failure are not available, but the death rate is much higher—about 60% for children and adults and over 80% for neonates.

B. Tracheostomy

There are a number of theoretical advantages of tracheostomy in tetanus. It reduces the dead space by about 100 ml and relieves laryngeal obstruction. The respiratory tract is isolated from the digestive system so that the chances of aspirating food or gastric juice are eliminated. Secretions which collect in the trachea and bronchi can readily be removed. The chances of atelectasis and aspiration pneumonia occurring would consequently appear to be less, and it should be possible to ensure proper pulmonary ventilation.

Tracheostomy has been advocated from the beginning of the illness for all cases of tetanus as a means of avoiding pulmonary complications and thus lowering the mortality rate. Although it seems to be such a logical procedure in this disease, there is no clear evidence that it makes any difference to the mortality rate when used in conjunction with a conservative regimen for controlling spasms (Creech et al., 1957; Adams et al., 1966). The reason appears to be that tracheostomy carries special risks of its own.

Tracheal secretions are increased; the tube may obstruct unless the inspired air is humidified; aberrant vessels are sometimes eroded and fatal hemorrhage may follow; sepsis occurs around the stoma and adds to the dangers of infection elsewhere. Tracheostomy does not eliminate the dangers of hypoxia after repeated or uncontrollable spasms and has only marginal advantages in the case of apneic attacks. Its main indication, when used with anticonvulsants such as chlorpromazine, is for those patients with excessive and tenacious secretions in the mouth and upper respiratory tract who do not fall into the category of severe tetanus because spasms are absent or occur very infrequently. Its main advantage is that it enables the full intermittent positive-pressure regimen to be applied immediately if respiratory failure occurs.

C. Intermittent Positive-Pressure Respiration

The method of treating patients with paralysis of the muscles of respiration by means of tracheostomy and intermittent positive-pressure respiration (IPPR), introduced by Danish workers during the severe poliomyelitis epidemic of 1952 in Copenhagen, was later successfully applied to the treatment of a patient with tetanus, the respiratory muscles being paralyzed by curare (Bjørnboe et al., 1953). Reports from Britain and Nigeria in the next few years were also encouraging (Ablett, 1956; Glossop and Low, 1957; Smith, 1958), but the death rate remained high. Nevertheless, since death in tetanus is usually the result of one or more of its respiratory complications and IPPR offered hope of avoiding most if not all of them, the method appeared full of promise. A randomized trial on infants with severe tetanus neonatorum in South Africa, comparing IPPR with a conservative regimen using chlorpromazine and phenobarbitone, showed that the death rate can be halved (Wright et al., 1961). Subsequent experience in a large series (184 cases) put the case fatality rate at 36% with IPPR, compared with more than double this death rate on conservative treatment (Adams et al., 1966). Lower rates of 25% (Thambiran, 1967) and 20% (Smythe, 1963) have been recorded, leaving no reasonable doubt that the method represents a real therapeutic advance in neonates. Similar proof based on controlled clinical trials does not exist in the case of children and adults, but the excellent results obtained in Britain (2 deaths in 59 consecutive patients treated by IPPR) puts the value of the method beyond doubt (Lancet, 1967).

After preliminary intubation tracheostomy is performed under local anesthesia in neonates and general anesthesia in older patients. The patient is kept paralyzed by repeated doses of curare and ventilated by mechanical means. The inspired air, enriched with oxygen, must be humidified. Regular physiotherapy, suction to clear the air passages, and changes of position are necessary.

Scrupulous attention to aseptic methods during IPPR is mandatory. Regular blood gas analyses are a useful guide to proper ventilation, and bacterial examination of aspirated secretions, should they become purulent, often helps in the choice of an antibiotic for pulmonary infections.

Ten days on this regimen suffices in most cases. To attempt to discontinue curare before this is often hazardous, since patients with severe tetanus, once they have been curarized, can seldom reestablish adequate spontaneous respiration before this time. Prolonging IPPR beyond 10 days is usually unnecessary in view of the natural history of the disease.

Removal of the tracheostomy tube, which can be tried 2 days after curare has been discontinued, is generally successful at the first attempt in children and adults. In neonates, a longer period is usually necessary and the first attempt is less often successful. Indeed, in some infants repeated attempts at weekly intervals for weeks or even months may be required before the patient can breathe normally.

Besides removal of the tube, other hazards are encountered during the IPPR regimen. Technical faults can be eliminated by vigilance and proper maintenance of machines, but they are an ever-present danger. Infection of the respiratory tract cannot always be prevented. Particular importance must be attached to aseptic measures and careful disinfection of respirators. The more common bacterial causes of pulmonary infection—hemolytic streptococci, pneumococci, and staphylococci—can usually be controlled by penicillin or cloxacillin, but gram-negative infections are difficult to treat and carry a high mortality rate. They are probably one of the causes of the shocklike syndrome to which reference has already been made.

These problems and the technical details of IPPR have been more fully discussed by Mann et al. (1963) and Adams et al. (1969). Since there are many pitfalls, it would be unwise to attempt to treat an occasional patient with severe tetanus by this method far from a fully equipped unit which is staffed by trained personnel.

VII. PREVENTION OF TETANUS

No account of the clinical aspects of tetanus would be complete without some comments on prevention. The subject has been fully discussed by Adams et al. (1969) and the main points are summarized below.

Simple measures for minor lesions and the proper surgical care of major wounds, with emphasis on early attention in both cases, go far towards the prevention of tetanus and are of the greatest importance. Despite these measures, some bacteria and dead tissue may remain in wounds. Added safeguards are therefore advisable. There is no finality to the question of whether chemoprophylaxis (using an antibiotic such as cloxacillin in a dose of 500 mg every 6 hr for 5 days) is preferable to passive immunization with antitoxin. Heterologous antitoxin (prepared from the horse and given in a dose of 1500 units by intramuscular injection) is in common use but has the disadvantage of hypersensitivity reactions which may be fatal. Preliminary testing for sensitivity is mandatory (0.05 ml subcutaneously). It is better to use antitoxin prepared from human sources, but this is unfortunately in short supply; a does of 250 units is recommended. Hypersensitivity reactions are not likely to occur.

Active immunization with toxoid is by far the surest way of preventing tetanus. Ample testimony is provided by a comparison of the high death rate from the disease among wounded soldiers in World War I, when active immunization was not practised, with the virtual absence of tetanus in the American and British Armies during World War II, when immunization with toxoid was routine (Long and Sartwell, 1947; Boyd, 1959). The full course consists of three injections of toxoid (0.5 ml) given intramuscularly, with six weeks between the first two injections and six months between the second and the third. Protection is absolute in the first year after this, so in the event of an injury possibly contaminated by tetanus spores, antitoxin or further doses of toxoid are not necessary. A booster dose of 0.5 ml toxoid is all that is required between one and ten years after a full course of toxoid injections. In areas where the incidence of tetanus neonatorum is high, two doses of toxoid during pregnancy will significantly reduce the chances of tetanus occurring in the infant after birth (Schofield *et al.*, 1961). There is generally insufficient time for all three injections of toxoid during pregnancy, but it is wise to ensure lasting protection in the mother by completing the course after delivery.

VIII.   REFERENCES

Ablett, J. J. L. (1956), *Brit. J. Anaesth.*, **28**:258.
Adams, E. B. (1968), *S. Afr. Med. J.*, **42**:739.
Adams, E. B., R. Holloway, A. K. Thambiran, and S. D. Desai (1966), *Lancet*, **2**:1176.
Adams, E. B., D. R. Laurence, and J. W. G. Smith (1969), "Tetanus," Blackwell, Oxford.
Adams, E. B., R. Wright, E. Berman, and D. R. Laurence (1959), *Lancet*, **1**:755.
Bjørnboe, M., B. Ibsen, and S. Johnsen (1953), *Ugeskrift Laeger*, **115**:1535.
Boyd, J. (1959), *Proc. Roy. Soc. Med.*, **52**:109.
Bytchenko, B. (1966), *Bull. World Health Organ*, **34**:71.
Clifton, B. (1964), *Lancet*, **1**:785.
Creech, O., A. Glover, and A. Ochsner (1957), *Ann. Surg.*, **146**:369.
Garcia-Palmieri, M. R. and R. Ramirez (1957), *Ann. Intern. Med.*, **47**:721.
Glossop, M. W. and M. D. W. Low (1957), *Brit. J. Anaesth*,. **29**:326.
Hendrickse, R. G. and P. M. Sherman (1966), *Brit. Med. J.*, **2**:860.
Lancet, 1967, Tetanus in Britain, **1**:886.
Laurence, D. R., E. Berman, J. N. Scragg, and E. B. Adams (1958), *Lancet*, **1**:987.
Long, A. P., P. E. Sartwell (1947), *Bull. U.S. Army Med. Dep.*, **7**:371.

Mann, N. M., B. G. Jackson, and R. Holloway (1963), *Arch. Disease Childhood*, **38**:251.

Patel, J. C., B. C. Mehta, and K. N. Modi (1965a), Prognosis in tetanus, *Proceedings of the First International Conference on Tetanus*, Nov. 1963, Bombay (J. C. Patel, ed.).

Patel, J. C., P. L. Goodluck, S. S. Sheshia, and D. H. Deshpande (1965b), Morbid Anatomical Lesions in Tetanus, *Proceedings of the First International Conference on Tetanus*, Nov. 1963, Bombay (J. C. Patel, ed.).

Prys-Roberts, C., J. L. Corbett, J. H. Kerr, A. C. Smith, and J. M. K. Spalding (1969), *Lancet*, **1**:542.

Schofield, F. D., V. M. Tucker, and G. R. Westbrook (1961), *Brit. Med. J.*, **2**:785.

Smith, A. C. (1958), *Proc. Roy. Soc. Med.*, **51**:1006.

Smythe, P. M. (1963), *Brit. Med. J.*, **1**:565.

Thambiran, A. K. (1967), Assisted respiration in the treatment of neonatal tetanus, M. D. thesis, University of Natal, Durban.

Torres Gost, J. and A. Figueroa-Egea (1965), Mortality in tetanus, *Proceedings of the First International Conference on Tetanus* Nov. 1963, Bombay (J. C. Patel, ed.).

Turner, T. B., E. A. Velasco-Joven, and S. Prudovsky (1958), *Bull. Johns Hopkins Hosp.*, **102**:71.

Vaishnava, H., M. N. Passey, C. N. Neogy, S. C. Gupta, N. S. Dixit, and N. Arora (1965), Clinical Study of Tetanus in Delhi for a period of 32 months, *Proceedings of the First International Conference on Tetanus*, Nov. 1963, Bombay (J. C. Patel, ed.).

Vakil, B. J., S. N. Aiyer, A. T. Tulpule, A. J. Mehta, and T. H. Tulpule (1965a), A study of 2130 cases of tetanus with special reference to incidence, clinical types, and prognosis, *Proceedings of the First International Conference on Tetanus*, Nov. 1963, Bombay (J. C. Patel, ed.).

Vakil, B. J., T. H. Tulpule, M. M. Rananvare (1965b), The causes of death in tetanus, *Proceedings of the First International Conference on Tetanus*, Nov. 1963, Bombay (J. C. Patel, ed.).

Wright, R. (1960), The treatment of tetanus, M. D. thesis, University of Cape Town.

Wright, R., M. K. Sykes, B. G. Jackson, N. M. Mann, E. B. Adams (1961), *Lancet*, **2**:678.

Chapter 11

Biochemical and Physiological Aspects of Tetanus Intoxication

Sumner I. Zacks and Michael F. Sheff

University of Pennsylvania School of Medicine, and
Pennsylvania Hospital
Philadelphia, Pennsylvania, U. S. A.

I. INTRODUCTION

Because of man's susceptibility to traumatic injury, plus the widespread disse,nination of tetanus spores, the syndrome of wounding followed by a delayed illness characterized by muscle spasms and agonizing death was well known to the ancients. Hippocrates described a triad of wounding, lockjaw, and death. The syndrome is characterized by spreading stiffness of striated muscle, usually beginning in the area immediately surrounding the wound, ultimately leading to generalized spastic rigidity and death. Death seems primarily due to interference with respiratory mechanisms. The course of the clinical syndrome can be very slow, lasting weeks or months. As a result, observations on the mechanism of intoxication and the cause of death are liable to confusion between the primary mechanism and the secondary pathology that is produced as a result of the generalized incapacity of the patient.

Modern research into the cause of this syndrome began with the discovery of the causative organism, *Clostridium tetani*, by Nicolaïer (1884). That the disease was caused by a substance produced by the bacteria was shown by Faber (1890), who produced the tetanus syndrome experimentally with bacteria-free filtrates. Kitasato (1891) and von Behring (1892) discovered that an antitoxin could be produced to neutralize the effects of the toxin. Most studies in the early period were concerned with the route of entry and dissemination of the toxin. Unfortunately, the controversy stimulated by the centripetal dissemination theory of Morax and Marie (1903) diverted attention of investigators from the basic mode of action of the toxin. Much of the controversy resulted from use of variable toxin preparations, because purified neurotoxin was unavailable.

Early attempts to purify tetanus toxin by Brieger and Cohn (1893) and London and Aristovsky (1917) yielded only a partially purified product. Crystalline toxin was first produced by Pillemer and his associates in 1946.

The history of the study of tetanus intoxication parallels the history of new concepts and new techniques as they were developed by experimental biologists. For example, there is an electrophysiological period, an early biochemical period, and later, a subcellular-particle biochemical period. Each of the techniques of these disciplines was applied to the study of tetanus intoxication. Most recently, sophisticated methods for protein separation, protein tracing, and protein binding have been applied to the tetanus problem. The present review will attempt to outline recent major advances in the investigation of the mode of action of tetanus toxin and to present current hypotheses concerning its mode of action.

II. THE TOXIN

A. Components of Culture Filtrates

Several early investigators recognized that crude tetanus culture filtrates contained many substances. In 1898, Ehrlich described a "tetanolysin" that lysed red cells and a neurotoxin that he called "tetanospasmin." Flemming (1927) stated that tetanolysin was formed during active growth of the bacteria, whereas tetanospasmin was found in the culture filtrates after cessation of the phase of active growth. While references to tetanolysin still occur, it has become apparent that this does not invariably accompany tetanospasmin in cultures of the organism, and that it has little to do with the process of intoxication. It is apparently produced only under specific conditions of growth by specific strains of the organism, none of which have so far been defined and may be omitted from a discussion of the mechanism of the action of tetanus toxin.

Other investigators found that culture filtrates contained proteases, esterases, and lipases (Imbriano, 1950). More recently, Parsons et al. (1966) described a nonspasmogenic tetanus neurotoxin.

B. Purification of Tetanus Toxin

Ferric ammonium sulfate and cadmium chloride were used by Eaton

(1936) and Eaton and Gronau (1938) to precipitate toxin from culture filtrates. A more satisfactory method, employing cold methanol at controlled pH and ionic strength, was used by Pillemer *et al.* (1946) to precipitate crystalline toxin. The fact of its crystallization was originally considered to be good evidence for the purity of the toxin, and no other characterization was carried out. More recent studies in a variety of systems have shown that proteins can co-crystallize, so crystallization alone is no longer an index of purity. The crystals obtained by Pillemer *et al.* (1946) were yellow. Later studies have indicated that this color is probably due to an impurity precipitated with the toxin.

More recently, a variety of column chromatographic techniques (Marr and Patterson, 1960; Hardegree and Wannamaker, 1965) have been employed on a variety of media to obtain various preparations of the toxin. We have previously reported a separation method involving the use of DEAE cellulose which yielded a purified material (Sheff *et al.*, 1965).

Murphy and Miller (1967) developed a procedure for separation of pure tetanus toxin by extraction of whole cells and chromatographic separation. An initial ammonium sulfate precipitation followed by sequential ion-exchange chromatography and gel filtration yielded a purified toxin with an average specific activity of 150×10^6 mouse MLD/mg of nitrogen. A single line resulted on immunoelectrophoresis and double diffusion on agar. A single band was obtained on gel electrophoresis and a single peak was obtained in the ultracentrifuge and on Sephadex G-100 chromatography. This material was interpreted to be the biologically active monomer, and no smaller or larger lethal fractions, could be obtained. An S value of 6.4 agrees with the figure obtained by Raynaud, Turpin, and Bizzini (1960) and with the material that we isolated.

The problem of definition of purity must be considered. The increase in our ability to resolve protein mixtures which has occurred during the change from free electrophoresis to electrophoresis with molecular sieving, has shown that criteria such as homogeneity on free electrophoresis, symmetry of the peaks on free electrophoresis, and homogeneity and symmetry of peaks on ultracentrifugation are not necessarily indicators of purity. On cellulose acetate, a supporting medium which gives greater resolution than free electrophoresis, tetanus toxin has but three components. Disk electropherograms, however, resolve the toxin into approximately fifteen components.

The maximum specific activity of the toxin may be used as a criterion of purification, providing it is known that the system contains no synergistic components. We have tested all the fractions obtained in the separation of tetanus toxin on DEAE cellulose columns and have found there is no appreciable activity in any of the components other than the one which we have designated as the neurotoxin. We have also tested for synergy between components by adding nontoxic components to the toxic fraction in various quantities. In no case could we detect any increase in toxicity by a sensitive bioassay. We ascribe all the toxic activity to a single component demonstrated by disk electrophoresis.

According to Hardegree and Wannamaker (1965), tetanospasmin is a single antigen regardless of bacterial strain. We currently define purified tetanus toxin as the material that migrates in a single narrow band on disk electrophoresis. This criterion has been accepted by others and used as the basis of differentiation in their work.

The position of the protein on migration both on cellulose acetate and on other supporting media is very similar to that of serum beta-globulins. This would be consistent with reports of a molecular weight of 90–150,000 and an isoelectric point of approximately pH 6.5. The consistency of electrophoretic running, in the sense that free electrophoresis, cellulose acetate electrophoresis, and disk gel electrophoresis all place tetanus toxin in the same area of the electropherogram, indicates very strongly that the overall configuration of the toxin molecule does not have any marked peculiarities. Otherwise, sieving effects would alter its relative mobility. There have been no reports of its being a conjugated protein, nor does the toxin give any abnormal staining after electrophoresis. Thus, the results of this type of investigation seem to indicate that the tetanus toxin molecule is a "typical" globulin.

C. Molecular Weight of Tetanus Toxin

Various investigators have reported different values for the sedimentation coefficient of purified toxin. Pillemer and Moore (1948) found sedimentation coefficients of 4.5, and 7, whereas Largier, (1956) reported coefficients of 3.9 and 7.5. Raynaud et al. (1960) described toxic proteins with coefficients of 2.3, 4.5, and 7. According to Lamanna and Carr (1967), interconversion of 2.3, 3.9 (4.5 and 7.0), and 7.5 forms yielding active toxin may occur, whereas some of the (7–7.5) proteins may be inactive. Initially, most investigators reported molecular weights in the range of 67,000, although recent data by Murphy et al. (1968), who isolated tetanus neurotoxin by sequential ion-exchange and gel filtration chromatography, demonstrated a protein peak at $S_{20,w} = 6.4$. Diffusion constants of 4.2 and 4.4 were obtained by chromatographic and immunodiffusion methods. They found average molecular weights of 120,000 to 140,000.

Mangalo et al. (1968) used a hypertonic extract of bacteria and gel filtration on Sephadex G-100 to obtain a single constituent on immunodiffusion testing and disk electrophoresis. This purified tetanus toxin was a 7.88S protein with a molecular weight of 150,000 ($\pm 8\%$). Tetanus toxin isolated from toxic filtrates by Dawson and Nichol (1969) had an average molecular weight of 176,000 $\pm$ 5000 without evidence of heterogeneity of the molecules.

Addition of sulfite produced partial cleavage of disulfide bonds linking toxin subunits, a procedure that destroyed toxicity. The authors concluded that disulfide bonds occur either at the toxic site or are placed in such a way as to maintain the integrity of the site. They believe that this accessible bond appears distinct from that responsible for holding the subunits together. When the toxin was treated with aldehydes, sedimentation studies revealed marked protein aggregation.

We have subjected an electrophoretically pure preparation of the toxin made in our laboratory to ultracentrifugation and found a sedimentation coefficient of 6.7.

Partial amino acid analysis by Dunn et al. (1949) demonstrated that 80% of the tetanus toxin molecule is composed of 13 amino acids. This composition is that of a simple protein without any striking clue to explain its remarkable biologic activity. However, because the extreme reactivity of the toxin towards its sites of binding in vivo must be due to the configuration of its active centers, it is apparent that the amino acid composition is an area requiring further study. Investigations using 8M urea and gel filtration demonstrated that the tetanus toxin molecule is a single polypeptide chain with no free N-terminal amino acids (Murphy et al., 1968).

D. The Relationship Between Dose and Response in Tetanus Intoxication

Tetanus toxin was originally assayed by the number of animal lethal doses which were found in the test solution. One measurement which is commonly used is the minimum lethal dose. This is the amount of toxin which, when injected into mice, produces death within a specified period, usually 4 days. This is related to the LD_{50}, a dose such that 50% of a group of mice injected with a given dose of toxin will die within the specified period. These measurements have been used to assay the number of defined doses contained in 1 ml of a culture filtrate. Other workers related the toxicity of the solution to its ability to react with antitoxin thus giving rise to the concept of the L_f and L_t dose. These assays have been reviewed and the methodology underlying them described by Wilson and Miles (1964). Crystallization of purified tetanus toxin by Pillemer et al. (1946) led to measurements of the number of micrograms of toxin represented by the minimum lethal dose or LD_{50}. Most recently, Bizzini et al. (1969) made an exhaustive study of the relationship between toxicity and flocculation using purified tetanus toxin.

In general, early investigations of the dose–response relationship showed increasing time for the appearance of signs of intoxication as the dose of the toxin decreased. Using purified tetanus toxin, Zacks and Sheff (1963) measured the dose–response relationship with high doses of purified toxin. They found that the relationship could be expressed by the formula

$$\text{survival time} = T + K \log 1/d$$

In this formula, d is the toxin dose actually given, K is a constant, and T is the absolute minimum time in which animals can be killed with any dose of toxin. Use of this formula has indicated a minimum saturation dose (SD_{min}) of 10 μg of toxin for a 20–25 g mouse. Presumably, T is the time needed for exhaustion of a stored metabolite or ion. It is curious, and probably coincidental, that this relationship in goldfish is similar to that in mice. The saturation dose for 20–25 g goldfish is similar to the saturation dose for a mouse of similar weight. Changes in the value of T in mice kept under conditions of environmental stress presumably are related to the effect of that stress on the rate of utilization of a necessary metabolite. A further conclusion which may be drawn from the shape of these curves is that, at least at high dose levels, the rate of utilization of stored material must be the rate-limiting process in the intoxication. Furthermore, its rate must be an order of magnitude less than the rates of the other phases of intoxication, namely dissemination of the toxin and its binding to sites of action. Otherwise, the curve would not approach a steady value at a finite time, but would instead become asymptotic to a survival time of zero minutes.

The equation describes the shape of the curve obtained and does not have functional significance. The survival time is actually the rate at which the animals die, and the relationship of this rate to the dose is a complex function involving the number of sites available, the rate at which the process of biochemical intoxication occurs at each of these sites, and the rate at which the toxin reaches and is bound at these sites. Model equations describing hypothetical systems can be set up and are currently being investigated by us.

III. BIOCHEMICAL MECHANISMS INVOLVED IN TETANUS INTOXICATION

A. General Considerations

As with many other aspects of tetanus intoxication, there are many reports on the biochemical changes which accompany the disease. Unfortunately, few of these observations are directly comparable one to another. Studies on patients have been made under a wide variety of therapeutic regimens, including patients in different nutritional states and in whom the process of intoxication has existed for unequal periods of time. Experimental models have used a great variety of animals, from the unicellular organisms such as paramecium through poikilothermic animals including frog, lizard, and tortoise, to birds and a number of mammalian species (mouse, rat, guinea pig, monkey, cat, and others). Some investigators have studied the changes which occur in local tetanus; others, the changes which occur in generalized tetanus induced by low doses of the toxin, and still others, the effects observed in animals which have been intoxicated with very large doses of toxin. There has been a similar variation among the preparations of toxin used, and in few cases the investigators have used a toxin defined neither in terms of its content of neurotoxic protein nor of the other components of the system. From the biochemical point of view, this last variation is of particular importance, because we have found, in at least one batch of toxin, evidence for the presence of a component capable of inhibiting the first coupling steps (NADH$^+$ oxidation) in oxidative phosphorylation. Later work with the *same material* showed that this inhibitor of oxidative phosphorylation played no role in intoxication. The biochemical changes which occur in tetanus intoxication must be further divided into those which are primary, that is, those that are due specifically to the action of the toxin at its binding sites, and those which are secondary. The toxin produces a profound neuromuscular dysfunction. In severe clinical cases, as well as in the experimental situation, the spastic rigidity finally induced affects striated muscles throughout the body, including the respiratory muscles. It is common practice to treat patients at this stage of intoxication by curarization and some form of artificial respiration. Such individuals also require intravenous feeding. In experimental animals which have been poisoned with small doses of the toxin, the course of the disease may progress over several days. These animals are left without respiratory aid and are not fed intravenously. It is not surprising that under these circumstances, various secondary pathological changes develop and that biochemical evidence of them can be found. For example, increases in serum aldolase, serum glutamic oxaloacetic transaminase, and creatinephosphokinase have been reported in patients. These are typical indicators of muscle damage. However, in attempts to confirm these changes in mice, we have found that the creatine phosphokinase rises only in chronic intoxication. For example, in mice poisoned with a sufficiently large dose of the toxin to kill them in 3 hr (10 μg), there is no elevation of serum creatine phosphokinase. However, if 1 % of this dose is given so that intoxication lasts from 48–72 hr, the serum creatine phosphokinase begins to rise after 24 hr. Changes such as these may be classified as nonspecific muscular damage due to chronic intoxication. Similar criteria apply to observations on the storage of metabolites in chronically poisoned animals. Such animals will, of necessity, be unable to eat efficiently, and it is, therefore, not surprising to find, as did Davenport and Ranson (1929) that the total glycogen content of the tissue is diminished. In experiments in our laboratory, using acutely intoxicated mice dying within a period of 3 hr, there were no changes in glycogen content of the skeletal muscles and liver as compared with control animals. Even when such intoxicated animals were made to do work by placing them on a treadmill during intoxication, there were no significant changes in glycogen stores as compared with control animals which had been on the treadmill for an equivalent time. Similarly, interference with the respiratory mechanism leading to retention of CO_2 and consequent fall of blood pH will lead typically to electrolyte changes. These have been described in patients. However, such reports of electrolyte changes immediately before death may have no relationship to the mechanism of intoxication. The cause of death in tetanus intoxication appears to be loss of mechanical *respiratory* function rather than any destructive effect of the toxin on any vital organ. It is not surprising that, as detailed elsewhere in this review, there are no specific morphological changes in the tissues at the light-microscopic level of resolution.

If loss of respiratory function due to muscular rigidity is the underlying cause of death in tetanus intoxication, then it follows that the operational definition of the primary biochemical lesion in intoxication is the process that causes the rigidity, a tautological argument. Furthermore, if the toxin is active primarily in the central nervous system, as has been claimed by Brooks, Curtis, and Eccles (1957), then the loss of respiratory function is due simply to the CNS lesion, producing what is in effect a physiological tetanus of the respiratory muscles. The biochemical problems of the primary lesion of tetanus intoxication would then be the problem of how the toxin acts at the inhibitory synapses and on motor neurons so as to lower the degree of central inhibition. Since in this concept the motor neuron may be normal, the biochemical lesion would be further limited to one which would not interfere with the generalized function of the nerve, but simply prevent the passage of inhibitory impulses.

B.   Direct Action of Tetanus Toxin on Skeletal Muscle

Evidence exists of the direct involvement of skeletal muscle in tetanus intoxication. Much of this evidence is neurophysiological and is considered elsewhere in this review. Evidence of the direct effect of the toxin on skeletal muscle has been obtained by Michelazzi *et al.* (1955) and confirmed by Patel and Rao (1966). These investigators have demonstrated that muscle ATPase activity is apparently lowered by the toxin. Kloetzel (1961) demonstrated interference with anerobic metabolism of diaphragm muscle. Our experiments (Zacks and Sheff, 1966) show that muscle isolated from mice which have been intoxicated with tetanus toxin have abnormal electrolyte flux. The observation by Zacks and Sheff (1968) that tetanus toxin is specifically bound at the junction of the T system and sarcoplasmic reticulum (SR) in mouse skeletal muscle is not direct evidence that the toxin serves a particular function at that site, but fits well with evidence on the altered calcium metabolism of the intoxicated muscle as described elsewhere in this review. A lesion at this site has been recently reported in a new clinical entity in which there is a transient tetanus developing on excitation (Brody, 1969). Careful investigation of this effect has shown that it lies solely at the periphery. Subfractionation of the muscle fibers revealed that the SR from the muscles of these individuals were incapable of accumulating calcium at the same rate as SR from normal muscles. Thus, despite a normal firing rate of the motor neuron and apparently normal neuromuscular transmission, the lowered rate of the calcium accumulating process in the SR so increased the time constant for the relaxation process, that the muscle went into physiological tetanus.

It is most useful to try to divide the available biochemical data into various systems. The first of these is the effect of toxin on overall metabolic pathways. As mentioned above, the evidence on the diminution of tissue glycogen is variable. It is our impression that there is no essential change in this component and that it is improbable that either the catabolic or anabolic processes involved in glycogen synthesis and breakdown are primarily affected. Wensink and his collaborators (1953a,b) claimed that there was a block in the pathway which led to the resynthesis of glycogen via the gluconeogenetic pathway. The particular enzymes which they claimed to be affected were triosephosphate dehydrogenase and aldolase. They demonstrated that the formation of lactate by tetanus-poisoned muscle was much lower than that formed by normal muscle when tissue homogenates were incubated with glucose 1-phosphate as the substrate. This was partially confirmed by Kloetzel (1962), who found that diaphragm muscle from mice poisoned with tetanus toxin had diminished anaerobic respiration. None of these authors used a highly purified tetanus toxin preparation. Therefore, it is possible that the inhibition of triosephosphate dehydrogenase postulated by Wensink, which would be a possible point of blockade in Kloetzel's experimental system as well, was caused by an impurity similar to that interfering with $NADH^+$ oxidation found in impure preparations of tetanus toxin. It is also noteworthy that Wensink's experiments were performed on starved animals. As against these results, we must mention that Muntz (1949), showed that lactic acid production was normal in the intoxicated animals. Histochemical estimations of enzyme activity by Zacks and Sheff (1964) and Frangini et al. (1956) are also contradictory.

At a higher level of metabolic resolution, Zacks and Sheff (1966) showed that oxidative phosphorylation proceeded normally in both brain and liver mitochondria. This was shown only after purifying the toxin from the as yet unidentified factor which inhibits the coupling of oxidative phosphorylation. A similar result was reported by Patel and Rao (1966).

Against these largely negative results concerning attempts to find a specific metabolic lesion must be set data from whole-organism studies. Kloetzel (1961) showed that normal rates of aerobic metabolism appeared to be associated with increased oxygen consumption by intoxicated animals as compared with normal animals. Kerr et al. (1968) showed that in tetanus-poisoned patients, there was a high CO_2 output that accompanied the increased metabolic rate (Macrae, 1967).

Sheff et al. (1963) showed that in the terminal phase of acute, generalized intoxication in mice poisoned with large doses of tetanus toxin, there was lessened metabolic activity in the sense that there was insufficient release of metabolic energy to maintain body temperature.

It is apparent from all of these results that there is some interference with the mechanism by which heat is produced in the body, but it is not clear whether this is a result of some primary action of the toxin on a metabolic pathway or a secondary effect resulting from the basic lesion. One possible biochemical site for a primary lesion that would produce, as a secondary effect, changes in both heat production and muscle function, would be interference with the degradation and resynthesis of high-energy phosphates.

Although the basic physiological data is unavailable, interference with a similar process in neurons may also occur. The evidence previously considered indicates that it is unlikely that there is interference with the synthetic pathway at the mitochondrial level, particularly in experiments with *isolated* mitochondria. As has been thoroughly studied in man, the proper maintenance of the high-energy phosphate level is dependent upon ionic movement in the whole tissue.

The emphasis on muscle work in the following section does not mean that the metabolic lesion occurs only in muscle. Unfortunately, insufficient data concerning the recycling of high-energy phosphates in nervous tissue is available for an adequate discussion of what might occur under conditions of tetanus intoxication. Furthermore, use of whole-tissue slices in studies of the biochemistry of the lesion are potentially misleading because of the apparent discreteness of the lesion. Thus, small metabolic changes in motor neurons might be undetectable against a background of normally respiring glial cells.

1. High-Energy Phosphate Metabolism

Attempts to study the metabolism of ATP and associated enzyme systems in skeletal muscle, like the studies on other enzyme systems, have yielded contradictory results. According to Gorini (1954), the only noticeable abnormality was a slight increase in the ATPase activity of isolated myofibrils from animals poisoned with tetanus toxin. A more extensive study was by Michelazzi *et al.* (1955), who used guinea pigs to study the content of high-energy phosphates in heart muscle, muscle with local tetanus intoxication, muscle from animals with generalized tetanus intoxication, and control animals. The use of heart muscle as an internal control on each animal was used because it is known that the heart is unaffected by tetanus intoxication. Zacks and Sheff (1965) have also demonstrated that the heart, in contrast to skeletal muscle, does not bind tetanus toxin. The studies by Michelazzi *et al.* on enzyme systems showed that the processes for synthesis of ATP were unaffected. Furthermore, they found no interference with the oxidative mechanism in muscle mitochondria. The only enzyme that they found to be affected to any significant degree was myofibrillar ATPase. They found that the ATPase activity in muscle from animals with generalized tetanus or muscle with local tetanus were both increased nearly 100% when compared to the controls. From the studies on the accumulation of ATP, ADP, AMP and other high-energy phosphate intermediates in muscle, these investigators concluded that ATP in muscle was greatly diminished when the muscle was poisoned by tetanus toxin, and that this was due to the increased myofibrillar ATPase activity. However, examination of the data reveals that while ATP was undoubtedly diminished, the "true" inorganic phosphate and total phosphate contents of the muscle were also considerably diminished. The decrease in "true" inorganic phosphate was sufficient to account for the decrease in muscle total phosphate. Zacks and Sheff (1964) and Zacks, Hall, and Sheff (1966) have shown that muscles from both experimental animals and patients contain accumulations of electron-dense granules in the matrix of skeletal muscle mitochondria that have been identified by others (Peachly, 1962; Weiss, 1955) to be accumulations of divalent cations, probably as phosphates. Similar changes in mitochondrial dense granules have been shown to occur in occasional CNS mitochondria during experimental tetanus intoxication. Because these granules are located in the matrix of the mitochondria, it is possible that they may not have been extracted by the techniques used by Michelazzi *et al.* (1955).

It may be noted that simple experiments by both Gorini (1954) and Sheff and Zacks (1966), in which mice in the late stages of tetanus intoxication were given intravenous injections of ATP and ADP to try to replace a supposed deficiency of these materials, were uniformly unsuccessful in altering the course of intoxication. The accumulation of dense granules within the matrix of muscle mitochondria, although not specific for tetanus intoxication, suggests that there may be some abnormality in electrolyte metabolism in the intoxicated muscle.

Recently, Lipskaya (1968) studied the effect of local tetanus in rat hind legs on oxidative phosphorylation and calcium transport in muscle mitochondria. These investigators interpreted their observations as support for the concept that isolated mitochondria from tetanus-poisoned rat muscles are loosely coupled and demonstrate increased capability of calcium accumulation. This would correlate with the observed increase in number and size of matrical dense granules in mouse muscle mitochondria (Zacks and Sheff, 1964).

2. *Electrolyte Metabolism*

Although it is difficult to separate primary from secondary effects, evidence has been obtained by Zacks and Sheff (1966a) that electrolyte changes are primary rather than secondary. In the experiments on toxin binding to be described, Sheff and Zacks (1966a) demonstrated that the binding of doses of 10 μg tetanus toxin to muscle occurs 15–20 min after intravenous injection of the toxin and is completed in approximately 30 min even though the animals live for another $2\frac{1}{2}$ hr and show no signs of intoxication for an additional 30–40 min after binding has occurred. Blood samples drawn from the mice during the period when the toxin is binding revealed that there was an increase in both serum calcium and magnesium during the binding period but before any signs of intoxication occurred. This is demonstrated in Fig. 1. The observed increase was approximately 0.5 mg% for

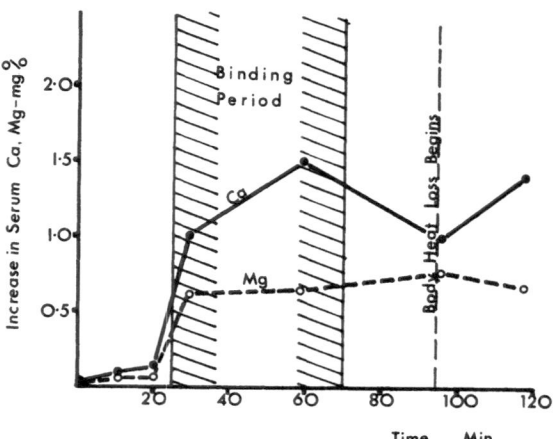

Fig. 1. The relationship, in mice with acute generalized tetanus intoxication, of the rise in serum calcium and magnesium to the time course of the intoxication. At zero time, 5 μg of purified tetanus toxin injected. Mice were sacrificed in groups of five at the times indicated in the curve, and serum Ca^{2+} and Mg^{2+} were estimated. The binding period was determined in a separate experiment as described in the text. The cations were measured by atomic absorption spectrophotometry.

Table I.
Rate of Entry of Calcium into Muscle in Tetanus Intoxication

Time after injection of toxin at which sample was withdrawn (min)	Relative uptake of calcium by muscle (percentage)
Control, no toxin	100
30	104
50	89
70	80
90	77

magnesium and 1.5 mg% for calcium. This indicates that the lesion in electrolyte metabolism in terms of these cations is one that is associated with the binding of tetanus toxin to its sites of action before effects of the toxin become evident. Therefore, these changes may be considered to be closely related to the biochemical lesion caused by the toxin. The small increase in serum magnesium is less interesting, because skeletal muscle contains more magnesium than does serum. The rise in calcium is against the concentration gradient and therefore cannot be due to a simple leakage of this cation from muscle. Rather, it suggests that some stage in the turnover of calcium has been altered so that acquisition of this cation by muscle no longer occurs normally. Calcium is known to be compartmentalized in muscle with different time constants for three hypothetical compartments.

Experimental data indicate that the rise in serum calcium occurs in a few minutes, suggesting that the fastest component of calcium movement with a time constant of $T_\frac{1}{2}=5$ min is the one that is affected by the toxin. Experiments with radioactive calcium in our laboratory confirm this hypothesis. The results are presented in Table 1. The table demonstrates that the rate of passage of intravenously injected radiocalcium into striated muscle is decreased in acutely intoxicated mice.

In these experiments 0.1 ml of an isotonic solution of ^{45}Ca in NaCl was injected into mice at intervals after the injection of 10 μg of toxin. The animals were killed 10 min later (at the time shown in the table). Serum and muscle samples were assayed for radioactivity, and the serum samples assayed for calcium. The relative specific activity of the serum and the counts per mg dry weight of muscle were calculated. The activity in muscle was not expressed in terms of relative specific activity (RSA) of Ca, since much muscle Ca does not exchange significantly with plasma. The relative uptake was found by dividing the cpm/mg dry weight in muscle by the RSA of the serum, and defining this to be 100% in the controls. No correction was made for Ca diffusing between plasma and the muscle intracellular space. Removal of this amount would considerably increase the differences between control and experimental animals. There were four animals in each group.

Changes in the flux of the other electrolytes (Na^+, K^+) have also been studied. Kloetzel (1963) measured serum potassium and sodium in patients with tetanus intoxication. His studies revealed that there was some diminution in the serum potassium, but apparently not in the sodium level. Experiments on brain tissue slices (Evans and MacIlwain, 1967), on neuromuscular junctions (Parsons *et al.*, 1966), and on isolated muscle from animals with acute generalized tetanus (Zacks and Sheff, 1966a) have also been concerned with electrolyte changes during intoxication. Evans and MacIlwain (1967) reported that there was no change in the electrolyte balance or metabolism of slices of cerebral cortex which had been incubated with tetanus toxin. However, these slices of cortical tissue contain a large number of glial cells that are unaffected by the toxin. Absence of electrolyte changes in these cells might obscure possible changes in electrolytes in poisoned neurons. Parsons *et al.* (1966) concluded that there were some changes in the conduction properties of poisoned nerve terminals with respect to sodium and potassium ions and that added calcium and magnesium would enhance the activity of the toxin. Zacks and Sheff (1966a) demonstrated that there were considerable changes in the movement of monovalent ions between skeletal muscle sheets and the incubating medium (Krebs–Henseleit–Ringer) when muscles from normal animals were compared with muscles from mice poisoned with tetanus toxin. For this purpose, we used very thin sheets of pectoral muscle from acutely poisoned mice, because these sheets can be prepared with minimum damage to the cells. Normal muscle incubated in Krebs–Henseleit–Ringer solution tends to lose potassium and gain sodium. Muscles from mice in the later stages of acute, generalized tetanus intoxication had a greater tendency to lose potassium and gain sodium than did the muscles from the control mice when exogenous ATP was omitted from the incubating mixture, even though the respiratory rates for both sets of muscle were comparable in terms of the oxygen uptake/ per mg of tissue. When exogenous ATP was included in the incubating medium, there was a marked effect on the electrolyte balance of the muscle sheets taken from the poisoned mice, but not on the muscle from the control mice. Sodium uptake was significantly less than in the experiments in which no ATP was added, and, similarly, the potassium loss was markedly reduced. This result should be contrasted with the consistent observations by Zacks and Sheff (1966a) and others that the sodium and potassium content of the tetanus-poisoned muscles before incubation in Ringer solution show no difference between control and poisoned animals. These results indicate that ability of the poisoned muscle to maintain ion equilibrium is considerably reduced in the poisoned animal. In the intact animal, metabolic adjustments are sufficient to maintain the monovalent cations at their normal levels. However, when the muscle is stressed by being removed from the animal and placed in an incubation medium, there is insufficient generation of high-energy phosphates to maintain ionic equilibrium. This data could be considered to confirm the studies of Michelazzi *et al.* (1955).

IV. EFFECT OF ENVIRONMENTAL TEMPERATURE ON TETANUS INTOXICATION

Another aspect of tetanus intoxication, yielding results important in studying the metabolic effects of the toxin, is the effect of environmental temperature on the course of intoxication. Data in mammals has been reported by Ipsen (1961) and Sheff *et al.* (1963), and there are several pertinent notations in the clinical literature. In patients, hyperpyrexia rather than hypopyrexia is more characteristic of advanced tetanus intoxication, unlike the pattern in rodents. The reasons for this difference are unknown. However, it is probably related to the small dose and lengthy time course common in human tetanus intoxication. Of interest is the observation (Vejss and Kozesnick, 1954) that decreased body temperature delays the *onset* of tetanus intoxication symptoms in man.

In none of these studies can the effect of temperature on the site of the lesion produced by the toxin be studied, because there is little variation in the internal body temperatures of mammals. A further complication is the metabolic response of mammals to temperature stress. The important variable in such studies in mammals is not the effect of temperature on intoxication, but its effect on the metabolic rate of the animal. Poikilothermic animals acclimated to a wide range of environmental temperatures may be used to study this problem, because there is little difference in their metabolic rate at various temperatures once they have been acclimated. A variety of animals has been studied. Cowles and Nelson (1949) studied the effect of cold on tetanus intoxication in lizards, and Rowson (1961), following up earlier studies, carried out a thorough investigation of the effect of environmental temperatures on the action of tetanus toxin in frogs. We have recently reported (Sheff and Zacks, 1968) the effects of changes of environmental temperature on tetanus intoxication in goldfish. In both the lizard and the goldfish, survival time after injection of the toxin is a simple linear function of the logarithm of the temperature. This does not appear to be the case in frogs, for which Rowson, following previous workers (Courmont and Doyon, 1893), found a critical temperature below which the frogs could not be intoxicated with the toxin. The frog is also unusual in the remarkably large dose of the toxin required to produce intoxication. Rowson (1961) calculated that the LD_{50} for frogs at room tenperature was 3000 times greater than for mice poisoned with the same toxin. Another difference between frogs and mammals was the inability of frog central nervous system tissue to bind toxin in the same way as mammalian CNS tissue. Analysis of Rowson's data indicates that between 23 and 28°C there is a $2\frac{1}{2}$-fold increase in the rate at which the toxin produces death, equivalent to a Q_{10} in this temperature range of 3.26. By contrast, further lowering of the temperature by 5°C from 23 to 18°C increases the duration of the survival time of the intoxicated frogs more than threefold, and at 15°C, the animals are unaffected by the toxin. Because he was able to recover active, circulating toxin from frogs incubated below 15°C, in the absence of signs of intoxication, Rowson suggested that in this temperature range, the toxin did not bind to active sites. A possible explanation is that there is a change in the overall nature of the active sites at the critical temperature. If the toxin binds to a particular membranous component, it is possible that at some temperature the lipid constituents of this component may undergo some kind of phase change (Luzzati and Husson, 1962), altering the configuration of the membrane.

In contrast to these results, Cowles and Nelson (1947) found that the desert iguana was sensitive to tetanus toxin at temperatures as low as 10–11°C, although they noted that the symptoms of intoxication were much less apparent. These investigators studied the animals over a temperature range from 10–38°C and obtained a Q_{10} value of 3–4.

Our studies have utilized both the goldfish and the mouse (Sheff and Zacks, 1963). In studies of temperature effects on intoxication in goldfish, the fish were acclimated in large tanks for several days at each of the chosen temperatures and were then injected intraperitoneally (1 cm anterior to the anal pore in the midline) with purified tetanus neurotoxin. Previous studies (Table II) revealed that there is a dose–response relationship in the goldfish that is similar to the relationship demonstrated in mice. Goldfish were acclimated at 31°C in large aquaria. They were injected with 0.1 ml. of solution containing either a known amount of purified tetanus toxin or saline. The fish were observed until they died. None of the controls showed any ill effects. Because our goldfish were similar in weight to the mice used in previous studies, the similarity of the dose–response relationship suggested

Table II.
Dose-Survival Time Relationships in Goldfish at 31°C

Dose	Number of animals dead in		
(μg)	9 hr	13 hr	26 hr
20	0/0	5/5	5/5
10	0/0	4/5	5/5
5	0/0	1/5	5/5

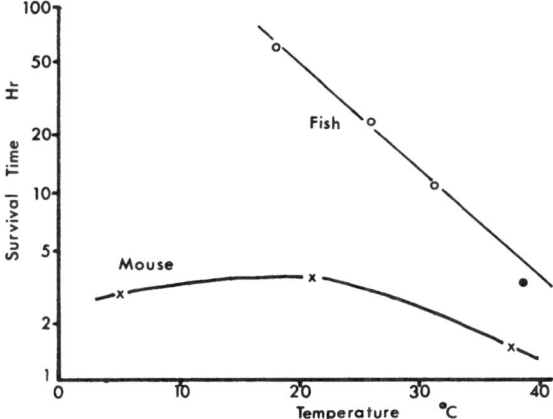

Fig. 2. The relationship between environmental temperature and time of survival for mice and goldfish. All animals were chosen to be of similar weight and all were poisoned with 10 μg of the same preparation of purified tetanus toxin. The filled-in circle is the survival time for acclimated mice plotted as though the "environmental temperature" of the tissues were the body temperature, 37°C. Five animals were used for each point.

that the number of binding sites per animal appeared to be more related to the body weight or possibly the muscle mass, than to the mass of nervous tissue. The results of experiments in which both mice and goldfish kept at various environmental temperatures were challenged with a saturating dose of the toxin (10 μg of purified neurotoxin) are presented in Fig. 2. The mouse data demonstrates a nonlinear response to the change in temperature, whereas the goldfish data has a log/linear relationship. The three points on the curve represent the three environmental temperatures at which the assay was carried out (18, 25, and 31 °C), and the filled circle represents the survival time of an acclimated mouse kept at room temperature. This is plotted at 37°C, because the internal temperature of the mouse corresponds to the environmental temperature of the binding sites of the animal. This plot yields a Q_{10} of 4.2 for the overall process of intoxication. We should emphasize that the value for the mouse rate lies close to the extrapolated curve for the goldfish. It seems likely that this Q_{10} value represents an important parameter of tetanus intoxication and is common to the lizard and goldfish and probably to the frog (in the temperature range where this animal is sensitive to the toxin) and by implication to the mouse. The significance of this parameter must now be considered.

A. Activation Energy for the Process

Crozier (1924) studied the effect of variations in temperature on several physiological processes in poikilothermic animals. He found that similar log/linear relationships could be developed for a variety of processes. Using the integrated form of Arrhenius' equation, he obtained a characteristic number μ which was expressed as calories. Later, development of a theory concerning such measurements suggested that μ is numerically equal to an activation energy A for an overall process. The appropriate equation is derived from the integrated form of the Arrhenius equation which relates reaction rate to absolute temperature. The relationship between A, the activation energy, and Q_{10} is shown in the following equation

$$\ln k_1/k_2 = A/R \times (1/T_1 - 1/T_2)$$

where A is the activation energy, R, the gas constant (1.98 cal/mole) and k_1 and k_2 are the reaction rates at temperatures T_1 and T_2 respectively. If T_1 and T_2 are ten degrees apart, then $k_1/k_2 = Q_{10}$. If we choose T_1 and T_2 to be 25°C and 35°C, values that occur in most experiments of this kind, then the numerical values can be inserted and the equation rearranged to yield the simple relationship

$$A = 1.82 \times 10^4 \quad (\ln Q_{10} \text{ cal/mole})$$

This relationship was employed in a study of binding of botulinum type A toxin in goldfish (Cartwright and Lauffer, 1952). These investigators obtained a figure for A of 60,000 cal/mole in their system, which resembles our experimental system of tetanus intoxication in goldfish. It may be significant that they also found that the appropriate value for A for the mouse on the same scale coincided with the extrapolation of the goldfish values. Calculations of an activation energy from our goldfish data yielded an A of 27,000 cal. A comparable figure can be calculated for the lizard and the frog, and, by implication, for the mouse. This energy was thought by Crozier to represent the characteristic energy of the rate-limiting process involved in a sequence of events. There is still too little data to be explicit as to the fundamental process of tetanus intoxication, but the following points may be considered. First, if more than one step is involved in the process, then the observed Q_{10} must be affected by the rate processes for the individual steps. Only under two circumstances will the observed value be a true quantitation. If all the processes are affected in exactly the same way by a change in temperature, then the observed value will be characteristic for all of them. Otherwise, the observed value will only be a good approximation of the coefficient of activation energy for the limiting process, if that process is extremely slow compared with all the other steps in the sequence. Thus, the characteristic value that we have obtained is likely to be the lower limit for the activation energy of the rate limiting steps.

The process of intoxication can be divided into three phases. The first of these is the dissemination of the toxin from the site of injection to the binding sites. This process will be governed by laws of diffusion and is likely to be rapid compared to the other processes. Rowson (1961), who measured blood levels of toxin in the frog, found that when doses which killed the animal in 7 days were injected, the maximum serum toxin level was reached after 3 hr. This process will have a small temperature coefficient in the temperature range studied, because it is directly proportional to the *absolute temperature*. The other two processes involved in intoxication are the binding of the toxin to its sites of action and its activity there.

For reasons that will be discussed in the section concerning the dose–response relationship, binding time is unlikely to be a limiting factor at the dose levels studied. Thus, one must conclude that the Q_{10} value that we have obtained most likely represents the third process, the activity of the toxin at its sites of action. The value calculated for A is large for most physiological processes. Crozier's (1924) collection of values for μ showed that for most physiological processes, μ has a value between 12,000 and 18,000 cal.

It is impossible to identify an enzyme system from its activation energy. For the enzymes involved in muscular contraction and relaxation, values from 7000 to 30–40,000 cal are found in the literature.

A speculative hypothesis that includes the observations reviewed here follows. The toxin is tightly bound to some morphological constituent of skeletal muscle and neurons. In the case of skeletal muscle, the principal site of binding appears to be at the junction between the SR and the T tubules. In the case of neurons, the specific site of binding may be at the inhibitory synapse. In general, biochemical evidence indicates that the primary lesion produced by the toxin interferes with neither the normal metabolic pathway nor with the energetic coupling of oxidation to phosphorylation. There is some measure of agreement that one of the effects of the toxin, presumably a primary one since it occurs very early in intoxication, is production of abnormal electrolyte balance. There is some evidence that this abnormality is associated with lack of high-energy phosphates. *In vivo*, there is a slight increase in the serum levels of divalent cations, with the increase of calcium more significant because it occurs against the normal gradient. Careful examination of the enzyme system in skeletal muscle indicates that there is also an increase in myofibrillar ATPase activity. In mice, these metabolic abnormalities appear to culminate in the animal's loss of its ability to maintain internal temperature. The factor controlling death rate appears to be related to the stores of some substrate rather than in the processes involved in dissemination or binding of the toxin. Thus, the death rate becomes independent of dose when the dose exceeds a certain value that we have called the minimum saturation dose (SD_{min}). Comparative evidence from other physiological systems indicates that muscles will go into rigid contraction under a number of circumstances. Two matters of particular importance to this discussion are the recently demonstrated inability of the SR to bind calcium in patients studied recently and the better known physiological tetanus produced by supramaximal firing of the motor nerve. The compartmentalization of calcium in skeletal muscle has been extensively studied and is reviewed by Daniel (1965) and also Nayler (1965). It appears that calcium is contained in three compartments within skeletal muscle. There is a very rapidly exchanging component, a second more slowly exchanging component, and finally a third, nonexchangeable store of calcium. The process of muscular excitation and relaxation is accompanied by movement of calcium ions in and out of the fast component compartment, a mechanism involving the "relaxing factor" associated with the SR, T-system and phosphates in various forms including pyrophosphate (Ebashi and Endo, 1964). Unfortunately, there are no available physiological data on a possibly comparable system in neurons that presumably might be analogous to the cyclic mechanism of skeletal muscle. The possible hypothetical scheme for the action of tetanus toxin in skeletal muscle would then be as in Fig. 3. Ca_a is calcium in the active form that can be used for muscular contraction. This can be obtained from three sources: the exchangeable calcium stored in muscle, calcium acquired from the plasma via the T-system, and the calcium cyclically regenerated by the relaxing system of skeletal muscle. Ca_p is calcium after its use in contraction. No assumptions are made concerning the particular form of calcium represented by Ca_a or Ca_p. Ca_p is in equilibrium with the plasma calcium, possibly by direct leakage, or, more probably, through the T-system and SR, and also with other calcium stores. Ca_{st1} is a calcium store that is capable of exchanging, and Ca_{st2} is the so-called unexchangeable calcium store. The nature of the reactions in steps 1, 2, 3, 4, and 5 need not be specified. Providing they have finite reaction rate constants, the mechanism will be cyclical. If tetanus toxin is introduced into skeletal muscle and binds in the junction of the T-system and SR, it could

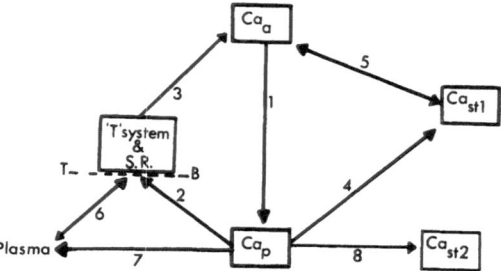

Fig. 3. A generalized hypothetical scheme for calcium movement in skeletal muscle showing where a possible block in tetanus intoxication might occur.

form a hypothetical block at the dotted line, TB, illustrated in Fig. 3. This would block reactions 2 and 6. The following events might then be expected to occur. Over a period of time, Ca_{st2} would increase if reaction 8 has a finite rate and, if reaction 7 is still operative, there would be a slight increase in the plasma calcium. It should be noted that the latter reaction would be the only absolute loss of skeletal muscle calcium. Our data shows that in the 20–25-g mouse with a plasma volume of 1–1.5 ml, changes in plasma calcium levels represent a loss of only 3–5 μg/g wet weight of muscle, an insignificant amount assuming that during the period of acute generalized intoxication the amount of calcium lost in the urine is negligible. If reaction 2 is rapid compared with reaction 4 and reaction 8 in normal muscle, blocking it in the poisoned muscle will result in accumulation of Ca_p. This is the calcium functionally defined as that which must be removed in order for relaxation to occur. Gradual rise in this component would result in muscular rigidity. The level of Ca_a would be partly maintained by means of the calcium in the exchangeable compartment Ca_{st1}. Thus, the muscle would continue to be able to contract. This hypothesis is compatible with the general picture of tetanus intoxication, but should not be considered as an explanation of the mechanism of tetanus intoxication. Depending upon the degree of blockade of the relaxing system and the relative rates of the reactions involved, this kind of mechanism might play a major or a subordinate role to the neural phase of tetanus intoxication. A block at this site would lead to the reaction mechanism involved in step 1, the reaction whose activation energy would be characterized for the value of Q_{10} which we have obtained. Whether such a system could be applied to central nervous tissue is not known. The only relevant studies are those of Luxoro and Yanez (1968) on the compartmentalization of calcium in the squid giant axon. This study extends the earlier work of Hodgkin and Keynes (1957) and demonstrates that if a suitable technique is chosen, two distinct exchangeable compartments for calcium can be demonstrated in the squid axon. However, without knowing whether calcium plays different roles at excitatory and inhibitory synapses, speculation on this point is inappropriate. Hyperexcitability of nerve is generally associated with hypocalcemia.

V. BINDING OF TETANUS TOXIN

Early students of the action of tetanus toxin were impressed by the strong affinity of tetanospasmin for nervous tissue. Wasserman and Takaki (1898) observed that homogenates of brain bound and inactivated tetanus toxin, but other organs did not. It was claimed by some (Marie, 1897) that cerebral gray matter bound more toxin than white matter. An important observation by Mayer and Ransom (1903) with great significance for clinical work was that once the toxin was bound it could no longer be neutralized by tetanus antitoxin. As early as 1908, Takaki attempted to isolate the material from brain which bound toxin. He isolated an alcohol-soluble mixture, most abundant in the white matter, that he called "cerebron." Earlier work by Landsteiner and Botteri (1906) had demonstrated that the fraction which bound toxin most strongly could be obtained by hot ethanol extraction of brain after prior acetone–ether extraction. This mixture, which he called "protagon," contained sphingolipids, cerebrosides, and sphingomyelin. More recently, in a series of investigations, van Heyningen and his associates attempted to identify the substances responsible for tetanus toxin binding in the central nervous system. These investigators found that both "protagon" and crude phrenosine fractions were active in binding the toxin, whereas sphingomyelin fractions were inactive (van Heyningen, 1959a). It was concluded that the tetanus toxin receptor was associated with the cerebroside fraction. In later work (1959b, 1961), it was stated that two components, gangliosides and cerebrosides, reacted together in the presence of calcium to bind the toxin. The ganglioside from gray matter was found to be an acidic, nondialysable, water-soluble glycolipid containing sialic acid, sphingosine, hexose, and hexosamine. Van Heyningen stated that toxin binding was dependent on free carboxyl and sialic acid residues. It should be stressed, however, that although the studies demonstrated that binding of the toxin to gangliosides occurred *in vitro*, there was no demonstration of a connecting link to the lethal action of the toxin.

This work was advanced by use of differential sedimentation to attempt to localize subcellular sites of tetanus toxin binding. Janoff (1964) reported that rabbit brain lysosomes and microsomes bound the toxin, probably due to their content of gangliosides. Patel and Rao (1966) reported that mitochondrial and microsomal fractions sedimented from rat and pigeon brain bound tetanus toxin and reduced its toxicity. Studies by Mellanby and Whittaker (1968), employing subfractionated, disrupted synaptosomes, disclosed that synaptic vesicles and mitochondria bound little toxin, whereas the synaptosome membrane fraction bound ten times the amount of the toxin bound by the synaptic vesicles and two times the amount bound by whole brain homogenates. It was concluded that little ganglioside is present in the synaptic vesicles and that earlier reports (Burton *et al.*, 1964) failed to reveal this.

Because of the technical problems of localizing minute quantities of protein at their sites of binding in disrupted tissue, an immunohistological method employing horseradish peroxidase was used by Zacks and Sheff (1968). Equine tetanus antitoxin was labelled with horseradish peroxidase by the method of Nakane and Pierce (1966) and used to localize sites of tetanus toxin binding in the fine structure of mouse brain and skeletal muscle. In skeletal muscle, the histochemical reaction product was found within the lumen of T-tubules and terminal sacs of the sarcoplasmic reticulum. Nonspecific binding of horseradish peroxidase within the gap substance filling synaptic clefts has complicated our work concerning toxin binding in mouse brain. The data from skeletal muscle suggests that tetanus toxin may produce a change in the ordinarily impermeable junction between the terminal sacs of the sarcoplasmic reticulum and the T-tubules in skeletal muscle.

A. The Rate of Binding of Tetanus Toxin *In Vivo*

1. Binding to Active Sites

It is generally agreed that the binding of tetanus toxin *in vivo* is a relatively irreversible process that takes place rapidly. The clinical observation supporting such a hypothesis is the fact that tetanus antitoxin is ineffective in altering the course of the intoxication once the signs have become visible. Wright (1954) showed, by giving antitoxin 30 min after the administration of intracerebral toxin to a guinea pig, that at least 50% of the 1 MLD dose was already bound.

Because of the extremely small amounts of toxin bound, it is not possible to use tracer substances attached to the toxin molecule as a means of measuring the rate of binding directly, and, consequently, indirect techniques must be used.

2. Toxin–Antitoxin Interaction

The most obvious method is to study the effectiveness of antitoxin in arresting intoxication. In all such models, the general technique of the experiment is as follows: A known dose of toxin is given at zero time; following this, a dose of antitoxin is given at specified time intervals after the toxin, and the development or lack of development of intoxication is noted. There are numerous variations which may be made on this simple technique. The site of injection of toxin or antitoxin can be intramuscular, intraperitoneal, intravenous, or any combination of these, and the amount of toxin injected can vary over a considerable range. The effects of these variations of techniques on the possible results are considerable, particularly because of the nature of the antigen–antibody reaction. A site of action for the toxin is, by definition, a site at which a molecule of toxin binds. Therefore, the process of binding at the site is, by definition, a bimolecular reaction. However, as has been noted by Eckmann (1963), the combination between toxin and antitoxin is a polymolecular process in which the combination between the molecules does not have a single value. This is characteristic of many antigen–antibody reactions and is the basis of the Danysz phenomenon (Danysz, 1899). In a given animal, the number of sites is finite, and if each is equally accessible to the toxin, the rate of binding should, to a first approximation, vary directly with the concentration of the toxin. However, for the reaction between toxin and antitoxin, the rate will vary exponentially with the concentration of the antitoxin. The exponent is the number of molecules of antibody bound by one toxin molecule. This is important in experimental situations where antitoxin is given to an animal to neutralize the circulating toxin, because this is a competitive situation in which the antitoxin is competing with the binding sites for the toxin. The proportion of the toxin which is bound to its sites of action in the presence of antitoxin will be partitioned according to the ratio between the velocities of the binding (v_b) and the neutralization (v_{nz}) reactions. If both these reactions are relatively irreversible, the fraction of the free toxin which will be bound in a short interval in the presence of antitoxin will be

$$\text{fraction bound} = \frac{v_b}{v_b + v_{nz}}$$

If the reaction with the binding site can be described as

$$T_f + S_f \rightarrow TS$$

where T_f is the free toxin, S_f is the number of free sites, and TS is toxin bound to sites, then

$$v_b = k_b\,(T_f) \cdot S_f \tag{1}$$

K_{nz} being the rate constant of binding.
If neutralization proceeds according to the reaction

$$T_f + nA_f \rightarrow TA_n$$

where A_f is the free antitoxin, n molecules of which react on an average with one molecule of toxin to yield the antibody–antigen complex TA_n, then

$$v_n = k_{nz}(T_f)\,(A_f)^n \tag{2}$$

k_{nz} being the rate constant of neutralization, and from this the fraction bound (F) will be

$$F = k_b/k_b + k_{nz}\,(A)^n/S_f \tag{3}$$

This relationship must be taken into account in all experiments in which antitoxin is given. The fact that a given dose of antitoxin will neutralize a particular quantity of toxin in the test tube does not necessarily mean that under competitive conditions, and the degree of dilution occurring *in vivo*, that that amount of antitoxin will have any effect. As a numerical example, 1 ml of a particular preparation of antitoxin may completely neutralize 5 μg of toxin in the test tube in 2 min. If however, 0.2 ml of this antitoxin preparation along with 1 μg of toxin (the same ratio between toxin and anti-toxin) are injected into a mouse with a plasma volume of 1.5 ml, there will be a dilution of 7.5 times. If the value of n is 2 (a low value for most anti-toxin–antigen combinations), the total rate of reaction between the two will be slowed by a factor of $1/7.5 \times 1/7.5^2$ or 422 times. Thus, in this example, complete neutralization requiring 2 min in the test tube would now require 844 min, a period of time more than adequate in the competetive situation to permit sufficient quantity of the toxin to bind and subsequently bring about death of the animal. It seems likely that some of the results obtained in the past by comparing the effectiveness of antitoxin against intravenous toxin with its effectiveness against intramuscular toxin have failed to consider the decreased rate of neutralization due to dilution. In experiments with very small intramuscular doses of toxin, the rate at which it diffuses from the muscle will keep the serum level of toxin low. In low dose experiments, antibody injected via the intravenous route will be excreted in a few days, which will tend to increase the partition of toxin between binding sites and neutralization so as to favor the binding sites. On the other hand, a large antitoxin/toxin ratio will favor a maximum number of antitoxin molecules being bound to each toxin molecule. The fact that antitoxin appears to be more effective against intravenous toxin than intramuscular toxin may be explained on a kinetic basis. However, Pillemer (1967) believes that the difference is due to reversible binding of toxin to a muscle component.

We have already given a preliminary report of our experiments on measuring the rate of binding of tetanus toxin in mice (Sheff and Zacks, 1966c). We began by incubating tetanus toxin and antitoxin together under the same conditions of osmolarity, pH, temperature, and concentration as we expected to use in *in vivo* experiments. Small aliquots were drawn from these incubation mixtures at various times and injected intravenously into mice. The volume of injection was 0.1 ml, giving a dilution factor of 15. We expected that the neutralization reaction would be greatly slowed and any residual toxin should be available for intoxication of the animals. We found that 80 units of commercially obtained tetanus antiserum of equine origin neutralized 10 μg of purified tetanus toxin in 2 min under these conditions. For this experiment, we used 0.1 ml of the solution containing 1500 units/ml of antitoxin so that, when diluted in the mouse, it would give a plasma concentration of approximately twice that in the test system. We gave groups of mice intravenous injections of known doses of tetanus toxin. At timed intervals, 0.1 ml of antitoxin was injected. The survival times of these groups of mice were recorded and compared with the survival times of a group of control mice which had received varying doses of the toxin. Comparison of the survival times of the mice receiving both toxin and antitoxin with those of the control animals yielded an "apparent dose." For example, an animal which had received 10 μg of toxin (known to be lethal in 120 min under these conditions) received antitoxin after 25 min and died 200 min after

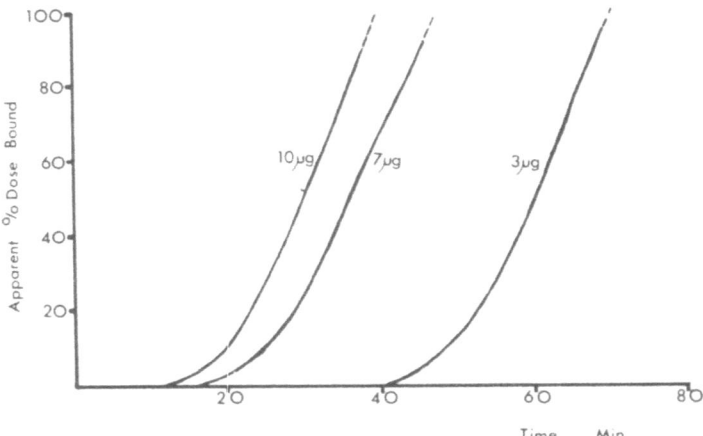

Fig. 4. Examples of the kinds of curves which are obtained when the rate of binding of large doses (as indicated on the curves) of purified tetanus neurotoxin is studied *in vivo* by the technique described in the text. The ordinate indicates the percentage of each dose which is apparently bound at the time of injection of antitoxin. Each curve represents the mean of 48 animals injected with each dose. The form of the time course of intoxication has been found in preliminary experiments. The 48 animals at each dose received their antitoxin on an individual, timed basis within the period covered by the binding curve. For this reason, the times of injection of antitoxin are not indicated.

receiving toxin. Examination of the survival time versus dose curve for the control animals shows that this is the expected survival time for a 5-μg dose. Thus, the "apparent dose" in this animal would be 5 μg or 50 % of the dose that was bound after 25 min.

The results of these experiments are shown graphically in Fig. 4, in which the apparent percentage of the dose bound is plotted against the time in minutes. The question arises as to the relationship between the apparent dose bound and the actual amount of toxin which was bound at the time the antitoxin was given. One obvious source of discrepancy would be if the toxin became unavailable to the antitoxin by passing through some barrier impermeable to the antitoxin without actually being bound. We do not think that this is likely. Tetanus toxin is an unremarkable molecule. The most recent figures for its molecular weight place it in the same range as those for the antitoxin. In addition, our experimental work on the localization of the toxin has never shown any appreciable quantities of the toxin free in the tissue spaces. Once the toxin leaves the circulation it is taken up at a rapid rate by the specific sites of action.

Other objections to these experiments are of a more technical nature. The two extremities of the curve are determined with maximum accuracy. It is easy to observe that within a certain time period, antitoxin is totally effective in inhibiting the reaction of the toxin, and it is equally easy to observe the point at which the antitoxin has no further effect upon the course of intoxication. The curves indicate that the whole of the 3 μg toxin dose is bound in approximately 75 min, whereas the first three 3 μg of the 10 μg dose is bound in 25 min. Taking these two figures alone, one would conclude that the initial rate of reaction between toxin and its site is directly proportional to the concentration of the toxin. If this were so, the rate of binding should diminish as more of the toxin is bound. However, the curves show that the rate of binding, based upon the apparent percentage dose bound, is either constant or may even increase with time. A second observable feature is that the time during which the antitoxin is totally effective, that is, the time before any of the toxin is bound, appears to be linearly proportional to the dose, and this again is inconsistent with the simple hypothesis that the rate of binding is directly proportional to the concentration of free toxin.

Although a definitive explanation of the shape of the binding curve is premature at this time, we suggest that curves of this shape might be expected if the binding of the toxin to its active sites is an irreversible process with a high activation energy and that the process involves cooperation between the binding sites as described by Ling (1969).

Figure 1 illustrates the results of experiments in which serum samples from mice poisoned with 5 μg of tetanus toxin were assayed for Ca^{2+} and Mg^{2+} content. The resulting curve indicates that changes in Ca^{2+} and Mg^{2+} occur during the binding period and that the binding period precedes the first of the overt physiological signs of intoxication in acutely intoxicated mice, the onset of body heat loss. Mice receiving 5 μg doses of toxin did not, under the conditions of these particular experiments, die in less than 250–300 min. The first signs of respiratory distress did not occur until 100–120 min. The binding period indicated in the curve covers the whole range of binding from 0–100%. It shows that 80% of the toxin is bound in approximately 30 min, or 10% of the entire time course of the intoxication. This is consistent with the previous discussion concerning the relative rates of development of the phases of intoxication, where it was concluded that the rate of binding of the toxin was not the limiting factor in the rate of development of the intoxication. Until some technique for stopping the action of tetanus toxin is found, the method described here appears to be the only one capable of yielding estimates of the rate of binding of the toxin. Although less than adequate, it offers opportunities for further experiments.

VI. PHYSIOLOGY OF TETANUS INTOXICATION

A. Effects of Tetanus Toxin on Neuromuscular Junctions

As with so many aspects of the physiology of tetanus toxin, there has

been considerable controversy about the action of the toxin on the neuromuscular junction. Lack of agreement between various investigators is
probably due to use of variably impure toxin preparations and to experimental techniques and type of equipment used. In 1939, Harvey reported
that he could produce transient local tetanus by intramuscular injections of
1/50–1/100 of a cat lethal dose. He used concentric needle electrodes placed
in the muscle to record electrical activity. Harvey observed that there was
persistence of electrical activity on voluntary movement and clonus on
dorsal flexure of the foot before evidence of muscular rigidity occurred.
When the peripheral nerve was cut, there was slight decrease in muscular
rigidity which was followed by complete relaxation over a period of 3–5 days.
Harvey interpreted this to be the result of the time required for complete
degeneration of the nerve endings. He claimed that no muscular rigidity
occured if the denervated muscle were injected with toxin. Injection of a
severed nerve 24 hr following injection of toxin into the muscle produced
signs of early rigidity that later subsided. Harvey found that skeletal muscle
injected with tetanus toxin gradually lost its ability to respond to maximal
stimulation of the motor nerve and that loss of twitch amplitude of 50–
60% occurred in approximately 5 days. In decerebrate animals, after cutting
the central connections of the motor nerves to the tibialis muscle, muscular
rigidity persisted. Electromyograms showed oscillatory potentials of various
frequencies and rhythms, and intermittent stimulation of the muscle produced outbursts of electrical activity and irregular twitching. Harvey stated
that curare, known to block acetylcholine receptors in neuromuscular
junctions, eliminated the toxin-induced spontaneous electrical activity and
rigidity. This occurred with doses of curare that did not eliminate the response of the muscle to stimuli arriving via the motor nerve. This partial
curarization reduced the duration of the repetitive action potentials and
resulted in decreased twitch tension. In addition, Harvey claimed that
physostigmine potentiated the oscillatory potentials that occurred during
the prolonged mechanical response of the muscle. It was concluded that the
site of toxin action was in the neuromuscular junction, not the muscle
itself. Several investigators (Schaeffer, 1944; Perdrup, 1946; Wright *et al.*,
1952; and Wright, 1955) were unable to repeat these experiments.

In more recent studies of toxin action at neuromuscular junctions,
Mackereth and Scott (1954) studied *in vivo* response of rat phrenic nerve–
diaphragm preparations. Following injection of toxin into the rat diaphragm, the local *in situ* electrical activity was recorded to indicate signs of
local tetanus. The *in vivo* diaphragm produced outbursts of potentials
proportional to the respiratory movements, whereas the intoxicated diaphragm produced continuous irregular potentials upon which were superimposed the respiratory potentials. When the diaphragms were studied *in*

vitro, the intoxicated diaphragm–phrenic nerve preparations did not produce spontaneous action potentials or nonrepetitive firing responses to a single stimulus, nor were there differences from the control in the sensitivity to curare. These findings, therefore, failed to confirm Harvey's observations. The Mackereth and Scott studies yielded no support for the peripheral action of the toxin and suggested that the *in situ* electrical hyperactivity of the intoxicated diaphragm–phrenic nerve preparation arose in the central nervous system.

The problem was further complicated by data obtained by Kobinger *et al.* (1956), who studied the release of potassium from skeletal muscle following intra-arterial injection of acetylcholine into cats with local tetanus. These studies revealed changes in the neuromuscular junctions that resembled those occurring following denervation. For example, there was no change in potassium release from the muscles 3 days after injection of the toxin; however, 6–8 days after injection, decreased amounts of acetylcholine were found necessary to obtain release of measurable quantities of potassium. Fourteen to 21 days following injection, there was a significant shift in the dose response curve to resemble the kind that occurs in chronic denervation of neuromuscular junctions.

In another study using electromyographic techniques (Prabhu and Oester, 1952), electrical activity was recorded from the tibialis anticus muscle of rabbits with local tetanus produced by injecting toxin either intramuscularly or intraneurally. These investigators found that early in local tetanus (1–5 days), there was constant stiffness and hyperreflexia, though there was also much normal motor activity. As intoxication progressed over a period of 5–8 days, polyphasic potentials, positive sharp waves, and fibrillation potentials appeared in the electromyograms. In the later period of 10–35 days, fibrillation potentials occurred that resembled the potentials observed in chronic denervation. As the muscle recovered from the effects of local tetanus intoxication, the sequence of electromyographic events was reversed. The investigators concluded that their data could only be explained by action of tetanus toxin at the muscle level as well as in the central nervous system.

More recent studies by Feigen *et al.* (1963) and Parsons *et al.* (1966) were concerned with the action of tetanus toxin on peripheral synapses. They measured these effects in isolated nerve–muscle preparations. These investigators found that impure toxin increased the frequency of random discharges of miniature endplate potentials recorded by microelectrodes from intoxicated skeletal muscle. Their interpretation of this data was that the toxin caused depolarization of the presynaptic terminal, an effect that was absent when calcium was excluded from the bathing medium. Thus, the action of toxin was potentiated by calcium. Depolarization by potassium blocked or reversed the peripheral affects of tetanus toxin, indicating that the toxin probably acted by lowering the presynaptic resting potential. Some of these studies (Feigen *et al.*, 1963) were concerned with a fraction of the purified toxin remaining after 98 % of what the authors termed "central acting" tetanospasmin was removed by absorption on "protagon." This procedure yielded a protein that was reported to have predominantly peripheral action. The nature of this peripherally acting toxin has not yet been studied by other investigators. Feigen *et al.* (1963) did not provide data to identify which toxin fraction they had isolated. These studies suggested that the toxin decreased the probability of transmitter release following nerve spikes, thereby decreasing the rate of initial transmitter depletion and the level of sustained transmitter output in neuromuscular junctions. Kowarzyk *et al.* (1965) studied the concurrent intoxication of mice with botulinum and tetanus toxins. Their results are difficult to interpret and do not seem to warrant the conclusion that two distinct receptors can be identified by this kind of experimentation.

A recent study by Muchnick and Rubinstein (1967) was concerned with the relative importance of the peripheral and central actions of tetanus toxin. Rat phrenic nerve–hemidiaphragm preparations were used in *in vitro* experiments and rats were injected intravenously with large quantities of toxin in *in vivo* experiments. These investigators found that large amounts of tetanus toxin applied to the phrenic nerve–diaphragm preparation produced progressive decrease in the amplitude of the mechanical response of the muscle to nerve stimulation. This effect was blocked by pretreatment of the toxin with antitoxin. *In situ* injections of the toxin resulted in fatigue of muscular contractions during low frequency stimulation. Tetanic fusion was obtained at lower stimulation frequency. When the rat moved its hind legs spontaneously, the stimulated leg was frequently placed in hyperextension. The authors concluded that tetanus toxin has direct local action on skeletal muscle but that central stimulation is necessary to bring out the complete syndrome. This contribution fails to state the degree of purity or the means of preparation of the toxin. It is likely that crude toxin was employed because of the large doses used.

It is clear that there is considerable difficulty in demonstrating a specific action of tetanus toxin on neuromuscular junctions in the presence of intact innervation. Possibly, various impure toxin preparations may have been the source of some of the discrepancies in this kind of data. The presence of nontoxic protein and uncontrolled quantities of cations may have been the source of the variable results obtained by electromyographic recordings from intoxicated skeletal muscle.

From the morphologic point of view, we have been unable to demonstrate either acute or long-range changes in the fine structure of neuromuscular junctions poisoned with tetanus toxin, nor have we been able to localize by light microscopy or electron microscopy binding of tetanus toxin within neuromuscular junctions.

B. Effects of Tetanus Toxin on the Physiology of Skeletal Muscle and the Problem of Local Tetanus

The majority of early investigators of tetanus intoxication believed that the central nervous system was primarily affected, although there was evidence for action at the neuromuscular junction. (*See* Chaps. 10 and 12 for discussions of central nervous system involvement.) There were several clinical and experimental observations that could not be explained by exclusive central action of the toxin (Klemm, 1889; Vaillard and Vincent; 1891, Abel *et al.*, 1938; and Penitschka, 1953). For example, universal clinical observations of transient local tetanus that did not proceed to descending tetanus suggested that a central site of action could not explain this aspect of the syndrome. Another phenomenon, not easily explained by a central lesion, was the observation that when tetanus intoxication had proceeded to muscle contracture, there was no muscular relaxation when the motor nerve was cut. This was regarded as a form of myostatic contracture, a nonspecific phenomenon known to occur following tenotomy.

When attention to the problem of changes in skeletal muscle during tetanus intoxication was investigated, distinct abnormalities were found. Ranson and Morris (1926), Ranson (1928), Ranson and Dickson (1928), and Ranson and Ranson (1929) observed reduced elasticity and inability to relax after repeated contractions of tetanus-poisoned skeletal muscles. Ranson (1928) described an "obscure alteration" in the muscle that was retained after section of the motor nerve. He measured a probably significant, decreased rate of relaxation in poisoned rat muscle, although this contradicted observations by Speigel (1923). Ranson also reported a questionably significant reduction in the degree of shortening during contraction of tetanus-poisoned muscle. Ranson suggested three possible explanations for the observed changes in the skeletal muscle during local tetanus. His results could be due to: (1) local effects on proprioceptors, (2) tonic impulses from other than ventral root sources, and (3) direct action of the toxin on skeletal muscle. He favored the last explanation because he observed that if 1 ml of toxin was injected into cat muscle and 6 days later the sciatic and femoral nerves were cut, pressure curves recorded from the muscle demonstrated resistance to flexion as if the muscle were a "viscous body." The muscle failed to return to rest length when stretched. Ranson emphasized that normal muscle is not ductile, whereas tetanus-intoxicated muscle shows an initial increase in ductility followed by a decrease as intoxication proceeds. A study by Schottelius and Schottelius (1959) reported increased tetanus twitch ratios, shortened twitch relaxation time, lower fusion frequency, and increased semidynamic stiffness with short stretch on tetanic stimulation in skeletal muscle poisoned with tetanus toxin. The twitch relaxation time in these studies was found to be 73% of the control value, and the peak twitch tension was 51% of the control. These data indicated that relaxation of intoxicated skeletal muscle was slowed.

Evidence from morphologic studies employing labelled antibodies (Zacks and Sheff, 1968) demonstrated that tetanus toxin is localized in the T-system and terminal sacs of the sarcoplasmic reticulum of skeletal muscle, sites involved in the excitation–relaxation process. It is possible that the toxin interferes with the movement of calcium to and from the sarcoplasmic reticulum, a mechanism known to be essential for muscle relaxation (Podolsky and Constantin, 1964). Binding of tetanus toxin in the location of the junction of T-system and the terminal sarcoplasmic reticulum could interfere with the exchange of calcium in this critical system. We have already shown in preliminary experiments with ^{45}Ca (Sheff and Zacks, 1968) an increased mobility of calcium in and out of the muscle at the time when binding of the toxin is complete and physical signs of intoxication are maximal.

C. Dual Target Sites of Toxin Actions: The Central Nervous System and the Skeletal Muscle

From the available evidence, it appears that the syndrome of tetanus intoxication is dependent upon tetanus toxin binding within the central nervous system, particularly in the spinal cord, as well as by skeletal muscle. This would explain many of the physiological data as well as morphologic findings using labelled antibodies. As we have pointed out, this concept of dual action has been common in the writings of many early students of tetanus intoxication. The major evidence for the muscular site of action includes the studies of Ranson and his associates, and, more recently, evidence of selective binding of purified tetanus neurotoxin labelled with fluorescein or horseradish peroxidase. Furthermore, biochemical abnormalities in potassium, sodium, and calcium in tetanus-intoxicated muscle have been obtained by Zacks and Sheff (1966).

We have previously described the controversy concerning toxin action at the neuromuscular junction. Although no direct evidence to resolve this point is available, an hypothesis that could account for several reports of abnormal neuromuscular function recorded electrophysiologically (Kobinger et al., 1956; Prabhu and Oester, 1962; Feigen et al., 1966) would be that the postsynaptic membrane or specific areas of contact of T-system with the subneural apparatus within the neuromuscular junction (Saito and Zacks, 1970) may be altered by the binding of toxin. This would lead to changes in electrolyte permeability that, by altering membrane potentials, would affect neuromuscular transmission without directly interfering with acetylcholine release or the action of acetylcholinesterase. Since binding of the toxin to T-system tubules and terminal sacs of the sarcoplasmic reticulum is temporarily associated with electrolyte changes that imply changes in membrane excitability, it is likely that similar changes in excitability may occur in central neurons or at inhibitory synapses where toxin is bound to these membranes. Many of the previous experiments designed to rule out peripheral sites of toxin action were inadequate because of serious errors of design and technique. For example, if a dual lesion involving a hyperexcitable muscle and hyperexcitable nerve is required for the full production of local tetanus, any experiments in which the nerve is interrupted by sectioning or by sclerosing solutions, thus eliminating the pathway by which central excitation reaches the hyperirritable muscle will, not surprisingly, eliminate signs of local tetanus intoxication. Experimental studies showing changes in neuromuscular junctions consistent with denervation are not in accord with the experimental or clinical tetanus syndrome.

VII. SUMMARY

It is curious that after 80 years of intensive investigation, we are still unable to describe the lesion in tetanus intoxication in more than general terms. The explanation seems to lie in the fact that tetanus intoxication is fundamentally a problem of molecular pathology. In order to understand the action of the toxin, it is first necessary to understand the normal molecular biology of its target organs, and also something of the chemistry of the toxin molecule itself. It is useful to remember that in the 1890s, when tetanus intoxication was shown to be due to a soluble substance found in cellfree culture filtrates, virtually nothing was known of the mechanisms involved in muscular contraction or in the initiation and transmission of the nerve impulse. Nothing was known of the movement of electrolytes in either muscle or nerve during activity and the relationships of the concentrations of these electrolytes to the processes of excitation and relaxation. Nor was anything known of the proximal–distal movement of proteins in axons. Knowledge of the microanatomy of nerve was also unknown, and the structure of the motor endplate with its special relationships between axonal and Schwann cell elements had not been described. The existence of central excitatory and central inhibitory states was beginning to be understood, but the existence of specific inhibitory and excitatory synapses on the neuron was unknown. There were, therefore, few objective physiological criteria which had to be satisfied by any hypothesis that would explain the action of the toxin. Hypotheses were made about its transport in the nerve "fiber" to act in some manner on neurons, without these postulates having to satisfy, either quantitatively or qualitatively, known physiological data. The only criterion for these hypotheses seemed to be that they should be logically complete descriptions of the intoxication at a relatively superficial level. The growth of purely mechanistic models of neuromuscular activity, in the early twentieth century, which gave complete descriptions at the macroscopic level without any biochemical constraints, did little to disturb these early hypotheses.

The situation today is very different. Both contraction and relaxation in skeletal muscle are known to be active processes involving the use of high-energy phosphates and the movement of ions, particularly the divalent ion, calcium. Many details still remain obscure, but enough is known to limit the number of hypotheses which can be made about the action of substances which prevent muscular relaxation. Less is known of the biochemical events in the central nervous system, since the nature of this tissue makes study of these events extraordinarily difficult. There is, therefore, a wide gap between the description of the events which occur at the motor neuron, in terms of electrical changes which can be recorded electrophysiologically, and the biochemistry of the movement of charged particles, which is the physical substratum from which the neural potentials arise. The microanatomy of the pathway from the neuron to skeletal muscles has been well described, though controversy still exists. There is considerable evidence for the passage of protein down the axon from the neuron cell body and considerable evidence against the passage of macromolecules of protein size up the entire length of the axon from muscle to the neuron cell body. These last observations, and the morphological description of the motor nerve at the electron microscope level of resolution, make the descriptions of the mechanism of tetanus intoxication by absorption of the toxin at the neuromuscular junction and passage up the nerve "fiber" extremely doubtful.

We must state that at the present time there is insufficient biochemical evidence about the mechanism by which the nerve impulse arises under normal circumstances, and insufficient evidence of the biochemical effects of tetanus toxin on these mechanisms under conditions of intoxication, to form a logically complete theory of tetanus intoxication. The bulk of the evidence seems to favor a dual site of action; that is, the toxin acts both within the central nervous system and also peripherally in skeletal muscle. The central nervous system lesion, which may be more important, remains virtually undescribed. The physiological evidence is clear that the toxin in some manner lowers the level of inhibition of motor neurons, possibly by inter-fering with the transmission of inhibitory impulses. In skeletal muscle, the toxin localizes at the site, the junction between the sarcoplasmic reticulum and the T-system, which is morphologically consistent with a biochemical lesion of the relaxing system. Independent evidence shows that, when bound to skeletal muscle, the toxin is capable of interfering with electrolyte balance, and in particular, with the mechanism concerning calcium movement within the muscle. The toxin does not appear to act directly upon any of the major metabolic systems, but instead changes in these appear to be secondary to toxin interference with the mechanism of respiration. Interference with respiratory movements are also visible in the goldfish, in which the signs of intoxication closely resemble those occurring in mammals.

There is a wide field for further research. Further data are required concerning the role the toxin plays in disturbing electrolyte balance in skeletal muscle, possibly by quantitating its effects on calcium uptake by sarcoplasmic reticulum. It would be of great interest to know precisely what enzymatic functions involved in electrolyte transport are either stimulated or inhibited by the toxin. At a deeper level of resolution, it would be of considerable interest to know the structure and location of the center where the toxin acts, and the mechanism by which it forms such a strong bond with its morphological substrate. The effects of the toxin on the central nervous system also provide an open field for investigation. Additional morphological studies on the exact site of localization of the toxin on or within the motor neuron are required. Beyond this, the student of tetanus intoxication must wait for future knowledge of the biochemistry of the nerve impulse and the biochemistry of inhibitory and excitatory transmitter substances before much progress can be made in studying the central action of the toxin. However, recent work by Johnston *et al.* (1969) and others indicates that biochemical knowledge in this area is increasing rapidly. It is possible that the use of purified toxin itself may facilitate the investigation of these important processes.

VIII. REFERENCES

Abel, J. J., W. M. Firor, and W. Chalian (1938), *Bull. Johns Hopkins Hosp.*, **63**:379.
Bizzini, B., A. Turpin, and M. Raynaud (1969), *Ann. Inst. Pasteur*, **116**:686.
Brieger, L. and G. Cohn (1893), *Z. Hyg. Infektions Krankh.*, **15**:1.
Brody, I. A. (1969), *New Eng. J. Med.*, **281**:187.
Brooks, V. B., D. R. Curtis, and J. C. Eccles (1957), *J. Physiol. (London)*, **135**:655.
Burton, R. M., R. E. Howard, S. Baer, and V. M. Balfour (1964), *Biochim. Biophys. Acta*, **84**:441.
Cartwright, T. E. and M. A. Lauffer (1952), *Proc. Soc. Exp. Biol. Med.*, **81**:508.
Courmont, J. and M. Doyon (1893), *Arch. Physiol.*, **25**:64.
Cowles, R. B. and N. B. Nelson (1947), *Proc. Soc. Exp. Biol. Med.*, **64**:220.
Crozier, W. J. (1924), *J. Gen. Physiol.*, **7**:189.
Daniel, E. E. (1965), Attempted synthesis of data regarding divalent ions in muscle function, *in* "Muscle" (W. M. Paul, E. E. Daniel, C. M. Kay, and G. Monckton, eds.), Pergamon Press, Oxford, pp. 295–313.
Danysz, J. (1899), *Ann. Inst. Pasteur*, **13**:156.
Davenport, H. A. and S. W. Ranson (1929), *Proc. Soc. Exp. Biol. Med.*, **26**:466.

Davies, J. R. and E. A. Wright (1955), *Br. J. Exp. Pathol.*, **36**:487.
Dawson, D. J. and L. W. Nichol (1969), *Austral. J. Biol. Sci.*, **22**:247.
Dunn, M. S., M. N. Camien, and L. Pillemer (1949), *Arch. Biochem.*, **22**:374.
Eaton, M. D. (1936), *Proc. Soc. Exp. Biol.*, **35**:16.
Eaton, M. D. and A. Gronau (1938), *J. Bact.*, **36**:423.
Ebashi, S. and M. Endo (1964), Further studies on the calcium-binding activity of the relaxing factor, *in* "Biochemistry of Muscle Contraction" (J. Gergeley, ed.), Little, Brown and Company, Boston, pp. 199–206.
Eckmann, L. (1963), "Tetanus prophylaxis and therapy," Grune and Stratton, New York.
Ehrlich, O. (1898), *Berlin Klin. Wochenschr.*, **35**:273.
Elis, J. and I. Janku (1961), *Cesk. Epidemiol. Mikrobiol. Imunol.*, **10**:296.
Evans, W. H. and H. MacIlwain (1967), *J. Neurochem.*, **14**:35.
Faber, K. (1890), *Berlin. Klin. Wochenschr.*, **27**:717.
Feigen, G. A., N. S. Peterson, W. W. Hofmann, G. H. Genther, and W. E. Van Heyningen (1963), *J. Gen. Microbiol.*, **33**:489.
Flemming, W. J. (1927), *J. Exp. Med.*, **46**:279.
Frangini, G., A. Comparini, and A. Dainelli (1956), *Lo Sperimentale*, **106**:316.
Gorini, L. (1954), *Boll. Ist. Sieroterap. Milan.*, **33**:488.
Hardegree, M. D. and L. W. Wannamaker (1965), *Proc. Soc. Exp. Biol. Med.*, **118**:692.
Harvey, A. M. (1939), *J. Physiol. (London)*, **96**:348.
Hodgkin, A. L. and R. D. Keynes (1957), *J. Physiol. (London)*, **138**:253.
Imbriano, A. E. (1950), *Sem. Méd. Buenos Aires*, **57**:185.
Ipsen, J. (1951), *J. Immunol.*, **66**:687.
Janoff, A. (1964), *Nature*, **202**:913.
Johnston, G. A. R., W. C. deGroat, and D. R. Curtis (1969), *J. Neurochem.*, **16**:797.
Kaeser, H. E. and A. Saner (1969), *Nature*, **223**:842.
Kerr, J. H., J. L. Corbett, C. Prys-Roberts, A. Crampton Smith, and J. M. K. Spalding (1968), *Lancet II*, 236.
Kitasato, S. (1891), *Z. Hyg. Infektions Krankh.*, **10**:267.
Klemm, P. (1889), *Deut. Z. Chir.*, **29**:168.
Kloetzel, K. (1961), *Rev. Inst. Med. Trop. Saõ Paulo*, **3**:290.
Kloetzel, K. (1962), *Rev. Inst. Med. Trop. Saõ Paulo*, **4**:29.
Kloetzel, K. (1963), *JAMA*, **185**:559.
Kobinger, W., O. Kraupp, H. Stormann, and P. H. Clodi (1956), *Arch. Exp. Path. Phamakol.*, **228**:425.
Kowarzyk, H., L. Czerchawski, and W. Fal (1965), *Arch. Immunol. Therap. Exp.*, **13**:426.
Lamanna, C. and C. J. Carr (1967), *Clin. Parm. Therap.*, **8**:286.
Landsteiner, K. and A. Botteri (1906), *Zbl. Bakt. I Abt. Orig.*, **42**:562.
Largier, J. F. (1956), *Biochim. Biophys. Acta*, **21**:433.
Ling, G. N. (1969), *Int. Rev. Cytol.*, **26**:1.
Lipskaya, T. Yu (1968), *Biokhimia*, **33**:867.
London, E. S. and V. M. Aristovsky, (1917), *C. R. Soc. de Biol.*, **80**:756.
Luxoro, M. and E. Yanez (1968), *J. Gen. Physiol.*, **51**:115.
Luzzati, V. and F. Husson (1962), *J. Cell. Biol.*, **12**:207.
Mackereth, M. B. and D. J. Scott (1954), *N. Z. U. Otago Med. Sch. Proc.*, **32**:13.
Macrae, J. (1967), *Proc. of a Symposium on Tetanus in Great Britain* (M. Ellis, ed.) Leeds, p. 11.
Mangalo, R., B. Bizzini, A. Turpin, and M. Raynaud (1968), *Biochim. Biophys. Acta*, **168**:583.
Marie, A. (1897), *Ann. Inst. Pasteur*, **11**:591.
Marr, A. G. M. and R. W. Patterson (1960), *Aust. J. Sci.*, **23**:131.
Mellanby, J. and V. P. Whittaker (1968), *J. Neurochem.*, **15**:205.
Meyer, H. and F. Ransom (1903), *Arch. f. Exp. Pathol. Pharmakol.*, **39**:369.
Michelazzi, L., M. D. Mor, and M. U. Dianzani (1955) *Experientia*, **11**:73.
Morganroth, J. (1900) *Arch. Intern. Pharmacodyn.*, **7**:265.

Morax, V. and A. Marie (1903), *Ann. Inst. Pasteur*, **17**:335.
Muchnik, S. and E. H. Rubinstein (1967), *Acta Physiol. Latino Amer.*, **17**:166.
Muntz, J. A., L. Pillemer, and K. C. Robbins, *Ann. Rev. Microbiol.*, **3**:265.
Murphy, S. G., T. H. Plummer, and K. D. Miller (1968), *Fed. Proc.*, **27**:268.
Murphy, S. M. and K. D. Miller (1967), *J. Bact.*, **94**:580.
Nakane, P. K. and G. B. Pierce, Jr., (1966), *J. Histochem. Cytochem.*, **14**:929.
Nayler, W. G. (1965), Calcium and other divalent ions in contraction of cardiac muscle, *in*, "Muscle" (W. M. Paul, E. E. Daniel, C. M. Kay, and G. Monckton, eds.), Pergamon Press, Oxford, pp. 167–184.
Nicolaiër, A. (1884), *Deut. Med. Wochenschr.*, **10**:842.
Parsons, R. L., W. W. Hofmann, and G. A. Feigen (1966), *Amer. J. Physiol.*, **210**:84.
Patel, A. A. and S. S. Rao (1966), *Brit. J. Pharm.*, **26**:730.
Peachey, L. D. (1962), Accumulation of divalent ions in mitochondrial granules of intact cells, *in*, "Electron Microscopy, Fifth International Congress, Philadelphia," vol. II, Academic Press, New York.
Penitschka, W. (1953), *Arch. Klin. Chir.*, **279**:434.
Perdrup, A. (1946), *Acta Pharmacol.*, **2**:121.
Pillemer, L., R. G. Wittler, and D. B. Grossberg (1946), *Science*, **103**:615.
Pillemer, L. and W. B. Wartman (1947), *J. Imunol.*, **55**:277.
Pillemer, L. and D. H. Moore (1948), *J. Biol. Chem.*, **173**:427.
Podolsky, R. J. and L. L. Costantin (1964), *Fed. Proc.*, **23**:933.
Prabhu, V. G. and Y. T. Oester (1962), *J. Pharm. Exp. Therap.*, **138**:241.
Ranson, S. W. (1928), *Arch. Neurol. Psychiat.*, **20**:663.
Ranson, S. W. and H. H. Dixon (1928), *Amer. J. Physiol.*, **86**:312.
Ranson, S. W. and A. L. Morris (1926), *J. Comp. Neurol.*, **42**:99.
Ranson, S. and S. W. Ranson (1929), *Arch. Pathol.*, **7**:949.
Raynaud, M., A. Turpin, and B. Bizzini (1960), *Ann. Inst. Pasteur*, **99**:167.
Rowson, K. E. K. (1961), *J. Gen. Microbiol.*, **25**:315.
Saito, A. and S. I. Zacks (1970), *J. Histochem Cytochem.*, **18**:302.
Schaefer, H. (1944), *Arch. Exp. Pathol. Pharmakol.*, **203**:59.
Schottelius, B. A. and D. D. Schottelius (1959), *Proc. Soc. Exp. Biol. Med.*, **100**:282.
Sheff, M. F., M. Perry, and S. I. Zacks (1963), *Proc. Soc. Exp. Biol. Med.*, **14**:96.
Sheff, M. F., B. Perry, and S. I. Zacks (1965), *Biochim. Biophys. Acta*, **100**:215.
Sheff, M. F. and S. I. Zacks (1966), unpublished observations.
Sheff, M. F. and S. I. Zacks (1966a), *J. Cell. Biol.*, **31**:105a.
Sehff, M. F. and S. I. Zacks (1968), *J. Cell. Biol.*, **39**:123a.
Sheff, M. F. and S. I. Zacks (1968a), unpublished observations.
Spiegel, E. A. (1923), "Zur physiologie u. pathologie des skelettmuskeltonus," Springer, Berlin.
Stevenson, J. W. (1958), *Amer. J. Med. Sci.*, **235**:317.
Takaki, K. (1908), *Beitr. Z. Chem. Physiol. Path.*, **11**:288.
Van Heyningen, W. E. (1959a), *J. Gen. Microbiol.*, **20**:291.
Van Heyningen, W. E. (1959b), *J. Gen. Microbiol.*, **20**:301.
Van Heyningen, W. E. and P. M. Miller (1961), *J. Gen. Microbiol.*, **24**:107.
Vaillard, L. and H. Vincent (1891), *Ann. Inst. Pasteur*, **5**:1.
Vejss, T. and B. Kozesnik (1954), *Chek. Fisiol.*, **3**:83.
Von Behring, E. (1892), *Z. Hyg. Infektionskrankh.*, **12**:45.
Wassermann, A. and J. Takaki (1898), *Berlin Klin. Wochschr.*, **35**:5.
Weiss, J. M. (1955), *J. Exp. Med.*, **102**:783.
Wensink, F. and J. A. Cohen (1953), *Biochim. Biophys. Acta*, **10**:184.
Wensinck, F., J. J. Boeve, and H. Renaud (1953), *Brit. J. Exp. Pathol.*, **34**:681.
Wilson, G. S. and A. A. Miles (1964), "Topley and Wilson's Principles of Bacteriology and Immunology," 5th ed., Williams and Wilkins Co., Baltimore, p. 278.
Wright, E. A., R. S. Morgan, and G. P. Wright (1952), *Lancet*, **2**:316.
Wright, E. A. (1954), *J. Path. Bact.*, **68**:131.
Wright, G. P. (1955), *Pharmacol. Rev.*, **7**:413.

Zacks, S. I. and M. F. Sheff (1964), *J. Neuropath. Exp. Neurol.*, **23**:306.

Zacks, S. I. and M. F. Sheff (1965), *Acta Neuropathol.*, **4**:267.

Zacks, S. I., J. A. S. Hall, and M. F. Sheff (1966), *Amer. J. Pathol.*, **48**:811.

Zacks, S. I. and M. F. Sheff (1966), Morphological and biochemical studies of tetanus intoxication in: *Proc. V. Internat. Congress of Neuropathology* (F. Lüthy and A. Bischoff, eds.), Excerpta Medica Found., Amsterdam, p. 673.

Zacks, S. I. and M. F. Sheff (1968), *Science*, **159**:643.

Chapter 12

Tetanus Toxin as a Neuropharmacological Tool

D. R. Curtis

Department of Physiology
Australian National University
Canberra, Australia

I. INTRODUCTION

The importance of the toxin of *Clostridium tetani* as a pharmacological tool is related to the suppression of certain types of central inhibition in vertebrates by both this toxin and strychnine. Although the actions of these substances on inhibitory synaptic transmission are not identical, both appear to affect the same type of synapse, which occurs predominantly in the spinal cord and which for convenience has been classified as "strychnine-sensitive."

Systemically administered strychnine affects the operation of neurons throughout the central nervous system. Although the alkaloid can be administered microelectrophoretically near a single neuron, the investigation of its effect on synaptic inhibition may be complicated by the inability to obtain a uniform concentration at all synapses upon that neuron, and by the complex concentration-dependent effects of strychnine on neuronal membrane. Tetanus toxin, after deposition of relatively small amounts near selected cells or nuclei, diffuses slowly through nervous tissue to produce a more or less uniform concentration around any one cell. As the action of the toxin is highly specific for inhibitory synapses, progressive changes in synaptic inhibition can be studied under conditions where at least initially there is minimal alteration in the afferent inhibitory volley, and little general disturbance to the rest of the nervous system. The following review is concerned mainly with the use of tetanus toxin in studying central inhibition, and in addition includes a discussion of its action at some peripheral cholinergic synapses.

II. TECHNIQUES OF ADMINISTRATION

Tetanus toxin (tetanospasmin, van Heyningen, 1950; Stevenson, 1962; Lamanna and Carr, 1967), isolated from filtrates of cultures of *Clostridium tetani*, can be obtained in crystalline form (Pillemer *et al.*, 1948) as a high-molecular weight protein (Pillemer and Robbins, 1949; Largier, 1956; Dawson and Mauritzen, 1967; Mangola *et al.*, 1968; Dawson and Nichol, 1969). Animals vary in their susceptibility to the toxin (Payling Wright, 1955), and for convenience assay is usually performed with mice (15–20 g). The MLD or LD_{50} is estimated from the proportion of animals dying with signs of tetanus within 96 hr of an intramuscular injection of toxin into the upper hind limb (Pillemer, 1946; Pillemer and Wartman, 1947). The purified toxin (2–20×10^{-7} MLD/mg nitrogen) is relatively unstable, but both highly pure and less-pure samples can be stored either in a dried form or at $-25°C$ dissolved in a buffered (pH 7.4) 0.3 M glycine solution. For assay and experimental purposes, dilutions are made with buffered saline or physiological solutions containing 1% peptone, 0.2% gelatin or 0.3 M glycine. It is important that the potency of stored toxin be checked before use, and that the presence of culture media products and other bacterial proteins does not complicate effects induced by relatively impure samples.

Because of its extreme toxicity (human lethal dose less than 10^{-4} mg, van Heyningen, 1968), tetanus toxin and all contaminated glassware, animals, etc. must be handled with great care. Detoxification is readily achieved by boiling in acidified water. All personnel must be protected both by prior immunization and the ready availability of antitetanus serum.

Although tetanus toxin can be injected peripherally into muscles or nerves, sites from which it eventually passes via the ventral roots into the spinal cord or brain stem, and thence into higher centers, direct microinjection into nervous tissue is usually a more convenient and rapid method of selective administration. Dosages are usually expressed in terms of the mouse MLD or LD_{50}. The volume of injected solution and the diameter of the micropipette are kept small to minimize tissue damage. Pressure injection into nervous tissue via fine ($<50\ \mu$) micropipettes may be complicated by leakage in the syringe system or by delayed ejection resulting from complete or partial occlusion of the pipette orifice by tissue components. Injection sites are usually determined visually on an anatomical basis. Assistance can be gained by electrical recording of multiple- or single-cell activity obtained by using either the fluid-containing micropipette as a recording electrode (Curtis, 1964; Keynes, 1964) or an attached microelectrode (Curtis and de Groat, 1968). The toxin has been estimated to diffuse through nervous tissue at a rate approximating 1 mm/hr (Brooks *et al.*, 1957; Brooks and Asanuma, 1965), the rate of spread along nerve trunks in the cat after intraneural or intramuscular injection being of the order of 4 mm/hr (Brooks, Curtis, and Eccles, unpublished observations). Tetanus toxin can also be administered electrophoretically from glass micropipettes (Curtis, 1964), although immediate effects may result from other components of the solution, particularly depressant amino acids such as glycine.

III. TETANUS TOXIN AND CENTRAL INHIBITION

Although similarities between the clinical effects of tetanus toxin and strychnine had been recognized for some time (Simpson, 1854; Nicolaïer, 1885; Payling Wright, 1955; van Heyningen, 1968), and Sherrington (1905) had demonstrated that both substances modified spinal reflexes and their inhibition by impulses of both segmental and supraspinal (cortical) origin, evidence has been provided only comparatively recently which equates the action of both tetanus toxin and strychnine to antagonism of spinal inhibition (Bradley *et al.*, 1953; Brooks *et al.*, 1957). In the intervening period much debate was concerned with the site of action of the toxin, and its means of distribution through the body. These arguments are not relevant to the present paper, but are discussed in detail in several reviews (Payling Wright, 1955; Stevenson, 1962; Laurence and Webster, 1963; Lamanna and Carr, 1967; as well as Chap. 11). It is believed that in mammals the toxin acts predominantly in the central nervous system after spreading along peripheral nerve trunks from the site of inoculation or toxin production (*see* Payling Wright, 1955; van Heyningen, 1968).

Experimental tetanus resulting from intramuscular or intraneural injection of the toxin can be outlined as follows: after injection of small amounts of toxin the effects remain restricted to spinal and brain stem segments anatomically related to the motor nerves carrying the toxin. "Local" tetanus is thus characterized by muscle rigidity, disturbed reflexes of limb or brain stem motor nuclei, and disturbances of sensory mechanisms. After larger doses of toxin, the effects are more widespread. The toxin travels cranially, caudally, and to contralateral segments ("ascending" tetanus), eventually involving brain stem neurons and reflexes. With extremely large doses, and presumably as a consequence of toxin reaching the nervous system via the blood stream, these manifestations may be preceded by the classical signs of generalized tetanus, the involvement of muscles of the face, head and neck, then of the limbs, and finally generalized convulsions—"descending" tetanus. Early involvement of the lower cranial motor nuclei by circulating toxin probably indicates penetration of the blood–brain barrier in the region of the floor of the fourth ventricle.

The clinical signs of the various forms of tetanus and their progression (see Courtois-Suffit and Giroux, 1918), are closely related to the site of toxin injection or production, the amount injected or produced, and its spread through the neural axis and blood stream. The initial effects of direct injection of the toxin into the nervous system are related to the site of injection: disturbances of segmental muscles and reflexes if into the spinal ventral horn (Meyer and Ranson, 1903; Firor and Jonas, 1938); hyperaesthesia and pain if into the dorsal root or dorsal horn—tetanus dolorosus (Fletcher, 1903); rapid death with signs ascribable to effects on brain stem nuclei after medullary injection (Wright et al., 1950); and alterations of cortical function after injection into the cerebral cortex (Brooks and Asanuma, 1962; Carrea and Lanari, 1962).

A. Spinal Cord

1. Inhibition of Spinal Afferent Origin

Whereas in his original experiments with strychnine and tetanus toxin Sherrington (1905) considered that spinal inhibition was converted into excitation, later work (Liddell and Sherrington, 1925) indicated that strychnine reduced and eventually abolished the inhibitory effect of certain spinal afferent volleys. Apparent reversal arose from the use of mixed excitatory and inhibitory volleys in the conditioning test. Subsequent investigations upon electrically recorded reflexes have confirmed this action of strychnine. The drug has been shown to suppress a variety of types of inhibition of spinal neurons generated by impulses either in spinal afferent or in descending pathways (see Bradley et al., 1953; Curtis, 1963, 1969). More recently, evidence has been offered that the spinal inhibitory transmitter is glycine, or a "glycine-like" amino acid, and that strychnine specifically and competitively competes with this amino acid for postsynaptic receptor sites (Curtis et al., 1968b; Curtis, 1969).

After intraneural or intraspinal injection of tetanus toxin in lumbar segments of the cat spinal cord, there is a progressive and eventually complete abolition of the "direct" and the recurrent inhibition of motoneurons (Brooks et al., 1957). Both of these inhibitory pathways involve one interneuron. The direct inhibitory interneuron is activated by impulses in the Group 1A muscle afferents, and Renshaw cells, which underlie recurrent inhibition, are excited monosynaptically by impulses in motor axon collaterals. Because the operation of these interneurons, as well as the magnitude of monosynaptic reflexes, remained virtually unaffected by the toxin, it was assumed that the toxin acted pre- or postsynaptically in the vicinity of spinal inhibitory nerve terminals. This proposal explained the reduction of the inhibitory effect upon motoneurons of volleys initiated in higher threshold afferent fibers of segmental muscle and cutaneous origin. Since such volleys have both excitatory and inhibitory effects on motoneurons, the eventual effects of the toxin are complex, as indeed are those of intravenously administered strychnine upon such mixed inhibitory–excitatory systems. In contrast, the inhibition of particular motoneurons by impulses in the largest afferent fibers from muscles of antagonistic function (direct inhibition), and recurrent inhibition, are reasonably "pure" inhibitions, uncomplicated by underlying excitation. Thus, the observation that both direct and recurrent inhibitions were abolished, and not converted into excitation (*see* Brooks *et al.*, 1957; Wilson *et al.*, 1960), indicated that the toxin either depressed inhibitory transmitter release or blocked postsynaptic action, without altering the *type* of transmitter action upon motoneurons.

The facilitation of polysynaptic reflexes (*see also* Webster, 1967), the increased "spontaneous" ventral root discharge, and the blocking of inhibition by Renshaw cells (Wilson *et al.*, 1960; Curtis and de Groat, 1968), indicate that the toxin influences inhibitory synapses upon spinal interneurons as well as those upon motoneurons. Modification of inhibitory influences on dorsal horn interneurons most probably accounts for the sensory abnormalities manifest in tetanus dolorosus. It is also very probable that tetanus toxin blocks the inhibition of gamma motoneurons (Erzina, 1961; Kano and Takano, 1969).

Clear evidence for the spread of tetanus toxin through spinal tissue was obtained by observing the rate at which the inhibition of various motonuclei was changed after injection of toxin just dorsolateral to the ventral horn. Results from this type of experiment are illustrated in Fig. 1. Tetanus toxin was injected, as indicated, at five sites several millimeters apart longitudinally and just lateral to the ventral horn within the seventh lumbar and first sacral segments of a cat anesthetized with pentobarbitone. From the investigation of Romanes (1951), the approximate relative locations of motoneurons supplying the flexor digitorum longus (FDL), the gastrocnemius (G), and biceps semitendinosus (BST) muscles are shown diagrammatically in Fig. 1. Before, and at various intervals after, the injection, a number of inhibitions were studied for each type of motoneurons, as indicated in the legend. Maximum monosynaptic reflexes were recorded from the appropriate muscle nerves in response to stimulation of the central ends of the transected seventh lumbar and first sacral dorsal roots. Because these roots were cut, conditioning volleys could reach the cord only via the sixth or higher lumbar dorsal roots, or the ventral roots. Hence a study was made of inhibitions resulting from stimulation of the ipsilateral saphenous and

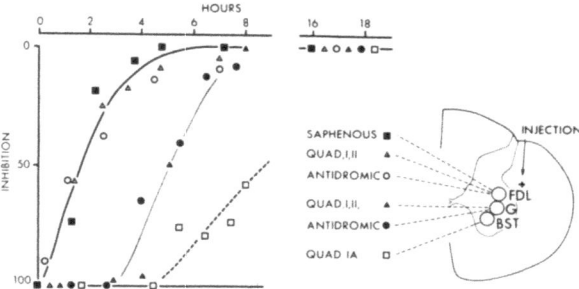

Fig. 1. The effect of tetanus toxin on the inhibition of different spinal motoneurons in the seventh lumbar and first sacral segments after injection of tetanus toxin at five sites, 1–2 mm apart, and at approximately the same location in the transverse section relative to the motonuclei, as shown in the inset diagram. Maximal monosynaptic reflexes evoked by stimulating dorsal roots were recorded from the nerves to FDL, G, and BST muscles, and were inhibited by stimulation of the saphenous nerve, group IA quadriceps fibers, groups I and II quadriceps fibers, and by volleys initiated in all other muscle nerves except that of the reflex being tested (antidromic), as indicated by the symbols. Ordinate: maximum inhibition plotted as a percentage of the values obtained before the toxin was administered. Abscissa: time in hours after the injection. Serial observations were made for the first 8 hr only. All inhibitions were abolished when further determinations were made 8–10 hr later.

quadriceps nerve (afferent fibers entering via the fifth and sixth lumbar dorsal roots) and of recurrent inhibitions resulting from volleys initiated in the muscle nerves and entering via the intact ventral roots.

For the sake of clarity, a number of inhibitions reported in the original paper have been deleted (*see* Brooks *et al.*, 1957). In each case, full inhibitory curves were constructed relating the inhibition of the reflex to the time interval between it and the inhibitory volley. The symbols of Fig. 1 plot the maximum inhibition observed at a particular time as a percentage of the inhibition observed prior to the toxin injection. The curves accordingly begin at 100% at zero time. It is quite clear from these results that inhibitions involving motoneurons located closest to the sites of toxin injection (FDL) were affected earlier than those located further away (G, BST). The inhibition of FDL motoneurons (solid line) was to a level of about 20% of their initial value within 4 hr, at which time inhibition of G motoneurons (dotted line) was beginning to be reduced. After a further 2–3 hr G inhibitions were reduced to 10–20%, and the direct inhibition of BST motoneurons (dashed line) was to approximately 60% of the control value. Frequent observations were made for only 8 hr, but all of the inhibitions studied were completely abolished 16–18 hr after the toxin had been injected.

Although a detailed analysis has not been made of the action of tetanus toxin in many mammalian species, the signs which follow administration of the toxin to the usual laboratory animals, including mice, rats, guinea pigs, rabbits, cats, and dogs, and their resemblance to the human disease, suggest that in all of these species tetanus toxin probably has the same central effect. Other vertebrates are also susceptible, including birds, reptiles, fish, and amphibia (Payling Wright, 1955; Rowson, 1961). It is relevant that strychnine blocks synaptic inhibition in the toad spinal cord (Kuno, 1957).

2. Presynaptic Inhibition

The experimental evidence described in the previous section was concerned with the action of tetanus toxin upon the *post*synaptic inhibition of spinal neurons, a inhibition associated with an increase in the membrane conductance of spinal neurones and a transient membrane hyperpolarization (Eccles, 1966, 1968). Spinal reflexes are also modified by another inhibitory process, considered to be presynaptic in nature (Eccles, 1966). In this case, the amount of excitatory transmitter released by excitatory synaptic terminals is depressed independently of a detectable change in postsynaptic membrane potential or conductance (Eide *et al.*, 1968). The basic mechanism has been proposed to be a depolarization of excitatory terminals, the depolarization of primary afferent terminals being detected both as a dorsal root potential and by changes in the electrical excitability of intraspinal fibers and terminals. Presynaptic inhibition in the spinal cord differs from postsynaptic inhibition in that the process is relatively insensitive to strychnine. Both the depolarization of afferent terminals and the inhibition of reflexes are reduced by picrotoxin, a substance which does not influence the conductance-type of postsynaptic inhibition (Eccles, 1966).

The effect of tetanus toxin on the presynaptic inhibition of extensor motoneurons has been determined in cats in which tetanus was localized by intramusclar injection to one hindlimb (Sverdlov and Alekseeva, 1965). The depolarization of the terminals of gastrocnemius primary afferent fibers by impulses in lower threshold posterior biceps–semitendinosus afferents was unaltered, yet the inhibitory effect of the latter impulses on the monosynaptic reflex of gastrocnemius motoneurons was considerably attenuated. The depolarization of spinal afferent terminals by impulses in cutaneous fibres was not reduced, but rather enhanced, by tetanus toxin (Kryzhanovsky and Lutsenko, 1969). Thus the prolonged depression of reflexes ascribed to presynaptic inhibition was apparently diminished, but the mechanism of depolarization of afferent terminals was not blocked by tetanus toxin.

3. "Descending" Inhibition

Tetanus toxin has been injected directly into the spinal cord as a means of studying the pharmacology of the inhibition of spinal motoneurons by volleys originating in supraspinal regions. The rationale for these experiments was that systemically injected strychnine could so modify the transmission of information through polysynaptic pathways, both at supraspinal and spinal sites, as to obscure any effect of the drug at inhibitory synapses upon motoneurons (*see* Curtis, 1968). However, alterations in the descending volley can be controlled to a considerable extent by allowing the toxin to ascend the spinal cord, either from injection sites caudal to the motoneurons producing the reflexes under study, or from peripheral sites of neural or muscular ejection. Subsequent study can be made of inhibitory synaptic action in cranial and contralateral segments as well as in areas affected by the toxin. A single drawback is that alterations in the final inhibitory effect of a volley of supraspinal origin could result from an action of the toxin both at inhibitory synapses on motoneurons and at synapses upon spinal interneurons through which the volley may be relayed.

In one investigation of this type (Curtis, 1959), the inhibition of lumbar motoneurons by repetitive stimulation of the anterior lobe of the cerebellum was reduced by tetanus toxin, in parallel with inhibitions of the same motoneurons produced by stimulating afferent fibers entering the cord close to the segments affected by the intraspinally injected toxin. Similarly, when tetanus toxin was injected intramuscularly into one hindlimb, the inhibitory effect upon the reflexes of this limb by repetitive stimulation of the medullary reticular formation was abolished, and the facilitory effect enhanced (Kryzhanovsky and Sheikhon, 1968).

B. Cerebral Cortex

Several studies have been made of the effects of tetanus toxin on the inhibition of neurons in the cat cerebral cortex. Depending on the amount of toxin injected into the pericruciate cortex, rigidity and eventually seizures were observed in the limb corresponding to the site of injection (Brooks and Asanuma, 1962, 1965). Correspondingly, the electrocorticogram showed irregularity and seizure patterns. (Similar observations were made in dogs; Carrea and Lanari, 1962.) Cortical inhibition was assessed as the reduction of cortical surface potentials, produced by repetitive stimulation of pyramidal tract fibers in the ipsilateral medullary pyramid. These potentials had been evoked by stimulating the contralateral forepaw, the neighboring, or the contralateral cortex. At a time when the electrocortigram exhibited abnormalities, "recurrent" inhibition was reduced, and was finally abolished over a period of hours. In the same study (Brooks and Asanuma, 1965), "recurrent" inhibition was not affected by strychnine administered intravenously, a finding in accordance with other reports of the lack of action of strychnine on recurrent and other types of inhibition of single cortical neurons (Crawford *et al.*, 1963; Krnjević *et al.*, 1966).

In contrast with these results, toxin injected into the suprasylvian and anterior ectosylvian gyri produced a change in excitability of neurons in the surrounding area of cortex. There was little or no consistent effect upon the inhibition of single cortical cells resulting from either electrical stimulation of the adjacent cortical surface or the electrophoretic administration of GABA (Krnjević *et al.*, 1966). This "local" inhibitory process, and the effects of GABA, were also unaffected by strychnine.

Both "recurrent" and "local" cortical inhibition appear to be insensitive to strychnine, and apparently involve an inhibitory transmitter different from that operating in the spinal cord. However, the reports of the effects of tetanus toxin on cortical inhibition are in conflict. Although it is conceivable, but most unlikely, that different transmission processes are involved in recurrent and local inhibition, it has been suggested (Krnjević *et al.*, 1966) that the apparent reduction in recurrent inhibition resulted more from increased excitability of cortical neurons as a consequence of mechanical, vascular, or chemical damage by material in the toxin solution, than from a specific abolition of inhibition. If this be so, the experimental evidence provides support for the proposal that tetanus toxin interrupts transmission only at inhibitory synapses influenced by strychnine. A number of other strychnine-resistant central inhibitions have been described (*see* Curtis, 1968), so it would be of interest to determine the effects of tetanus toxin upon these.

IV. TETANUS TOXIN AND CHOLINERGIC TRANSMISSION

The position is no longer tenable that local tetanus results solely from a peripheral effect of the toxin at proprioceptive nerve endings or at the neuromuscular junction (Payling Wright, 1955; Laurence and Webster, 1963). Nevertheless, there is still controversy regarding the action of the toxin at the latter synaptic junction. Muscles in the late stages of local tetanus remain contracted, and it is not clear whether this is a direct effect of the toxin on the contractile mechanism of muscle fibers, or merely the result of changes in this mechanism after a prolonged disturbance of spinal reflexes (*see* Chap. 11 for a detailed discussion of this problem.) Furthermore, flaccid paralysis has been noted to follow spasticity in severe generalized human and experimental tetanus (Courtois-Suffit and Giroux, 1918; Kaiser, Muller, and Friedrich, 1968), although the findings in humans may be complicated to some extent by the prior long-term administration of neuromuscular blocking agents.

These investigations are not all relevant to the use of tetanus toxin as a pharmacological tool, except those that indicate an action at cholinergic synapses not unlike that of botulinum toxin.

A. Sphincter Pupillae

A presynaptic action of tetanus toxin has been demonstrated at cholinergic synapses in the eye. Within 1–2 days of injecting crude toxin (Ambache et al., 1948a) or purified tetanospasmin (Mellanby et al., 1968) into the anterior chamber of the rabbit eye, the pupil became dilated and unresponsive to light. This condition persisted for 2–5 weeks after 300–1000 LD_{50} of toxin. The dilation was not reduced by sympathetic denervation, and the dilator pupillae muscle responded to stimulation of the cervical sympathetic nerves. The sphincter pupillae muscle did not contract when the oculomotor nerve was stimulated, except after administration of physostigmine, but fibers did contract readily when acetylcholine was injected into the eye (Ambache et al., 1948a). In subsequent experiments the sphincter pupillae was shown to be supersensitive to carbamylcholine (Ambache et al., 1948b). Furthermore, the level of acetylcholinesterase in the eye was normal, but the acetylcholine content of the aqueous humour was reduced, as was true of the iris, but to a lesser extent.

The selective impairment of cholinergic but not of adrenergic transmission by tetanus toxin is identical to that resulting from the intraocular injection of type A botulinum toxin (Ambache, 1949). The selectivity of action suggests a utility of these toxins in the study of cholinergic function (see Chap. 15).

B. Peripheral Neuromuscular Junction

Although no abnormality of neuromuscular transmission could be found in vitro in diaphragms removed from rats 6–12 days after intradiaphragmatic injection of tetanus toxin (Mackereth and Scott, 1954), very high levels of the toxin have been reported to reduce the mechanical response of isolated rat diaphragms progressively (Muchnik and Rubinstein, 1967). Some 8–10 days after injection into the tibialis anterior muscle of the rabbit, tetanus toxin produces fibrillation potentials and changes in the sensitivity of the muscle to cholinomimetics similar to those observed after denervation (Prabhu et al., 1962). A failure of acetylcholine release was advanced as a possible mechanism. A similar conclusion was drawn to explain the synergism between tubocurarine and tetanus toxin at the neuromuscular junction of the gastrocnemius muscle after earlier injection of the toxin (Kryzhanovsky and Kasymov, 1964). A block of neuromuscular transmission has been suggested in severe local tetanus in the rat (Kaeser and Saner, 1969), but an interference with contraction coupling or mechanisms of contraction–relaxation, rather than an action at the synaptic junction, has been indicated by the distribution of tetanus toxin within the mouse muscular sarcotubular system (Zacks and Sheff, 1968).

In part, some of these apparently different findings may have resulted from the different doses of toxin used, and the different toxin preparations. It is significant that the acute effects of partially purified tetanus toxin on mouse intercostal muscle *in vitro* appeared not to be associated with tetanospasmin (Feigen *et al.*, 1963). The increased spontaneous leakage of acetylcholine, indicated by an increased frequency but not amplitude of miniature endplate potentials, is difficult to correlate with other suggestions that the toxin blocks acetylcholine release, except perhaps as an early indication of a presynaptic phenomenon. This effect seemed to be concentrated in the fraction of toxin which remained after removal of tetanospasmin by adsorption upon protagon. In contrast, this nonspasmogenic fraction had little or no effect upon the sphincter muscles of the pupil (Mellanby *et al.*, 1968).

Although some material present in impure tetanus toxin clearly affects peripheral neuromuscular transmission, further research is required to relate this to the effects of tetanospasmin at cholinergic junctions in the eye.

C. Central Cholinergic Junction

The reduction of the "antidromic" or recurrent inhibition of spinal motoneurons by intraspinally or intraneurally injected toxin was not accompanied by any reduction in the synaptic excitation of the inhibitory interneurons of this pathway, the Renshaw cells (Brooks *et al.*, 1947). These cells are excited monosynaptically by impulses in cholinergic axon collateral fibers. After the toxin reduced spinal synaptic inhibition, transmission at these cholinergic junctions remained unaffected for at least 18 hr. This observation has been confirmed by injecting tetanus toxin close to individual Renshaw cells (Curtis and de Groat, 1968): the synaptic inhibition of these cells was suppressed, but the cholinergic excitation was unimpaired over several hours. It is possible that sufficient time was not allowed in these investigations for tetanus toxin to affect cholinergic transmission, 24–48 hr being required for the toxin to influence the cholinergic innervation of the sphincter pupillae, and even longer for peripheral skeletal muscle.

No definitive evidence is available for an action of tetanus toxin at central cholinergic synapses. Furthermore, such an effect does not account for its highly selective action at strychnine-sensitive synapses, since acetylcholine is not the transmitter at these junctions (Curtis and Crawford, 1969).

V. MODE OF ACTION

Although it is difficult to ascribe many of the structural changes which have been reported in both experimental and clinical tetanus (Baker, 1942; Yates and Yates, 1966) to a direct effect of the toxin on nervous tissues, marked changes have been observed in synapses located on spinal moto-neurons. Local tetanus confined to the hindlimb of the white rat produces a significant reduction in the number of silver-impregnated ring-like synapses on the bodies of these cells, and an increase in the number visible on den-drites (Geinismann et al., 1967). Assuming that silver impregnation depends on the "degree of activity" of the terminals, these findings were interpreted as indicating relative inactivity of axosomatic terminals and increased activity of axodendritic synapses. These observations are of considerable significance when considered in conjunction with physiological evidence that inhibitory terminals are located predominantly on the soma of motoneurons, whereas excitatory synapses are mainly axodendritic (Uchizono, 1966; Smith et al., 1967). The findings are compatible with a reduction of synaptic inhibition, and a consequent enhancement of intraspinal excitatory systems.

The toxin has been localized within the central nervous system by means of fluoroscein-labeled antitoxin (Zacks and Sheff, 1966), but technical difficulties have so far prevented detailed studies of its precise localization in the vicinity of synapses. However, recent investigations have shown tetanus toxin fixation by isolated synaptosomal membrane (Mellanby et al., 1965; Mellanby and Whittaker, 1968), presumably because of its specific binding to membrane gangliosides in association with cerebrosides (van Heyningen and Miller, 1961; van Heyningen and Mellanby, 1968). This may be relevant to a recent investigation which indicates that the toxin reduces the amount of transmitter released from spinal inhibitory terminals. It is conceivable that the selective binding of tetanus toxin to inhibitory terminals could provide a means for demonstrating these structures histochemically with high-resolution electron microscopy. However the toxin has apparently little or no effect on inhibitory transmission in the cerebrum, so the binding by synaptosomes prepared from guinea pig brain could be a nonspecific mechanism.

Since tetanus toxin reduces and finally abolishes the same types of spinal inhibition as does strychnine, the recent demonstration that glycine is most probably the transmitter at strychnine-sensitive inhibitory synapses (Curtis, 1969) provided an opportunity for determining the mode of action of tetanus toxin upon inhibition. Strychnine abolishes the inhibitory effect of both synaptically released transmitter and electrophoretically adminis-tered glycine. Hence, it seems likely that the alkaloid blocks the inhibitory mechanism at a postsynaptic site (see Curtis et al., 1968b). In contrast, tetanus toxin blocks the inhibitory process without affecting the sensitivity of spinal neurons to the amino acid (Curtis and de Groat, 1968; Gushchin et al., 1969), and thus probably has a presynaptic action.

Experimental observations in support of this proposal are illustrated in

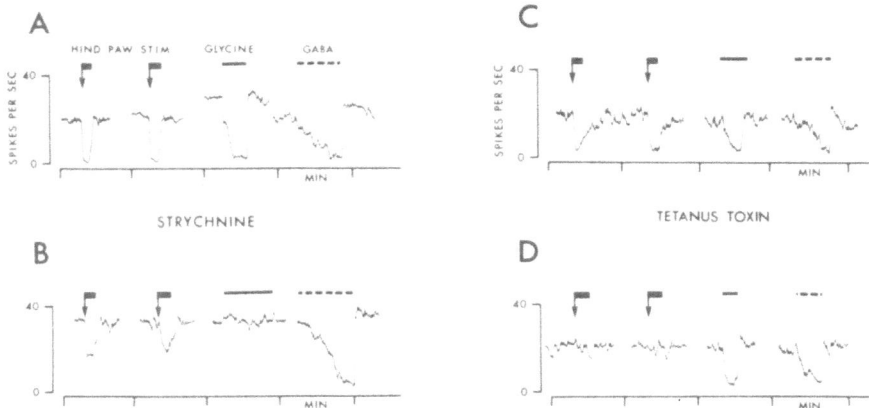

Fig. 2. A comparison of the effects of strychnine (A, B) and tetanus toxin (C, D) on the inhibition of two Renshaw cells resulting from mechanical stimulation of the ipsilateral hind paw (hind paw stim). Firing rates were maintained where necessary with electrophoretically administered acetylcholine, and the amino acids glycine and gamma-aminobutyric acid (GABA) were similarly ejected, over the times indicated by the horizontal solid and broken lines respectively, with currents which remained constant during each investigation: A, B. Glycine 4.5 nA, GABA 5 nA, C, D: glycine 5 nA, GABA 5 nA. A, before and B, during the electrophoretic ejection of strychnine (10 nA, 2 mM solution of strychnine hydrochloride in 165 mM NaCl). C, before, and D, 49 min after, tetanus toxin was administered with a maintained pressure of 300 mm Hg from a glass micropipette approximately 100 μm from the cell. Ordinates: rate of firing. Extracellular action potentials were recorded by the center barrel of seven (A, B) and five (C, D) barrel micropipettes. Abscissas: time in minutes.

Fig. 2, the investigations having been carried out on Renshaw cells in the lumbar segments of anaesthetized cats. The firing of these cells can be maintained at a reasonably constant level by administering acetylcholine electrophoretically from one barrel of a multibarrel micropipette (Curtis, 1964). Inhibition is observed as a reduction in firing as a result of either the administration of a depressant amino acid or the stimulation of certain hindlimb afferent fibers (Wilson *et al.*, 1964). This "afferent" inhibition is most easily achieved by squeezing the hindpaw mechanically (Fig. 2A, C). Electrophoretically administered strychnine abolishes the inhibitory effect of glycine (Fig. 2B), but not that of another depressant amino acid, gamma-aminobutyric. The afferent inhibition is reduced (Fig. 2B) and can be abolished by strychnine (Curtis *et al.*, 1968a). The apparent relative insensitivity of synaptic inhibition of these neurons to strychnine has been attributed to the widespread location of inhibitory synapses over the surface of the neurons, in relation to the restricted distribution of strychnine in the vicinity of the ejecting micropipette. In contrast, when tetanus toxin is administered by pressure ejection of approximately 100 μm from a single Renshaw cell, the afferent inhibition is slowly reduced and finally abolished after approximately 50 min. There is no alteration in sensitivity of the neuron to either inhibitory amino acid (Fig. 2D). The conclusion was drawn that if glycine is the transmitter at these strychnine-sensitive inhibitory synapses, and also at other spinal inhibitory synapses similarly blocked by strychnine, tetanus toxin probably suppresses synaptic inhibition by interfering with transmitter synthesis or release. This proposal gains support from the finding that spinal motoneurons affected by tetanus toxin remain sensitive to glycine (Gushchin *et al.*, 1969). Concentrations of tetanus toxin adequate to block the inhibition of Renshaw cells did not affect the cholinergic synaptic excitation of these neurons by impulses in motor axon collaterals. The monosynaptic excitation of spinal motoneurons is not blocked by the toxin (Brooks *et al.*, 1957; Gushchin *et al.*, 1969). It is unlikely that the highly selective depression of synaptic inhibition results from interference with transmission in preterminal fibers, since such a process would be expected to be rather nonselective.

In spite of the slow time course of the depression of spinal inhibition by tetanus toxin, even when administered relatively close to Renshaw cells, suggesting that there is an interference with transmitter synthesis, much of the latency of toxin action is probably concerned with its diffusion through spinal tissue. Furthermore, glycine levels within the grey matter of lumbar segments of the spinal cord of cats previously inoculated intramuscularly with tetanus toxin were considered not to be significantly lower than the normal values (Johnston *et al.*, 1969). However, in cats in which local tetanus was confined to one hindlimb, the levels of glycine in the grey matter of ipsilateral lumbar segments were considered to be significantly lower (approximately 8%) than those of the contralateral segments (Semba and Kano, 1969).

These results appear to be conflicting, but the two investigations are not strictly comparable, and there may indeed be a small reduction in spinal glycine levels in the initial stages of tetanus which would not be detectable by comparing tissue from different animals (Johnston *et al.*, 1969). The actual proportion of free glycine in spinal gray matter which is directly concerned with synaptic inhibition is unknown, and thus the physiological significance of alterations of the level of this amino acid is hard to evaluate. A reduction in the glycine concentration may indicate that tetanus toxin interferes with transmitter synthesis, and as a consequence reduces the amount released by each impulse. Unaltered glycine levels may indicate a failure of the actual release process. On the other hand, alterations in glycine levels may be produced or obscured because of the association of this amino acid in other processes, particularly of metabolic nature, in the tissue affected by the toxin. While the levels of gamma-aminobutyrate remain unaffected (Johnston *et al.*, 1969; Semba and Kano, 1969), the levels of aspartate in the gray matter were significantly elevated (approximately 50%, Johnston *et al.*, 1969). Such an effect could result from a possible relationship between glycine and aspartate metabolism in inhibitory neurons, interference with glycine release resulting in an elevation of the levels of a precursor. Alternatively, if aspartate is an excitatory transmitter in the spinal cord (Davidoff *et al.*, 1967), then the increased levels may reflect the increased activity of spinal neurons following suppression of inhibitory synaptic action. Further investigations of the effects of tetanus toxin on spinal amino acids are required, but an important clinical implication of the findings so far is the possibility of developing therapeutic procedures based on the administration of glycine precursors or analogs which, after penetrating the blood–brain barrier, enhance the production or effectiveness of this amino acid at inhibitory synapses influenced by tetanus toxin.

At the present time, although a major site of action of tetanus toxin is at certain spinal inhibitory synapses, the mechanism of action remains uncertain: perhaps there is a reduction in transmitter availability or a block of transmitter release. By analogy with the action of hemicholinium at central cholinergic synapses (Quastel and Curtis, 1965), suppression of transmitter synthesis would be expected to have a delayed effect on synaptic inhibition, depending upon the amount of transmitter stored within the terminal and its rate of use. The actual time at which the toxin reaches a particular neuron cannot be determined accurately, and exclusion of this mechanism would require a study of toxin action on two totally independent inhibitory pathways converging on a single neuron, and activated at different rates. The time course of abolition of inhibition should depend on the number of stimuli releasing transmitter, and thus be more prolonged for the pathway activated less frequently, given approximate equivalence of transmitter stores. Interference with transmitter release, perhaps as a result of the binding of the toxin by inhibitory presynaptic membrane, may also be relatively slow to completely suppress transmitter release. This type of process is similar to that proposed for the toxin of *Clostridium botulinum* (type A) at cholinergic junctions (Brooks, 1956; Thesleff, 1960). Furthermore, it has been found that paralysis by botulinum toxin develops more slowly if the junction is inactive (Hughes and Whaler, 1962).

Other similarities between tetanus and botulinum toxin may have a bearing on the action of these substances at cholinergic synapses. The toxins are produced by related anaerobic organisms, and may have common chemical characteristics, particularly in their content of amino acids (Pillimer and Robbins, 1949), although these analyses were not carried out on pure neurotoxins. The acute action of tetanus toxin seems to be predominantly a block of strychnine-sensitive inhibition, but it is possible that this toxin is slowly converted in the eye and peripheral muscle to a molecule similar to that moiety of botulinum toxin which is responsible for its specific effect at cholinergic junctions.

VI. CONCLUSION

Strychnine and tetanus toxin are of considerable importance in the analysis of central inhibitory mechanisms. Both agents interfere with transmission at certain central inhibitory synapses, which in the mammal occur mainly in the spinal cord and brain stem. Tetanus toxin interferes with the synthesis and/or release of the transmitter, whereas strychnine probably hinders its access to postsynaptic receptors.

Both strychnine and tetanus toxin are highly selective antagonists of "strychnine-sensitive" inhibition, but their experimental use may be complicated by the apparent enhancement of excitatory synaptic activity, consequent upon the suppression of inhibition. Systemically administered strychnine influences the whole nervous system, often rendering difficult the assessment of the sensitivity of a particular inhibitory pathway to this substance. Difficulties also exist when strychnine is administered microelectrophoretically since all synapses on a cell cannot be exposed to a uniform concentration. On the other hand, after direct injection of tetanus toxin into the nervous system, inhibitory processes in the vicinity can be studied because the toxin diffuses slowly towards selected nuclei or even single neurons. By such a method it may be possible to localize the inhibitory synapses in complex multineuronal pathways without major interference to the overall operation of the pathways, provided that the inhibition is of the strychnine-sensitive type. If, as appears probable, glycine is the transmitter at this type of inhibitory synapse, tetanus toxin may be of considerable assistance in determining whether the depressant effects of glycine on neurons in the cerebral cortex (Curtis *et al.*, 1968a; Kelly and Krnjević, 1968) and vestibular nuclei (Bruggencate and Engberg, 1969) are in fact related to the presence of glycine-releasing inhibitory synapses in these regions: the major inhibitory mechanisms which have been studied in the cortex and vestibular nuclei are not suppressed by strychnine (Krnjević *et al.*, 1966; Obata *et al.*, 1967).

Tetanus toxin also has a postsynaptic action at peripheral cholinergic synapses. This has not been demonstrated in the central nervous system, and seems to be of minor pharmacological importance when compared with the action of the toxin of *Clostridium botulinum*.

ACKNOWLEDGMENT

It is a pleasure to thank Mrs. H. Walsh for her assistance in the preparation of this manuscript.

VII. REFERENCES

Ambache, N. (1949), *J. Physiol. Lond.*, **108**:127.
Ambache, N., R. S. Morgan, and G. Payling Wright (1948a), *J. Physiol. Lond.*, **107**:45.
Ambache, N., R. S. Morgan, and G. Payling Wright (1948b), *Brit. J. Exp. Pathol.*, **29**:408.
Baker, A. B. (1942), *J. Neuropathol.*, **1**:394.
Bradley, K., D. M. Easton, and J. C. Eccles (1953), *J. Physiol. Lond.*, **122**:474.
Brooks, V. B. (1956), *J. Physiol. Lond.*, **134**:264.
Brooks, V. B. and H. Asanuma (1962), *Science (New York)*, **137**:674.
Brooks, V. B. and H. Asanuma (1965), *Amer. J. Physiol.*, **208**:674.
Brooks, V. B., D. R. Curtis, and J. C. Eccles (1957), *J. Physiol. London*, **135**:655.
Bruggencate, G. Ten and I. Engberg (1969), *Brain Res.*, **14**:533.
Carrea, R. and A. Lanari (1962), *Science (New York)*, **137**:342.
Courtois-Suffit, M. and R. Giroux (1918), "The abnormal forms of tetanus," University Press Ltd., London.
Crawford, J. M., D. R. Curtis, P. E. Voorhoeve, and V. J. Wilson (1963), *Nature (London)*, **200**:845.
Curtis, D. R. (1959), *J. Physiol. London*, **145**:175.
Curtis, D. R. (1963), *Pharmacol. Rev.*, **15**:333.
Curtis, D. R. (1964), Microelectrophoresis, *in* "Physical Techniques in Biological Research," vol. 5 (W. L. Nastuk, ed.), Academic Press, New York, pp. 144–190.
Curtis, D. R. (1968), Pharmacology and neurochemistry of mammalian central inhibitory processes, *in* "Structure and function of inhibitory mechanisms" (C. von Euler, S. Skoglund, and U. Söderberg, eds.), Pergamon Press, Oxford, pp. 429–456.
Curtis, D. R. (1969), *Prog. Brain Res.*, **31**:171.
Curtis, D. R. and J. M. Crawford (1969), *Ann. Rev. Pharmacol.*, **9**:209.
Curtis, D. R. and W. C. de Groat (1968), *Brain Res.*, **10**:208.
Curtis, D. R., L. Hösli, and G. A. R. Johnston (1968a), *Exp. Brain Res.*, **6**:1.
Curtis, D. R., L. Hösli, G. A. R. Johnston, and I. H. Johnston (1968b), *Exp. Brain Res.*, **5**:235.
Davidoff, R. A., L. T. Graham, Jr., R. P. Shank, R. Werman, and M. H. Aprison (1967), *J. Neurochem.*, **14**:1025.
Dawson, D. J. and C. M. Mauritzen (1967), *Aust. J. Biol. Sci.*, **20**:253.
Dawson, D. J. and L. W. Nichol (1969), *Aust. J. Biol. Sci.*, **22**:247.
Eccles, J. C. (1966), *Ann. N.Y. Acad. Sci.*, **137**:473.
Eccles, J. C. (1968), Postsynaptic inhibition in the central nervous system, *in* "Structure and Function of Inhibitory Neuronal Mechanisms" (C. von Euler, S. Skoglund, and U. Söderberg, eds.), Pergamon Press, Oxford, pp. 291–308.
Eide, E., I. Jurna, and A. Lundberg (1968), Conductance measurements from motoneurons during presynaptic inhibition, *in* "Structure and Functions of Inhibitory Neuronal Mechanisms" (C. von Euler, S. Skoglund and U. Söderberg, eds.), Pergamon Press, Oxford, pp. 215–219.
Erzina, G. A. (1961), *Sechenov. J. Physiol.*, **47**:1062.
Feigen, G. A., N. S. Peterson, W. W. Hofmann, G. H. Genther, and W. E. van Heyningen (1963), *J. Gen. Microbiol.*, **33**:489.
Firor, W. M. and A. F. Jonas, Jr. (1938), *Bull. Johns Hopkins Hosp.*, **62**:90.
Fletcher, W. M. (1903), *Brain*, **26**:383.
Geinismann, Y. Y., M. V. Dyakonova, and G. N. Kryzhanovsky (1967), *Bull. Exp. Biol. Med. (USSR)*, **11**:71.

Gushchin, I. S., S. N. Kozhechkin, and Y. S. Sverdlov (1969), *Doklady Akad. Nauk* (*U.S.S.R.*), **187**, No. 3:685.
Hughes, R. and B. C. Whaler (1962), *J. Physiol. London*, **160**:221.
Johnston, G. A. R., W. C. de Groat, and D. R. Curtis (1969), *J. Neurochem.*, **16**:797.
Kaeser, H. E., H. E. Müller, and B. Friedrich (1968), *Europ. Neurol.*, **1**:17.
Kaeser, H. E. and A. Saner (1969), *Nature (London)*, **223**:842.
Kano, M. and K. Takano (1969), *Jap. J. Physiol.*, **19**:1.
Kelly, J. S. and K. Krnjević (1968), *Nature (London)*, **219**:1380.
Keynes, R. D. (1964), Microinjection, in "Physical Techniques in Biological Research," vol. 5 (W. L. Nastuk, ed.), Academic Press, New York, pp. 183–190.
Krnjević, K., M. Randić, and D. W. Straughan (1966), *J. Physiol. London*, **184**:78.
Kryzhanovsky, G. N. and A. Kh. Kasymov (1964), *Bull. Exp. Biol. Med.* (*USSR*), **58**:1199.
Kryzhanovsky, G. N. and V. K. Lutsenko (1969), *Bull. Exp. Biol. Med.* (*USSR*), **2**:15.
Kryzhanovsky, G. N. and F. D. Sheikhon (1968), *Bull. Exp. Biol.*, **9**, No. 11:9.
Kuno, M. (1957), *Jap. J. Physiol.*, **7**:42.
Lamanna, C. and C. J. Carr (1967), *Clin. Pharmac. Ther.*, **8**:286.
Largier, J. F. (1956), *J. Immunol.*, **76**:393.
Laurence, D. R. and R. A. Webster (1963), *Clin. Pharmac. Ther.*, **4**:36.
Liddell, E. G. T. and C. S. Sherrington (1925), *Proc. Roy. Soc. B*, **97**:267.
Lundberg, A. (1967), *Electroen. Neurophysiol. Suppl.*, **25**:35.
Mackereth, M. B. and D. J. Scott (1954), *Proc. Univ. Otago Med. Sch.*, **32**:13.
Mangalo, R., B. Bizzini, A. Turpin, and M. Raynaud (1968), *Biochim. Biophys. Acta*, **168**:583.
Mellanby, J., D. Pope, and N. Ambache (1968), *J. Gen. Microbiol.*, **50**:479.
Mellanby, J., W. E. van Heyningen, and V. P. Whittaker (1965), *J. Neurochem.*, **12**:77.
Mellanby, J. and V. P. Whittaker (1968), *J. Neurochem.*, **15**:205.
Meyer, H. and F. Ransom (1903), *Arch. Exp. Pathol. Pharmak.*, **49**:367.
Muchnik, S. and E. H. Rubinstein (1967), *Acta Physiol. Latin Amer.*, **17**:166.
Nicolaiër, A. (1884), *Deut. Med. Wohnschr.*, **10**:842.
Obata, K., M. Ito, R. Ochi, and N. Sato (1967), *Exp. Brain Res.*, **4**:43.
Payling Wright, G. (1955), *Pharmacol. Rev.*, **7**:413.
Pillemer, L. (1946), *J. Immunol.*, **53**:237.
Pillemer, L. and K. C. Robbins (1949), *Ann. Rev. Microbiol.*, **3**:265.
Pillemer, L. and W. B. Wartman (1947), *J. Immunol.*, **55**:277.
Pillemer, L., R. G. Wittler, J. I. Burrell, and D. B. Grossberg (1948), *J. Exp. Med.*, **88**:205.
Prabhu, V. G., Y. T. Oester, and A. G. Karczmar (1962), *Int. J. Neuropharmacol.*, **1**:371.
Quastel, D. M. J. and D. R. Curtis (1965), *Nature (London)*, **208**:192.
Romanes, G. J. (1951), *J. Comp. Neurol.*, **94**:313.
Rowson, K. E. K. (1961), *J. Gen. Microbiol.*, **25**:315.
Semba, T. and M. Kano (1969), *Science (New York)*, **164**:571.
Simpson, J. Y. (1854), *Month. J. Med. Sci.*, **18**:97.
Sherrington, C. S. (1905), *Proc. Roy. Soc. B*, **76**:269.
Smith, T. G., R. B. Wuerker, and K. Frank (1967), *J. Neurophysiol.*, **30**:1072.
Stevenson, J. W. (1962), Bacterial neurotoxins, in "Neurochemistry" (K. A. C. Elliott, I. H. Page, and J. H. Quastel, eds.), Charles C. Thomas, Springfield, pp. 813–839.
Sverdlov, Yu. S. and V. I. Alekseeva (1966), *Fed. Proc.*, **25**:T931.
Thesleff, S. (1960), *J. Physiol. (London)*, **151**:598.
Uchizono, K. (1966), *Jap. J. Physiol.*, **16**:570.
van Heyningen, W. E. (1950), "Bacterial Toxins," Blackwell Scientific Publications, Oxford.
van Heyningen, W. E. (1968), *Sci. Amer.*, **218**, No. 4:69.
van Heyningen, W. E. and J. Mellanby (1968), *J. Gen. Microbiol.*, **52**:447.
van Heyningen, W. E. and P. M. Miller (1961), *J. Gen. Microbiol.*, **24**:107.
Webster, R. A. (1967), *Int. J. Neuropharmacol.*, **6**:207.

Wilson, V. J., F. P. J. Diecke, and W. H. Talbot (1960), *J. Neurophysiol.*, **23**:659.
Wilson, V. J., W. H. Talbot, and M. Kato (1964), *J. Neurophysiol.*, **27**:1063.
Wright, E. A., R. S. Morgan, and G. Payling Wright (1950), *J. Path. Bact.*, **62**:569.
Yates, J. C. and R. D. Yates (1966), *J. Ultrastruc. Res.*, **16**:382.
Zacks, S. I. and S. I. Sheff (1966), *J. Neuropath. Exp. Neurol.*, **25**:422.
Zacks, S. I. and M. F. Sheff (1968), *Science* (*New York*), **159**:643.

Chapter 13

The Clinical Aspects of Botulism

M. Glenn Koenig

Department of Medicine
Vanderbilt University School of Medicine
Nashville, Tennessee, U.S.A.

I. HISTORY

Botulism may have been known to antiquity. K. F. Meyer (1928) suggests that Emperor Leo VI of Byzantium (886–911 A.D.) earned the sobriquet, "The Wise," or "The Philosopher," possibly because of an edict that forbade the eating of blood sausage due to its harmfulness to health. Nine centuries later physicians of southern Germany recognized the disease as the often fatal syndrome that sometimes followed the consumption of a regionally popular blood sausage. As a consequence the manufacture of that dangerous food product came under strict government surveillance, and the term botulism (*botulus* is Latin for sausage) was applied to the illness. In 1895 an outbreak of a strange neuroparalytic disorder occurred among 34 members of a musical society who, after performing at a funeral in the Belgium village of Ellezelles, had eaten some raw, salted ham. Three of the musicians died, while 10 became critically ill. The Belgian bacteriologist van Ermengem investigated the outbreak and, in a paper that remains a classic in the annals of bacteriology, showed that a spore-forming anaerobic bacillus produced a toxin responsible for the disease in the sick musicians and caused the illness previously termed botulism (van Ermengem, 1897).

The frequency of reported cases of botulism increased in the first two decades of the twentieth century, spurred on by the growth of home canning and the commercial canning industry which developed during World War I. It soon became apparent that foods other than meats caused botulism, because ingestion of fish, cheese, and various vegetable products were all associated with the disease. Interest and concern regarding botulism reached a peak in the early 1920s, and the future of the commercial canning industry was seriously threatened. At that time Meyer and his associates undertook a series of investigations dealing with the species *Clostridium botulinum* which produced toxin, the distribution of spores in the soil, the conditions under which spores could survive and toxin be produced, and the manner in which the microorganism might be demonstrated in soil, suspected food or clinical material (Coleman and Meyer, 1922; Dubovsky and Meyer, 1922; Esty and Meyer, 1922; Meyer and Dubovsky, 1922a; Meyer and Dubovsky, 1922b). This work led to the technological advances which virtually eliminated botulism in the commercial canning industry in the United States and to the formulation of guidelines for the preparation of canned foods in the home.

Reported cases of botulism reached their peak in the United States in the mid-1930s and over the next three decades steadily declined. Interest in the disease lagged and a generation of physicians emerged who knew little about botulism. However, in 1963, 46 cases were reported in the United States, the largest number in 34 years. This increase was largely due to cases of type E disease which followed the ingestion of commercially packaged smoked whitefish. Interest in botulism was thus suddenly and dramatically rekindled and has remained at a high level since that time.

II. BOTULISM AS WORLD HEALTH PROBLEM

A. The Disease in Humans

Compared to other diseases caused by microbial parasites, the morbidity and mortality produced by botulism is trifling. Meyer (1956) reported that botulism had accounted for disease in 5635 individuals and had killed 1714 throughout the world in the preceding 50 years. During the years 1899 through 1967, 640 outbreaks of botulism with 1669 cases and 948 fatalities were reported in the United States (Gangarosa, 1969). Reported cases reached their peak in the decade 1930–1939, and the death-to-case ratio was highest during that period (*see* Fig. 1). Outbreaks of the disease have been reported in all states with the exception of Vermont, New Hampshire, Rhode Island, Delaware, South Carolina, and Hawaii. The incidence of botulism in this country has declined at a fairly steady rate during the past four decades with the exception of the 46 cases reported in 1963.

Botulism has been equally rare in other countries. Great Britain, from 1922 through 1963, recorded only 11 outbreaks with 21 cases and 16 deaths, though their first outbreak at Loch Maree in 1922 was a particularly dra-

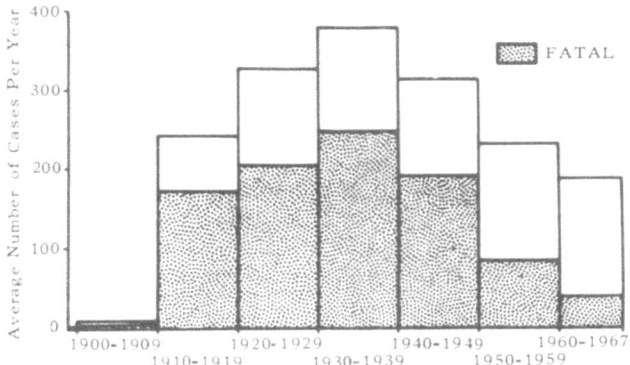

Fig. 1. Cases and deaths due to botulism, by 10-year periods, 1899–1967. (Reprinted from E. J. Gangarosa (1969), *J. Infect. Diseases*, **119**:308, with permission of the author and the University of Chicago Press.)

matic one (Dolman, 1964). Our Canadian neighbors reported 36 outbreaks, 110 cases, and 62 deaths from 1919 through 1963; the Soviet Union 163 outbreaks, 1283 cases, and 459 deaths from 1818 through 1939; Germany 434 outbreaks, 1294 cases, and 179 deaths from 1898 through 1948, and France during the war years 1940 through 1944, 500 outbreaks, over 1000 cases, and 15 deaths (Dolman, 1964). Japan has reported 62 outbreaks involving 347 individuals and 97 deaths from 1930 to 1963 (Dolman, 1964).

The rather infrequent occurrence of botulism throughout the world might appropriately prompt one to ask what stimulus has given rise to the extensive literature on botulism which developed during the first four decades of this century, and why this interest has remained high since 1963. The answer may lie in several areas. The toxin produced by *Clostridium botulinum* is the most potent biological poison known. The fact that tiny microbes can produce enough toxin to kill millions of humans has held a strange fascination for physicians, scientists, military men, journalists, and science fiction writers. As Dolman (1964) has pointed out, outbreaks of botulism have often had dramatic impact on the communities in which they occurred. They have often followed occasions of rejoicing or celebration or ironically followed funeral feasts. They have been frequently surrounded by an aura of mystery or unreality and have always received considerable attention in the press and other news media. Finally, the potential has and continues to exist that a widely distributed, commercially prepared food product may, through a technological slip, become contaminated with botulinum toxin and produce disease in hundreds or thousands of individuals in widely separated geographic areas.

B. The Disease in Animals

While botulism in humans is distinctly rare, the disease annually kills hundreds of thousands of animals. In some countries the loss of livestock due to botulism has been of major economic importance. The disease has posed a threat to the mink industry and has been known to decimate local waterfowl populations.

In South Africa thousands of cattle die annually from an illness locally designated *lamziekte*. The deaths are due to the ingestion of forage or animal carcasses contaminated with type D or less frequently type C botulinum toxin. The same illness, termed Midland cattle disease, kills thousands of cattle and sheep in Australia, and has been traced to intoxication with types C and D toxin, the source of which has often been traced to soil-contaminated rabbit carcasses.

Forage poisoning in horses and mules has been reported in America, Europe, Egypt, Australia, and South Africa. The mortality rate may be high and in many cases is due to ingestion of hay and ensilage contaminated with type B (America) or type C botulinum toxin (Europe, Africa, and Australia).

Botulism produces the syndrome termed "limberneck" in chickens and other domestic fowl. Affected birds often exhibit muscular incoordination and drooping necks. In the United States the disease has often followed the consumption of home-canned string beans by the afflicted fowl, and has been caused by type A toxin and occasionally type C toxin. Botulism in ducks and other waterfowl has been known to occur annually in certain lakes and mud flats in the western United States, Canada, several South American countries, Australia, Germany, and South Africa. Alkaline water conditions and oxygen deficiency caused by the growth of aquatic plants, algae, aerobic bacteria, and rotting vegetation provide appropriate conditions for toxin production. Type C strains of *Clostridium botulinum* have been most frequently implicated in avian disease.

Finally, type C botulism has produced significant morbidity and mortality among mink and other fur-producing mammals. Breeders of these animals often go to considerable expense to prevent the disease.

III. EPIDEMIOLOGIC CONSIDERATIONS

Six immunologically distinct strains of *Clostridium botulinum* have been described (designated types A, B, C, D, E, and F), each elaborating an antigenically specific toxin. While serologic cross-reaction between type A and type B toxins and antitoxins has been described (Johnson *et al.*, 1966) no cross-protection between the various antitoxins has been convincingly demonstrated. Type A, B, E, and F toxins have been implicated in human disease, while types C and D have produced illness almost exclusively in animals.

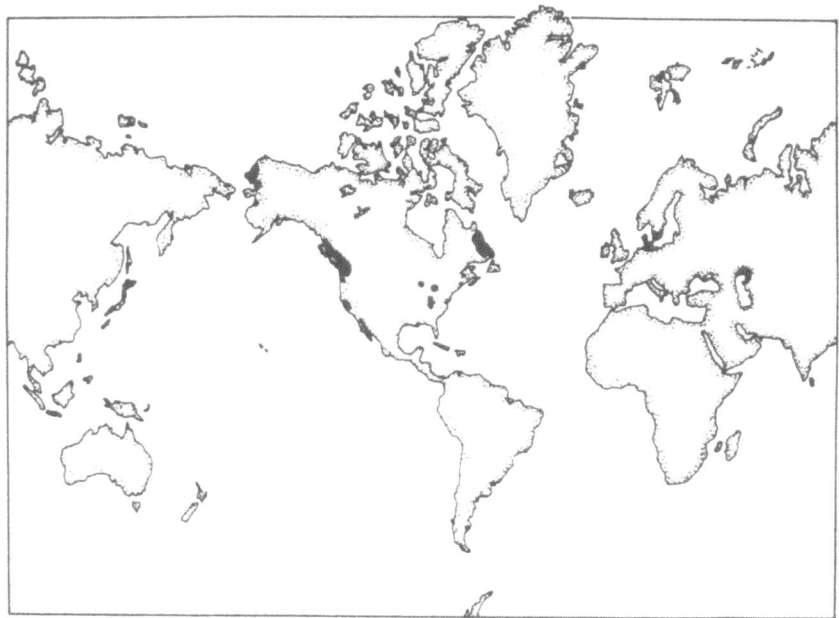

Fig. 2. The world-wide distribution of reported outbreaks of type E botulism. The geographic regions from which type E disease has been reported are shown in black. These areas are in the northern hemisphere and are generally located along sea coasts. The outbreaks shown in the central United States resulted from consumption of white-fish caught in the Great Lakes.

Type A and B spores are widely distributed in soil. Type A spores appear to be most common in the United States, especially along the Pacific Coast and in the Rocky Mountain States. Type B spores are common in the eastern half of the United States and in Europe. Type E spores have been frequently demonstrated in lakeshore mud, coastal sand, and marine sediments in northern latitudes, thus accounting for the high incidence with which fish products have been associated with type E botulism (*see* Fig. 2). However, it should be emphasized that canned mushrooms have been implicated in one outbreak of type E botulism, and in 23 reported outbreaks of fish-borne botulism, type A toxin has been demonstrated five times and type B toxin twice (Gangarosa, 1969).

Type F toxin was described as an immunologically unique type following an outbreak of human botulism traced to the ingestion of homemade liver paste on the Danish island of Langeland in 1960. Subsequently, type F strains have been recovered from marine sediments off the coasts of California and Oregon and from a salmon in the Columbia River. A single outbreak of type F botulism was reported from California in 1966, and involved three individuals who had ingested home-prepared venison jerky (National Communicable Disease Center, 1968).

The vast majority of human botulism has been caused by the consumption of improperly home-processed foods. Of the 640 reported outbreaks in the United States, only 60 have been traced to commercially processed products which have included: canned liver paste, type A; ham from Germany, type B; smoked ciscoes, smoked whitefish, smoked whitefish chubs, and canned tuna fish, type E; and cheese, frozen lobster tail, frozen chicken pie, and luncheon meat, type unknown. In the United States, vegetables, fruit, fish, and condiments have been the most frequent vehicles for botulism when the implicated food source has been identified (*see* Table I). Home-canned string beans, corn, beets, spinach, asparagus, chili peppers, olives, tomatoes, figs, apricots, okra, mushrooms, and peaches have been foods frequently involved.

While most strains of types A and B *Clostridium botulinum* are proteolytic, and food contaminated with them becomes putrid during their growth, type E strains (and at least rare type B strains) do not elaborate proteolytic enzymes. Consequently, foodstuffs containing lethal quantities of toxin may appear and taste perfectly normal.

IV. PATHOGENESIS

A series of rather fortuitous events must occur before clinical botulism develops (*see* Table II). A break at any point in this chain of events prevents the disease. A food product must become contaminated with viable *Clostridium botulinum* bacilli or spores. The spores can remain viable over a wide

Table I.
Foods Implicated in Botulism Outbreaks in the United States (1899–1967[a])

Food source	Percentage of total
Unknown	69.8
Vegetables	17.8
Fruit	4.1
Fish	3.6
Condiments	2.2
Beef	0.8
Milk	0.6
Pork	0.5
Poultry	0.1
Other	0.5
Total of 640 reported outbreaks	

[a] Data from National Communicable Disease Center, 1968.

Table II.
The Pathogenesis of Botulism

Food contaminated by *Clostridium botulinum* bacilli or spores.

Proper conditions for germination of spores must exist.
  Spores:
    Survive for several months at 6°C (42.8°F)
    Withstand boiling for hours
    Destroyed at 120°C (248°F) after 30 min

Time and conditions must allow toxin production before food is consumed.
  Toxin production:
    Strict anaerobiasis not always required
    Can occur at temperature as low as 6°C (42.8°F)
    Optimal temperature 30°C (80°F)
    Reduced at low pH

Toxin is not destroyed before food is consumed.
  Toxin:
    Destroyed at 80°C (176°F) after 30 min or 100°C for 10 min
    Unstable at high pH
    Type E toxin activated by trypsin

Toxin-containing food ingested by a susceptible host.

---

temperature range. They may survive at 6°C (42.8°F) for several months, and can withstand boiling temperatures for several hours. They are killed at temperatures of 120°C (248°F) after 30 min.

Sufficient time and proper conditions must exist for toxin production. While growth of *Clostridium botulinum* with subsequent toxin production occurs best under anaerobic conditions, strict anaerobiasis is not essential. Optimum toxin production occurs around 30°C (86°F), but toxin production has been demonstrated at temperatures as low as 6°C (42.8°F) with type E strains. It is somewhat disconcerting to note that such temperatures have been found on "refrigerated" shelves in food stores in this country. While toxin production is reduced at low pH, botulism has occurred after the ingestion of "acidic" foods. When conditions are optimal, lethal quantities of toxin may be produced in 12 to 24 hr; given less than optimal conditions many days may be required.

While the spores of *Clostridium botulinum* are quite resistant to heat, the toxin is considerably more heat-labile. It is destroyed by heating to 80°C (176°F) for 30 min or to 100°C for 10 min. Thus, regardless of the toxin content of a contaminated food, it can be rendered harmless if it is properly heated before consumption.

Botulinum toxins are unstable at high pH. But despite their protein nature, they are not destroyed in the gastrointestinal tract. In fact, type E toxin is actually activated by trypsin and is considerably more lethal when administered orally than parenterally.

Finally, the contaminated food must be ingested by a susceptible host. Animals differ widely in their susceptibility to the various botulinum toxins. There is indirect evidence that some humans may also be inherently resistant to these toxins. One of the more intriguing aspects of many botulism outbreaks is the question of why many individuals consuming foods known to contain lethal quantities of toxin fail to develop signs of illness. Of even greater interest are the two reports suggesting that botulinum toxin has been found in the circulation of individuals who had consumed contaminated foods (in one instance in considerable quantity) but who remained completely free of signs or symptoms of botulism (Koenig et al., 1964; Koenig, et al., 1967). These observations suggest that not all humans are equally susceptible to the action of botulinum toxins.

Some controversy exists as to whether botulism in humans is exclusively an intoxication, or whether the bacilli may actually produce toxin in the gastrointestinal tract. The latter concept is supported by some experimental animal data from Russian workers, but there is no evidence that such "toxico-infection" occurs naturally in humans or animals. The majority of investigators agree that botulism is caused by the ingestion of preformed toxin in contaminated foods, though it is accepted that rare cases have followed the contamination of wounds with *Clostridium botulinum* (Lamanna and Carr, 1967).

Studies by Dack and Gibard (1926) have shown that botulinum toxin is probably absorbed primarily in the stomach and upper small bowel. Toxin reaching the lower small bowel or colon is not destroyed and may be slowly absorbed from these sites (Haerem et al., 1938; Dack and Hoskins, 1942). This may account for the delayed onset and the prolonged symptomatology noted in many patients with botulism and may explain the fact that toxin has been demonstrated in the blood stream as long as 25 days after the ingestion of contaminated food (Semerau and Noack, 1919).

V. CLINICAL FEATURES OF BOTULISM

The clinical symptoms and signs of botulism follow from the mechanism of action of botulinum toxins in blocking acetylcholine release from the cholinergic nervous system (*see* Chap. 14, Sec. V). The manifestations of intoxication are generally most evident in the peripheral nervous system. However, limited clinical observation and some animal data suggest that botulinum toxins do act on the central nervous system (Tyler, 1963a; Tyler, 1963b; Simpson et al., 1967). The clinical disease may vary from an extremely

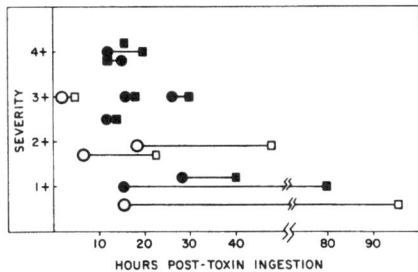

Fig. 3. The relationship between the time of onset of gastrointestinal symptoms (circles) and neuromuscular symptoms (squares) and the severity of clinical botulism. Note the disease tends to be more severe if neuromuscular symptoms occur early and if the interval between the onset of gastrointestinal and neuromuscular symptoms is short. The black figures represent patients with type E and the white figures with type B botulism.

mild illness, which is often overlooked or viewed as a minor disability such as indigestion, to a fulminant disease which may be fatal within 24 hr. The onset of symptoms may be insidious or abrupt. They usually begin within 12–36 hr after ingestion of toxin, though extremes of 2 hr to 14 days have been reported. In general, the earlier that neuromuscular symptoms or signs appear, or the shorter the interval between the onset of gastrointestinal and neuromuscular symptoms, the more serious the disease (*see* Fig. 3). However, the early onset of gastrointestinal symptoms *per se* does not indicate a poor prognosis (Koenig *et al.*, 1967).

Table III.
Symptoms of Botulism

Symptoms	Number affected[a]
Systemic	
Nausea and vomiting	11
Dry mouth	11
Weakness, lassitude	10
Dizziness, vertigo	9
Sore throat	5
Neuromuscular	
Ocular	
Blurred vision	9
Diplopia	7
Pharyngeal–laryngeal	
Dysphagia	9
Dysphonia	8
Respiratory difficulty	9
Other	
Constipation	7
Urinary retention	7
Abdominal fullness	3

[a] Of a total of eight patients with type E and four patients with type B disease.

The symptoms noted in eight patients with type E botulism seen in Nashville in 1963, and in four patients with type B disease seen in 1965 are listed in Table III. Nausea and vomiting usually occur early in the course of the disease and may be quite severe though usually short-lived. These symptoms may be more common in type B and type E intoxications than in type A disease. Weakness, a peculiar lassitude, dizziness (often with a postural component), and vertigo are frequent early complaints. Severe dryness of the mouth and throat, often accompanied by pharyngeal pain are frequently noted. Neuromuscular complaints may occur simultaneously or may be delayed for hours or even days. Ocular disturbances such as blurred vision or frank diplopia are often followed by dysphagia and dysphonia. Constipation may be severe and difficulty in voiding and urinary retention may occur. Abdominal fullness and distension may be marked, particularly in type E disease. As the disease progresses, many patients will complain of difficulty in breathing or weakness in their extremities or necks.

The physical signs noted in the Nashville patients with type E and type B botulism are listed in Table IV. On examination, patients are mentally clear and oriented, though marked sommolence has been noted—possibly a manifestation of central nervous system involvement. Hypotension, with or without a postural component, is often observed. Dryness of the tongue and mucous membranes of the mouth and pharynx may be marked (*see* Fig. 4). Dilated, unreactive pupils are frequently seen. Accommodation is impaired and the eyes are dry. Ptosis of the lids and facial muscle weakness may be noted (*see* Fig. 5). Extraocular muscle paresis is less common. Difficulties in articulation, deglutition, and swallowing are often obvious.

Table IV.
Signs of Botulism

Symptoms	Number affected[a]
Dry mouth and tongue	11
Dilated, fixed pupils	10
Respiratory impairment	8
Muscle weakness (soft palate, tongue, diaphragm, neck, extremities)	7
Pharyngeal erythema	6
Hypotension	5
Ptosis	5
Extraocular muscle paresis	4
Abdominal distension	4
Somnolence	4
Fever	1

[a] Of a total of eight patients with type E and four patients with type B disease.

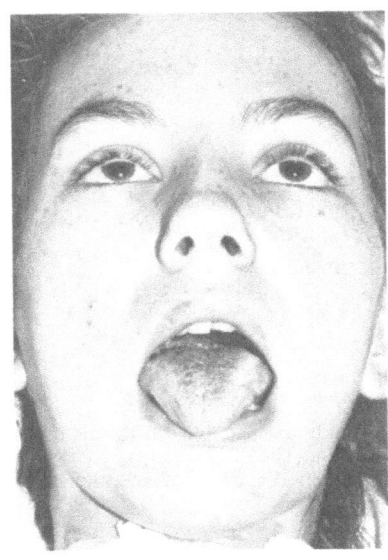

Fig. 4. Patient with type B botulism. Note the dry and coated tongue, ptosis, and the dilated pupils which remained fixed despite the photographer's bright lights. The patient was unable to wrinkle her forehead. (Reprinted from Koenig *et al.*, 1967, *Amer. J. Med.*, **42**:208, with permission of the publisher.)

Abdominal distension with absent bowel sounds may be marked, especially in patients with type E intoxication (*see* Fig. 6). Urinary retention is common. As the disease progresses, weakness of striated muscle groups, particularly in the neck and respiratory apparatus, appears. However, superficial

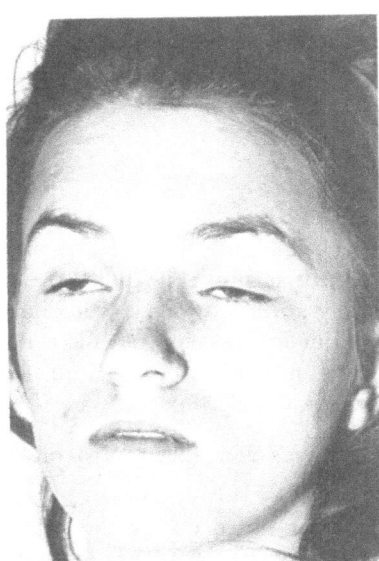

Fig. 5. Patient with type B botulism. Note the marked ptosis and weakness of the facial musculature. The patient had been asked to smile and wrinkle her forehead. (Reprinted from Koenig *et al.*, 1967, *Amer. J. Med.*, **42**:208, with permission of the publisher.)

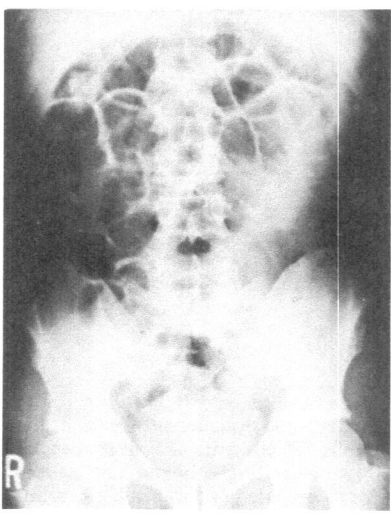

Fig. 6. Abdominal flat film of a patient with type E botulism. The dilated loops of bowel led to the mistaken diagnosis of mechanical intestinal obstruction.

and deep tendon reflexes usually remain intact. Fever is not observed in the uncomplicated disease, and when present suggests a secondary infection or alternative diagnosis.

Sudden respiratory or cardiac arrests occur in botulism. Whether these most often result from anoxia or are due to a primary action of botulinum toxin is at present unknown. Respiratory failure, airway obstruction, pulmonary infection, and cardiac arrest are the major causes of death.

VI. DIAGNOSIS

A. Routine Laboratory Studies

Routine laboratory studies are of no aid in the diagnosis of botulism. No characteristic changes in red cell or white cell counts are noted. A mild leukocytosis has been observed, but if marked, is probably indicative of secondary infection. The urinalysis is generally normal, though proteinuria is occasionally noted. No specific changes occur in the cerebrospinal fluid. Electrolyte disturbances may be observed if vomiting has been severe. No characteristic changes are noted in renal or hepatic function.

B. Electrocardiographic, Electroencephalographic, and Electromyographic Studies

Changes in the electrocardiogram have been noted during the course of several botulism outbreaks (Koenig *et al.*, 1967). These have usually consisted of minor T-wave and S-T segment changes, incomplete right bundle branch blocks, or disturbances in cardiac rhythm (Koenig *et al.*, 1964; Koenig *et al.*, 1967). None of these changes can be considered to be diagnostic, and it is not clear whether they result from a direct effect of botulinum toxins on the heart or from anoxia due to respiratory depression. There is, however, experimental data in animals to suggest that botulinum toxins may have a direct toxic effect on cardiac muscle (Bishop and Bronfenbrenner, 1936; Erzina and Mikhailov, 1956).

Electroencephalographic abnormalities have been seen in animals poisoned with botulinum toxins (Polley *et al.*, 1965; Simpson *et al.*, 1967). However, electroencephalograms obtained in three patients with type B disease failed to show any abnormality other than some increased slow-wave activity during periods of drowsiness (Koenig *et al.*, 1967).

Electromyographic changes consisting of abnormal potentials of short duration, fibrillation potentials, and fasciculations have been observed in patients with clinical botulism (Petersén and Broman, 1961; Tyler, 1963b). In addition, Tyler (1963a) demonstrated a slightly reduced conduction time in the ulnar nerve and exaggerated "H" reflexes, which he felt were indicative of some effect of botulinum toxin on the spinal cord. It should be emphasized that these abnormalities are in no way specific, and that electromyograms have been completely normal during the course of clinical botulism (Koenig *et al.*, 1967).

C. Specific Diagnosis

The diagnosis of botulism rests primarily on clinical grounds. If the index of suspicion of the physician attending a patient with the disease is not high, the diagnosis often will not be made. Definitive diagnosis rests on the identification of toxin in the body of the patient or in the incriminated food. As circulating toxin has been demonstrated up to 25 days after its ingestion (Koenig *et al.*, 1964; Koenig *et al.*, 1967; Semerau and Noack, 1919), 1.0 ml of fresh serum from patients suspected of having botulism should be injected intraperitoneally into mice, regardless of how long symptoms have been present. Other mice receiving the patient's serum should receive univalent types A, B, E, and F antisera. If toxin is present in sufficient quantity, the animals unprotected by specific antiserum will usually die, within 24 hr, of symptoms typical of botulism. Occasionally, death will be delayed for several days. This procedure has been particularly useful in making the diagnosis of type E and type B intoxications (Koenig *et al.*, 1964; Koenig *et al.*, 1967). The detection of type A toxemia is a rare occurrence—possibly due to its greater avidity for tissue binding sites—but has been reported on two occasions (Schneider and Fisk, 1939; National Communicable Disease Center,·1964).

If available, portions of the suspected food should be suspended in saline and injected intraperitoneally into mice with and without specific antisera. This will permit one to detect and identify botulinum toxin.

D. Differential Diagnosis

When the full clinical syndrome of botulism is present in an individual who gives a history of having consumed a home-canned food product, the diagnosis may not pose any difficulties. However, the history of ingestion of a suspicious food product is often not obtained, and the sequential appearance of symptoms and physical findings may be a source of considerable confusion. Even an extremely competent physician may fail to consider the diagnosis of botulism. The rarity of the disease may cause him to think of a process more familiar to him. The incorrect initial diagnoses made by the physicians first attending eight patients with type E botulism in Nashville in 1963 are shown in Table V.

The cranial nerve paresis, muscle weakness, and respiratory paralysis noted in botulism often lead to confusion with myasthenia gravis, Guillain–Barré syndrome, acute poliomyelitis, or a cerebral vascular accident. A negative edrophonium (Tensilon) test, the normal cerebrospinal fluid, the lack of sensory abnormalities, the preservation of deep tendon reflexes, the mental clarity, and the absence of corticospinal tract signs characteristic of botulism help to exclude these possibilities.

Other symptoms and signs observed in patients with botulism have led to misdiagnoses. The pharyngeal pain, erythema, and dysphagia have often suggested streptococcal or viral pharyngitis. The widely dilated, nonreactive pupils, together with the extremely dry mucous membranes seen in botulism, have frequently suggested the diagnosis of atropine, belladonna, or Jimson

Table V.
Incorrect Diagnoses Considered in Eight Patients with Type E Botulism

Cerebral vascular accident
Basilar artery thrombosis
Acute labyrinthitis
Acute Guillain–Barré syndrome
Acute poliomyelitis
Myasthenia gravis
Acute intoxication with an unknown poison
Food poisoning
Porphyria
Streptococcal pharyngitis
Viral pharyngitis
Small bowel obstruction
Coronary occlusion

weed poisoning. The absence of nervous system excitement and hallucinations and the delay in onset of symptoms usually observed in botulism should help to exclude these other intoxications.

Nausea and vomiting often observed in botulism have frequently suggested the diagnosis of other bacterial food poisonings. The development of neuromuscular symptoms should help point to botulism as the correct diagnosis. Finally, the abdominal distension, constipation, and ileus seen in botulism have been confused with mechanical intestinal obstruction and have even led to exploratory surgery (Koenig et al., 1964).

To summarize: the appearance of unexplained hypotension (often accentuated by upright posture), dilated, unreactive or slowly reactive pupils, extremely dry mucous membranes of the tongue, mouth, and pharynx, and progressive muscle paresis often involving the neck and respiratory musculature, in a previously healthy, afebrile patient who is mentally clear, should strongly suggest the diagnosis of botulism. It should be emphasized that in mild to moderately severe clinical disease, these symptoms and signs must, on occasion, be searched for with considerable care.

VII. TREATMENT

Respiratory and/or sudden cardiac arrest are the most likely causes of death in patients with botulism. Thus, *early* tracheostomy and the prompt use of the tank respirator or other mechanical aids to respiration are critically important steps in reducing mortality from the disease. Careful monitoring of respiratory and cardiac function are mandatory.

If the time from ingestion of toxin to the time when the patient is first examined is short, gastric lavage and oral administration of sodium bicarbonate may be useful in removing or inactivating the toxin. Because toxin may remain in the colon, and may be slowly absorbed over a period of many days, high colonic, cleansing enemas should be administered to remove unabsorbed toxin.

As most investigators do not subscribe to the "toxico-infection" theory of the pathogenesis of botulism in naturally occurring disease, it is generally felt that antimicrobials should be reserved only for the infectious complications that are often encountered; e.g., hypostatic or aspiration pneumonias. A minority of investigators do recommend the routine administration of penicillin to kill any *Clostridium botulinum* which may reside in the bowel.

The therapeutic efficacy of botulinum antitoxin has been a subject of controversy. Older studies by Burke and Elder (1921) and Dack (1962) have suggested that antitoxin does not alter the course of type A botulism. However, more recent data indicate that the gloomy reports regarding the efficacy of botulinum antitoxins should be revised. The Japanese experience reviewed by Dolman and Iida (1963), and the recent American experience (Koenig *et al.*, 1964; Whittaker *et al.*, 1964) with type E disease point strongly to the efficacy of antitoxin in reducing mortality from type E botulism. These patients often improve within hours of receiving type E antitoxin. The situation is less clear in regard to type B intoxication. However, because "unfixed" botulinum toxin has been observed to circulate for many days, it would appear that antitoxin should be administered to all patients with moderate or severe botulism regardless of the duration of the illness at the time of diagnosis.

A recently licensed trivalent A, B, E antitoxin is now available from the National Communicable Disease Center in Atlanta, Georgia, and is stockpiled at several locations in the United States. This antitoxin is manufactured by Connaught Laboratories, Toronto, Canada, and contains 7500 international units of type A, 5500 international units of type B, and 8500 international units of type E antitoxin per vial. The recommended initial dose is two vials, and this dose may be repeated in 2 to 4 hr. It has been shown that botulinum antitoxin may remain detectable in the circulation for over 40 days (Koenig *et al.*, 1964). As a result it seems reasonable to administer antitoxin in one course rather than to prolong its administration over several days. The latter program may increase the likelihood of allergic reactions. The antitoxin is of equine origin, and serum sensitivity must be ruled out before it is given. Lederle Laboratories still manufactures bivalent A, B antitoxin. However, this preparation should be utilized only in patients known to have intoxication with A or B toxin, or if there will be a delay in obtaining the trivalent preparation.

Recently, Cherington and Ryan (1968) have reported the use of guanidine—an agent known to increase the release of acetylcholine from nerve endings—in treating a patient with supposed botulism. Transient improvement was noted. However, their patient was not proven to have botulism. Further careful studies are necessary before guanidine can be recommended for therapy of botulism in humans.

VIII. PROGNOSIS AND RECOVERY

Since 1899 the mortality rate in recorded outbreaks of botulism in the United States has been 56% (National Communicable Disease Center, 1968). Formerly, type A strains caused the highest mortality—with rates reaching over 70% in some outbreaks. Type B and type E intoxications have generally had a better prognosis. Interestingly, from 1960–1967 mortality from type A disease within the United States has been 20%, from type B disease 10.5%, and type E disease 44.1%. Conceivably this may reflect the greater availability of types A and B antitoxin during that period. Hopefully, more rapid methods of diagnosis, more improved measures for the management of respiratory failure, and the greater availability of botulinum antitoxin will continue to improve survival rates.

In patients surviving the disease, complete recovery without residual symptoms may be expected. Return of function of the muscles of respiration, deglutition, and speech may be rapid—often within a week. However, generalized weakness, postural hypotension and constipation may persist for weeks. Ocular abnormalities involving the pupils, accommodation, and lacrimation may persist for months.

IX. REMAINING PROBLEMS

Several problems remain in the area of clinical botulism. Foremost is the need for the medical profession to maintain a high state of awareness regarding the signs and symptoms which may indicate the disease. We cannot afford to let another generation of physicians emerge from their training with little or no exposure to the perils of botulism.

Secondly, efforts must continue to devise methods which will make the diagnosis of botulism in man more rapid. The mouse-innoculation test is slow, and specific antitoxins are not widely available. Possibly, pharmacologic agents may be utilized to increase the sensitivity of the mouse to small quantities of toxin, and thus may lead to more accurate and rapid diagnosis. Immunologic techniques may be developed to facilitate the diagnosis.

Thirdly, further studies are needed to determine why certain individuals consuming toxin-containing foods fail to develop clinical disease. Differences in toxin distribution throughout the contaminated food product have often been offered as an explanation. In certain cases this explanation is not tenable. It is also clear that immunity does not play a role in resistance to the disease. Antitoxic immunity does not result from clinical botulism (Koenig et al., 1964; Koenig et al., 1967), and has been observed only in patients who have been immunized with botulism toxoids, or received botulinum antitoxin. The fascinating observation that patients *may* have botulinum toxin circulating in their blood streams and yet be free of clinical symptoms (Koenig et al., 1964; Koenig et al., 1967), suggests that certain individuals may have biochemical or structural differences at tissue-binding sites which account for their inherent resistance to botulinum toxins. Elucidation of these differences would provide a major advance to our understanding and therapy of botulism and other neuromuscular diseases.

Finally, the occurrence of type F botulism in humans in Denmark and the United States suggests that we may see more botulism of this type. It would appear that serious thought should now be given to the licensing of a quadrivalent A, B, E, F antitoxin in the United States. Such a preparation is currently made in Denmark and only available in limited supply from the National Communicable Disease Center.

ACKNOWLEDGMENTS

This work was supported in part by USPHS Grants Al-03082 and Al-00323. The author is the recipient of a Research Career Development Award from the National Institute of Allergy and Infectious Diseases.

X. REFERENCES

Bishop, G. H. and J. J. Bronfenbrenner (1936), *Amer. J. Physiol.*, **117**:393.
Burke, V. and J. C. Elder (1921), *Arch. Internal Med.*, **27**:265.
Cherington, M. and D. W. Ryan (1968), *New Engl. J. Med.*, **278**:931.
Coleman, G. E. and K. F. Meyer (1922), *J. Infect. Diseases*, **31**:622.
Dack, G. M. (1962), "Food Poisoning," 3rd ed., The University of Chicago Press, Chicago.
Dack, G. M. and J. Gibbard (1926), *J. Infect. Diseases*, **39**:173.
Dack, G. M. and D. Hoskins (1942), *J. Infect. Diseases*, **71**:260.
Dolman, C. E. (1964), Botulism as a world health problem, *in* "Botulism. Proceedings of a Symposium" (K. H. Lewis and K. Cassel, Jr., eds.), Public Health Service Publication # 999-FP-1, Public Health Service, Cincinnati, pp. 5–30.
Dolman, C. E. and H. Iida (1963), *Can. J. Public Health*, **54**:293.
Dubovsky, B. J. and K. F. Meyer (1922), *J. Infect. Diseases*, **31**:501.
Erzina, G. A. and V. V. Mikhailov (1956), *Bull. Exp. Biol. Med. (USSR)*, **41**:129.
Esty, J. R. and K. F. Meyer (1922), *J. Infect. Diseases*, **31**:650.
Gangarosa, E. J. (1969), *J. Infect. Diseases*, **119**:308.
Haerem, S., G. M. Dack, and L. R. Dragstedt (1938), *Surgery*, **3**:339.
Johnson, H. M., K. Brenner, R. Angelotti, and H. E. Hall (1966), *J. Bacteriol.*, **91**:967.
Koenig, M. G., A. Spickard, M. A. Cardella, and D. E. Rogers (1964), *Medicine*, **43**:517.
Koenig, M. G., D. J. Drutz, A. I. Mushlin, W. Schaffner, and D. E. Rogers (1967), *Amer. J. Med.*, **42**:208.
Lamanna, C. and C. J. Carr (1967), *Clini. Pharmacol. Therap.*, **8**:286.
Meyer, K. F. (1928), Ueber Botulismus, *in* "Handbook der pathog. Mikroorganismen" (W. Kolle, R. Kraus, and P. Uhlenhuth, eds.), vol. 4, Gustav Fischer and Urban Schwarzenberg, Berlin and Vienna, pp. 1269–1365.
Meyer, K. F. (1956), *Bull. World Health Organ.*, **15**:281.
Meyer, K. F. and B. J. Dubovsky (1922a), *J. Infect. Diseases*, **31**:541.
Meyer, K. F. and B. J. Dubovsky (1922b), *J. Infect. Diseases*, **31**:559.
National Communicable Disease Center (1964), *Morbidity and Mortality Weekly Report*, **13**:423.
National Communicable Disease Center (1968), "Botulism in the United States," U.S. Department of Health, Education, and Welfare, Government Printing Office, Washington, D.C., p. 3.
Polley, E. H., J. A. Vick, H. P. Ciuchta, D. A. Fischetti, F. J. Macchitelli, and N. Montanarelli (1965), *Science*, **147**:1036.
Schneider, H. J. and R. Fisk (1939), *J. Amer. Med. Assoc.*, **113**:2299.
Semerau, M. and K. Noack (1919), *Z. Klin. Med.*, **88**:304.

Simpson, L. L., F. de Balbian Verster, and J. T. Tapp (1967), *Exp. Neurol.*, **19**:199.
Tyler, H. R. (1963a), *Science*, **139**:847.
Tyler, H. R. (1963b), *Arch. Neurol.*, **9**:661.
van Ermengem, E. (1897), *Z. Hyg. Infektionshrankh.*, **26**:1.
Whittaker, R. L., R. B. Gilbertson, and A. S. Garrett (1964), *Ann. Internal Med.*, **61**:448.

Chapter 14

The Neuroparalytic and Hemagglutinating Activities of Botulinum Toxin

Lance L. Simpson

Laboratory of Chemical Biodynamics
University of California, Berkeley, California, and
Division of Neuroscience
New York State Psychiatric Institute
New York, New York, U.S.A.

I. INTRODUCTION

Were any investigator of botulinum toxin asked to describe the poison's taste, he would indeed be faced with a challenging question. It is unlikely there are surviving witnesses who could testify concerning the taste of toxin. Because the agent is so exceptionally lethal, a quantity sufficient to stimulate the palate would surely be fatal to an unprotected individual or animal. If the approximation of 0.5–5.0 μg toxin per human oral lethal dose is correct (Lamanna and Carr, 1967; Zacks *et al.*, 1968), then a 5-ml volume of ingested fluid need contain only 10^{-9} M toxin. A molarity of 10^{-9} is several orders of magnitude beneath that needed to stimulate even the most sensitive of taste receptors.

This observation is, in one sense, revealing; and in another sense, curious. Administration of botulinum toxin to experimental animals via intraperitoneal, intrasystemic, as well as oral routes, has revealed the toxin as the most deadly of all biological poisons. Beyond this, it is curious that such a deadly poison, lethal at doses far lower than necessary to alert oral senses, is a food poison.

Botulinum toxin is produced by the organism *Clostridium botulinum,* an organism ubiquitous in soil. Contaminated food preparations stored in vacuum but not sufficiently heat-treated to destroy the clostridia provide an ample environment for toxin production. The toxin is not known to serve any function in the economy of the organism. It is frequently spoken of as an exotoxin, but more likely it is a product of the organism's membrane (Boroff, 1955; Duda and Slack, 1969). In any event, a contaminated food-stuff does not need to harbor a large culture in order for subsequent ingestion of the foodstuff to be calamitous. (*see* Chap. 13). Current belief is that poisoning, as a clinical phenomenon, is entirely related to ingestion of preformed toxin; botulism is a form of intoxication and not a bacterial infection (*see* Chap. 13).

The reasons for delving into the mode of action of botulinum toxin are obvious. The potential for accidentally incurring the ailment is ever-present, and protective and therapeutic measures rest partly on identifying the agents and actions involved. Furthermore, the poison is a source of intrigue to the pathophysiologist, because such small quantities are potentially lethal. Finally, the toxin is now coming into use as an experimental tool in neuroresearch (*see* Chap. 15). It behooves the researcher to know, as precisely as possible, the molecular and biochemical events in which botulinum toxin participates.

II. CHARACTERIZATION OF THE BOTULINUM TOXIN MOLECULE

A. Purification of Botulinum Toxin

Botulinum toxin has two distinct and independent actions; it paralyzes cholinergic synaptic transmission and it agglutinates red blood cells. Only recently have these two properties been separated and made available for independent study. Many original investigations designed to characterize the botulinum molecule dealt with the heterogeneous neurotoxin–hemagglutinin aggregate. Although the hemagglutinin property appears to be a more homogeneous entity, the neurotoxin is produced in several immunologically distinct forms and designated types—A, B, Cα and Cβ, D, E, and F. With the possible exceptions of types Cα and Cβ, there appears to be little cross-reactivity between type-specific antitoxin and heterologous type toxin. Organisms are not totipotential in their ability to produce toxins. A single strain produces but one type, this being true also for Cα and Cβ.

Studies specific in their intention of describing the chemical nature of botulinum toxin have come principally from four groups of investigators, and have occurred in a tenuously chronological order. The aggregate molecule from type A toxin was first crystallized in 1946 by Abrams *et al.*

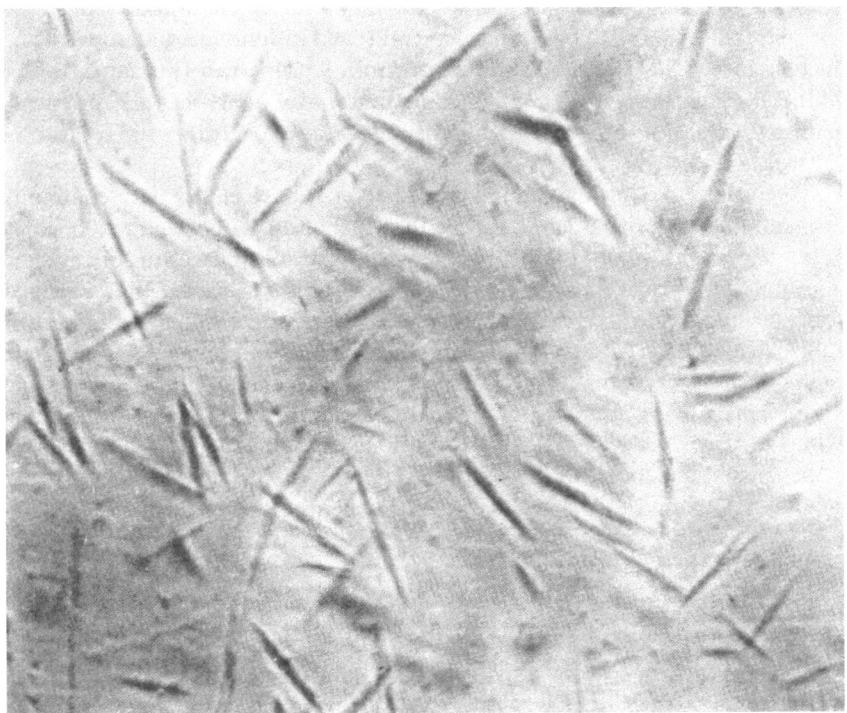

Fig. 1. Photomicrograph of the first crystals obtained from the toxin of *Clostridium botulinum*. The crystals are type A, and magnification is 225×. (Reprinted by permission, Abrams *et al.*, 1946.)

and Lamanna *et al.*, both in the Army Biolabs at Fort Detrick (*see* Fig. 1). The work was momentous for several reasons, namely: (1) crystallization of the toxin suggests a definable molecule upon which to conduct investigations; (2) the work represented the first successful crystallization of a supposed bacterial exotoxin; and (3) these investigations, in concert with those on diphtheria toxin and tetanus toxin, were bulwarks in verifying the protein nature of bacterial toxins. Botulinum crystals were reported as needle-shaped, homogeneous in appearance and in electrophoretic mobility, and lethal to the extent of approximately 2×10^8 LD_{50} (mouse) per mg nitrogen. A molecular weight estimation of about 1,000,000 was given. Types B (Lamanna and Glassman, 1947; Duff *et al.*, 1957), D (Cardella *et al.*, 1960), and E (Gordon *et al.*, 1957; Gerwing *et al.*, 1964) toxin have subsequently been isolated to rather high purity, but not crystallized.

The Fort Detrick group, having purified the botulinum type A molecule, proceeded to describe its molecular weight and homogeneity of size (Kegeles, 1946; Putnam *et al.*, 1947), its elemental and amino acid composition (Buehler *et al.*, 1947), and its physicochemical properties (Putnam *et al.*, 1948). The data, though very enlightening in terms of analytical and physical chemistry, did not provide any immediate clues regarding the poison's mode of action.

According to what Lamanna and Carr (1967) have called the "common sense notion," one would not expect that a molecule of weight 1,000,000 could survive the rigors of the gastrointestinal tract, plus diffusion across membranous barriers, intact. Indeed, this question was raised by a second group of investigators, also at the Army Biolabs, who commenced a series of ultracentrifugal analyses of the crystalline type A molecule (Wagman and Bateman, 1951; Wagman and Bateman, 1953; Wagman, 1954, 1963). In altering both the pH and the ionic strength of solutions containing botulinum toxin, they provided centrifugal observations pointing to the heterogeneity of the crystalline molecule. Moreover, it was possible tentatively to underscore a low-molecular-weight fraction as being neurotoxin, and a high-molecular-weight fraction as being hemagglutinin. These data were closely in keeping with *in vivo* studies. Both Heckly *et al.* (1960) and Hildebrand *et al.* (1961) demonstrated that neurotoxin present in the body fluids of poisoned animals was markedly smaller than the crystalline aggregate.

On the weight of evidence gathered by the two groups at Detrick, the first isolating and describing crystalline toxin and the second fractionating the crystals into their component properties, several comments seem justified: botulinum toxin is isolatable; the crystalline molecule is composed of neurotoxic and hemagglutinating fractions; neither fraction seems dependent upon the other to exert its pathologic influence. In deference to this evidence, it seems appropriate to clarify nomenclature. Thus, botulinum toxin refers to the crystalline aggregate molecule; botulinum neurotoxin refers to the component which paralyzes cholinergic synaptic transmission but does not lyse or clump red blood cells; botulinum hemagglutinin refers to the component which agglutinates erythrocytes.

B. Attempts to Separate Neurotoxin and Hemagglutinin

An ambitious attempt to isolate and to characterize botulinum neurotoxin has been undertaken by a third group, that of Dr. Gerwing and her associates in Canada. Working initially with type E toxin, and subsequently with types A and B, this group reports having separated neurotoxin from other contaminants. Using DEAE cellulose columns for separation of the aggregate molecule, and ultracentrifugal analyses for homogeneity estimates, these workers have "purified" neurotoxins E, A, and B and have suggested molecular weights of 18,600, 12,200, and 9000–10,000, respectively (Gerwing *et al.*, 1964, 1965, 1966). Certainly these molecular weights are more promising in terms of amino acid sequence analysis and tertiary structure determination than the aggregate of weight 1,000,000. Indeed, attempts have already been made at deciphering which amino acids contribute to the reactive portion of the molecule, and what may be an amino acid sequence in a portion of the molecule (Gerwing *et al.*, 1966, 1967).

In spite of this attractive beginning, several stern criticisms have been raised about the foregoing work. Most frequently noted is that it is not apparent from publications of the Canadian group that the fraction tested for centrifugal homogeneity, and concomitantly for molecular weight, was tested for toxicity. Toxicity testing was done with samples other than those identified in the ultracentrifuge. Besides, a study undertaken specifically to evaluate Gerwing's data produced profoundly different observations (Boroff *et al.*, 1968). Notably, the latter investigation, in studying supposedly homogeneous type B toxin supplied by Dr. Gerwing, as well as material prepared by Gerwing's methods, found the "purified" neurotoxin to contain several fractions. This was evident both in column chromatographic fractionation and in Ouchterlongy gel double-diffusion tests. The toxic component was shown to weigh more in the order of 100,000 than 10,000. In view of these criticisms, little confidence can yet be given to the reports of a small-molecular-weight botulinum neurotoxin.

The fourth group to invest itself in unraveling the botulinum toxin molecule is that of Boroff and DasGupta. Their initial report (DasGupta *et al.*, 1966) demonstrated that botulinum toxin type A could be chromatographically fractionated, and that by altering the ionic strength of chloride ions on a DEAE Sephadex column, two components were obtained. The components were labeled α, with an approximate molecular weight of 150,000, and β, with an approximate molecular weight of 500,000. The α fraction was highly toxic, being nearly five times as lethal on a mg-protein basis as the unfractionated botulinum toxin. The β fraction appeared to contain the botulinum hemagglutinin activity. An alternative technique has since been developed for separating the components, this using a linear gradient of phosphate buffer as eluent (DasGupta and Boroff, 1967). Data were comparable to those obtained using a chloride gradient. Ultracentrifugal analysis has reasonably verified the group's earlier estimates of botulinum neurotoxin weight, the centrifugal value being about 128,000 (Boroff *et al.*, 1966).

This line of research appears to be very encouraging. Although several techniques for isolating and estimating the molecular weight of botulinum neurotoxin were employed, the data have been quite compatible. Other laboratories have detected neurotoxin fractions which closely approximate the 128,000–150,000 figure (Freiman *et al.*, 1967; Zacks *et al.*, 1968). Particularly fascinating was the estimate of the neurotoxin's dimensions (Das-Gupta and Boroff, 1968). A physicochemical determination produced a mean diameter of 96 Å, a number in almost complete agreement with histological data (Zacks *et al.*, 1962).

Similar lines of investigation have recently been undertaken to characterize the neurotoxin of type B (DasGupta *et al.*, 1968) and type E (Kitamura *et al.*, 1967, 1968) botulinum toxin. The results have been closely analagous to those obtained in the studies on type A toxin.

III. BOTULINUM HEMAGGLUTININ

The ability of botulinum toxin to agglutinate red blood cells was first characterized by Lamanna (1948). The work successfully demonstrated that the hemagglutinating titer and neurotoxin titer of a preparation could be independently manipulated, thereby anticipating later fractionation of botulinum toxin. The demonstration was straightforward. Chicken erythrocytes were exposed to botulinum toxin, the agglutinated cells were centrifuged off, and the remaining suspension was tested for toxicity. The resulting neuroparalytic titer was not diminished.

In distinction to neurotoxin, the hemagglutinating property shows degrees of cross-reactivity. Antisera specific to type A or B botulinum toxin will cross-neutralize heterologous hemagglutinin (Lamanna and Lowenthal, 1951). The situation is analagous for types C and D toxin (Sterne, 1954). Type E antiserum has not been shown to react with any other than homologous type toxin, and therefore seems to be specific to E hemagglutinin (Lamanna, 1959). Type F has not been investigated thoroughly. Antiserum to type F produced several precipitation lines common to antisera for types A and B when type F botulinum toxin was tested. However, the possibility that this represented hemagglutinin cross-reactivity was not explored (Rezepov, 1967).

Hemagglutinin has not been isolated for physiological study. Investigations have employed either supernatant from clostridia cultures or crystalline botulinum toxin. The agent has been shown effective against red blood cells of all animals tested, except the cat (Simpson *et al.*, 1968). This observation was produced using the β fraction. It is not yet clear if the β fraction represents hemagglutinin exclusively.

The activity of hemagglutinin is stable at salt concentrations of 0.107–0.243 M and at pH values of 6.0–8.5. (Lowenthal and Lamanna, 1951). It is unlikely that any physiological situation would perturb red cell clumping. Hemagglutinin is more heat-stable but less pH-stable than neurotoxin.

Apparently cohesion of the aggregate botulinum molecule is pH-dependent (Lowenthal and Lamanna, 1953). At acid pH, agglutination of red cells will cause a companion loss of toxicity. At alkaline pH, toxicity is not lost in the clumping process. Although no mention is made, earlier successful separation of hemagglutinin and neurotoxin (*see* above) must have been conducted in an alkaline environment.

The mechanism of agglutination is not known, though suggestive experiments are available (Lowenthal and Lamanna, 1953). Hemagglutinin binds reversibly to red blood cells; the consequence is that a clumped preparation may be washed and subsequently reclumped by different hemagglutinin. Proteolytic enzymes destroy the binding capacity of red cells, and the binding is influenced by the nature and concentration of ions present. The data point to an adsorption phenomenon.

The capacity of botulinum toxin to bind to erythrocytes is of marginal importance to the pathologist, because it is not contributory to the disease state of botulism. However, it may be worthwhile to examine the efficacy of hemagglutinin in several animal species. The single unaffected species is the cat, and this animal is remarkably resistant to botulinal poisoning. If neurotoxin must be separated from the parent molecule before it paralyzes cholinergic synapses, as dimension studies cited above suggest, then a reasonable question occurs. Can resistance be partially explained by the sluggish separation of the two components of botulinum toxin? Even if the answer were negative, the research producing the answer would contribute to our understanding of hemagglutinin–neurotoxin binding *in vivo*.

IV. TARGET ORGANS OF BOTULINUM NEUROTOXIN

Clinical symptoms are a first index for the experimentalist attempting to decipher a poison's mode of action. Dizziness and lethargy, general locomotor dysfunction, and eventual respiratory collapse were taken as signs that botulinum toxin could produce a severe central nervous system (CNS) lesion. Accordingly, initial explorations by pathologists sought defects within the brain or neuraxis. As reviewed by Wright (1955), the various searches were fruitless. In retrospect, one might comment that even if there were a CNS defect, the initial explorers were not equipped with methods adequate for detection of such.

Although preceded by other reports, the manuscripts of Dickson and Shevky (1923a,b) were incisive in unveiling the site of action of botulinum neurotoxin. (Little physiological research has been conducted using purified neurotoxin. However, the author will use this term because the studies included in this and the following section clearly deal with neuroparalysis and not with hemagglutination.) Dissatisfied with attempts at correlating

CNS histological abnormalities and botulinal symptoms, Dickson and Shevky examined the peripheral nervous system (PNS) for possible labile sites. Using cats, dogs, and rabbits, they reported a series of unified findings. Several organs, innervated by what is now classified as the parasympathetic division of the autonomic nervous system, were found defective in their responsiveness to neurogenic stimuli during experimental poisoning. Specifically, there was a deficit in: (1) cardiac inhibition following vagal stimulation, (2) intestinal augmentation following vagal stimulation, (3) salivation following stimulation of the chorda tympani, (4) bladder contraction and penis erection after stimulation of the nervous erigens, and (5) pupillary constriction following oculomotor nerve stimulation. All experiments were performed on decerebrate preparations. The relation between these findings and clinical botulism were clear, because onset of illness and onset of failures were simultaneous. Efforts designed to reveal defects in the sympathetic system met with negative results.

In their second report (1923b), Dickson and Shevky pointed out several sites at which botulism was not producing anomalies. It became clear that the CNS, sensory fibers, and peripheral organs themselves were not affected. Nevertheless, striated muscle showed diminished responsiveness after neurogenic stimuli. From these findings there emerged the dual concept that neuroparalysis was occurring at the region of the end-organ, or synaptic junction, and that only cholinergic end-organs were susceptible to poisoning. Virtually all symptoms, both clinical and experimental, can be accommodated by the concepts just mentioned, including death due to paralysis of the phrenic nerve–diaphragm junction.

Later reports were confirmatory in citing the cholinergic end-organ as the target of botulinal poisoning (Bishop and Bronfenbrenner, 1936; Guyton and MacDonald, 1947; Burgen et al., 1949). It rapidly became clear that no concentration of toxin could disrupt nervous propagation except at the synapse. Burgen et al. (1949) therefore proceeded to examine the kinetics of botulinal activity on an isolated neuromuscular preparation, the so-called isolated rat phrenic nerve–diaphragm preparation of Bülbring (1946). Several of the findings are extremely interesting (see Fig. 2). It was noted that the Q_{10} of paralysis reflected an underlying chemical reaction. Together with this, it was found that binding of toxin is quite rapid and remarkably firm. Nerve–diaphragms exposed to poison for at least 5 min could be washed without altering the onset of synaptic failure. Corollary to these data was the observation that tissue bathed for a short time in a toxic medium could not be protected by addition of antiserum. Probably antiserum can neutralize free toxin, but it is inactive against toxin bound to tissue. Perhaps as helpful as the data, was the introduction of the phrenic nerve–diaphragm as a preparation for studying paralysis. In addition to the convenience and

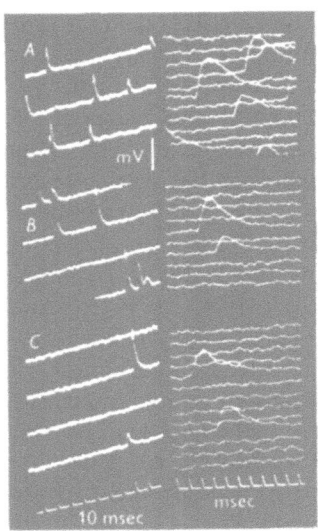

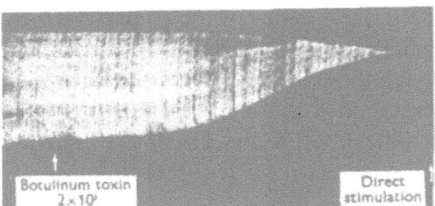

Fig. 2 Left: Recording of the twitch of an isolated rat phrenic nerve–diaphragm preparation. The time elapsed between addition of poison and resulting paralysis is about 90 min. Note that even after complete loss of responsiveness to neurogenic stimuli, the muscle continues to respond to direct stimulation. (Reprinted by permission, Burgen *et al.*, 1949.) Right: Recording of mepp's before and after addition of botulinum toxin. A microelectrode has been positioned near the muscle endplate, and electrophysiological events are tabulated in the absence of overt muscle movement. Trace A was obtained 8 min prior to addition of poison; trace B, 20 min after poison; and trace C, 41 min after poison. Clearly the frequency of mepp's is reduced. (Reprinted by permission, Brooks, 1956.)

hardiness of the tissue, it seems appropriate to be working at the site whose ultimate failure is often the cause of death in botulism.

Due to a series of electrophysiological studies, the tips of the cholinergic fibers were identified as the target for neurotoxin (Stover *et al.*, 1953; Brooks, 1954, 1956). The literature has not progressed beyond this point in terms of defining the nature of a site to which the poison can bind. The study of Zacks *et al.* (1962), localizing injected conjugates of botulinum toxin and ferritin by electron microscopy, confirmed little other than that toxin specifically situates itself within the cholinergic synaptic interspace. The bulk of research has tended to expand the number of cholinergic synapses at which a neuroparalytic effect has been witnessed. Ambache (1949, 1951) has studied the poisoned ocular apparatus extensively. Movements of external ocular muscles plus pupillary constriction could not be elicited by nervous stimulation in intoxicated animals. In contradistinction, adrenergic fibers, as evidenced by pupillary dilation, were resistant. Both Ambache (1951) and

Kupfer (1958) demonstrated a toxic influence on ganglionic transmission. Hilton and Lewis (1955) confirmed earlier work by showing chorda tympani stimulation to be ineffective at the distal organ after neurotoxin. Likewise, Ambache and Lessin (1955) witnessed partial intestinomotor difficulty. It becomes obvious that a number of cholinergic junctions have been tested, and none has proven resistant to paralysis by neurotoxin.

It should be mentioned that neurotoxin produces conspicuous changes in the physiology of cholinergically innervated organs, particularly muscle, but this is due to an indirect rather than to a direct action (*see* review by Guth, 1968). In 1959, Axelsson and Thesleff described the phenomenon of supersensitivity in skeletal muscle. The term "supersensitivity" refers to the fact that in a chronically denervated mammalian skeletal muscle, the area of muscle membrane sensitive to acetylcholine (ACh) is widespread beyond the endplate region. In the normally innervated muscle, the endplate region is exclusively receptive to minute quantities of ACh. Thesleff (1960) has experimentally demonstrated supersensitivity to ensue in botulinum-poisoned skeletal muscle. It would seem that both denervation and neurotoxin can remove a trophic factor by which the nerve contains and restricts the area of muscle fiber exquisitely receptive to ACh. Presumably ACh, or some substance released in the company of ACh, is the trophic factor (*see* Chap. 15, Sec. III).

When observation of poisoned skeletal muscle is followed for a considerable length of time (>14 days), atrophy is prominent (Jirmanova *et al.*, 1964). Both wet weight of the whole muscle and diameter of extrafusal fibers decreases to approximately 60% of controls. There may be a proliferation in the number of muscle cell nuclei. Since the total number of fibers is lessened in the experimental animals, complete degeneration must occur. Throughout the process of muscle atrophy, nerve bundles and individual nerve fibers survive without detectable histological damage (Thesleff, 1960). The preserved integrity of nervous tissue is also true in the clinical situation (Tyler, 1963b).

Supersensitivity of salivary gland resulting from treatment with neurotoxin has been reported by Emmelin (1961). This is not surprising, for denervation will also produce the effect.

V. MECHANISM OF NEUROTOXIN ACTION

A. Peripheral Cholinergic System

In scanning the literature pertinent to the mode of neurotoxin action, one is struck by what appears to be a collective application of the exclusion principle. The overwhelming bulk of data reflects what the poison is *not* doing, rather than what it is doing. Undoubtedly this is true for any pharmacological agent whose mechanism of action has long eluded experimenters.

As reported above, neurotoxin does not block propagation of the nerve impulse, for the phrenic nerve trunk will fire even when respiration has ceased (Bishop and Bronfenbrenner, 1936). Many workers have recorded that organs continue to respond to direct stimulation even though stimulation via the nervous supply is curtailed. The first proposal which took into account that neurotoxin acts at cholinergic synapses came from Torda and Wolff (1947). They proposed that choline acetylase can be strongly inhibited; cholinergic transmission cannot long persist when a synthesizing enzyme of ACh is inhibited. Burgen et al. (1949) investigated this possibility and quickly refuted it. However, the latter workers did observe that in paralyzed preparations there was a diminution in ACh output. From this observation, the idea was advanced that toxin prevents the extrusion of transmitter substance by causing failure of transmission in the fine, unmyelinated nerve terminals. Both Ambache (1951) and Brooks (1956) experimentally discounted this alternative. Brooks favored the proposal that release of ACh is prevented at the terminal of the nerve fiber.

In addition to the possibilities of inhibiting synthesis of ACh or inhibiting release of ACh, the possibility of postsynaptic activity was considered. Data did not support a curariform action, nor were postsynaptic receptors desensitized (Guyton and MacDonald, 1947; Masland and Gammon, 1949; Burgen et al., 1949). Neither is there evidence that acetylcholinesterase (AChE) is affected. Workers who have recorded endplate potentials (epp) or miniature endplate potentials (mepp) did not observe alterations in the amplitude or duration of such during the onset of synaptic blockade (Brooks, 1956; Thesleff, 1960). The mepp especially should be increased in amplitude and lengthened in duration were AChE inhibited. Marshall and Quinn (1967) claimed AChE inhibition by toxin in an in vitro system. The observation could not be reproduced by Sumyk and Yocum (1968) or Simpson and Morimoto (1969).

The hypothesis now given credence is that neurotoxin paralyzes cholinergic synaptic transmission by interfering with some as yet unspecified step in the release mechanism of ACh.

Only two hypotheses have been advanced which were aimed at explaining the means by which neurotoxin could suppress transmitter release. In a series of publications (Boroff, 1959; Boroff et al., 1963; Boroff and Fleck, 1967), Boroff has favored the idea that neurotoxin could prevent 5-hydroxytryptamine (5-HT) from fulfilling a possible role in cholinergic transmission. This hypothesis was derived from the postulated role of 5-HT in membrane transport of calcium (Woolley, 1958), from the observation that 5-HT is an *in vivo* antagonist of intoxication (Boroff, 1959) and from the reported importance of tryptophan in the botulinum toxin molecule (Boroff and Das Gupta, 1964). Calcium, of course, is an obligatory intermediate in the neurogenic release of ACh. Data have not favored the hypothesis. Isolated rat phrenic nerve–diaphragm preparations were not protected by 5-HT (Simpson and Tapp, 1967b). The protective effect of the indolealkylamine is manifest only in the *in vivo* situation. Furthermore, the *in vivo* protective activity is not specific to botulinum neurotoxin, for animals poisoned with nereistoxin, curare, or hemicholinium show the 5-HT effect (Simpson, 1968b, Simpson and Morimoto, 1970). Evidence points to a nonspecific protective event that is removed from the synaptic environment (Simpson, 1970) and denies a role for 5-HT in cholinergic transmission.

Thesleff (1960) observed an epp in a previously unresponsive preparation after addition of twice normal concentrations of calcium. This observation allowed the hypothesis that neurotoxin could act in a magnesium-like manner, competitively inhibiting calcium from promoting ACh release. It has been shown that calcium will partially protect isolated neuromuscular preparations (Simpson and Tapp, 1967a). However, kinetic analyses showed calcium and neurotoxin to be acting at different mechanistic sites. Also, the ion effect was best expressed in terms of the calcium : magnesium ratio rather than in terms of either ion singly. Calcium seems to increase the probability of ACh release, and thereby indirectly antagonizes neurotoxin (Simpson and Tapp, 1967a; Thesleff, personal communication). This conclusion has received both direct and indirect support. Hubbard *et al.* (1968) found that there exist two distinct categories of mepp's, one of which is calcium-dependent and one of which is calcium-independent. Electrophysiological studies reviewed above have witnessed a complete cessation of neuromuscular activity during paralysis. Clearly inhibition of calcium could not account for the ability of neurotoxin to interrupt all activity, since one fraction of the mepp's is calcium-independent. Drachman and Fanburg (1969) measured the uptake of calcium by isolated synaptosomal preparations. The calcium sequestering power of synaptosomes from nervous tissue is impervious to toxin.

B. Central Nervous System

Much to the embarrassment of workers in the field, the author included, the area of CNS research is surely more replete with confusion and contradiction than any other aspect of neurotoxin research. Not only is there disagreement among several investigators, but single individuals also have contradicted the trend of their own data.

Earliest attempts at proving the CNS susceptible to malfunction during botulism looked for histological damage (*see* Dickson and Shevky, 1923a;

and Wright, 1955, for literature cited). Tissue samples were frequently taken from patients who expired due to intoxication. Data emerged and so did two camps of thought—those who were able to detect tissue abnormalities, and those who were not. Neither camp held a clear experimental edge. In their studies on the PNS, Dickson and Shevky made the salient introductory remark that although some did claim to see CNS abnormalities, the abnormalities were in places obscurely related to nervous dysfunctions. Armed with the findings of Dickson and Shevky, Cowdry and Nicholson (1924) performed a detailed histological study of the CNS from experimentally poisoned animals. Their findings were uniformly negative. Due to these experiments, as well as PNS work which points to a biochemical rather than anatomical lesion, the specter of CNS histological derangement has not been revived.

Contemporary work from the clinic has not been so easily resolved. Tyler (1963a) reported the occurrence of an "H reflex" in a case of human botulism. Supposedly the H reflex, which is dependent upon damage within the neuraxis before it becomes manifest, suggests a CNS effect. Koenig *et al.* (1967) did not witness exaggerated H reflexes in patients with type B botulism (Tyler's study did not determine the type botulism involved). They did, though, report conspicuous patient somnolence. Peripheral cholinergic blockade is an unsatisfactory explanation for sleepiness, so the clinical situation is still open to question. Fortunately for humanity, botulism is sufficiently rare to preclude detailed clinical study.

Efforts to localize botulinum toxin histologically within the CNS have not been unequivocal. Pak and Bulatova (1962) prepared ^{35}S-labeled type B toxin. The unfractionated molecule was injected intravenously into mice. Many organs, including brain, showed subsequent radioactivity, but the relation between these findings and the possibility of selective binding at cholinergic synapses is remote. Zacks (1965) examined the distribution of fluorescein-labeled botulinum toxin on *in vitro* sections. Unfractionated type A toxin did not show preferential localization in central nervous tissue. More recent *in vivo* work was similarly unencouraging in showing CNS deposition, while the neuromuscular apparatus was nicely labeled (Zacks *et al.*, 1968).

These findings raise at least one crucial question. Why are *in vitro* sections of spinal cord not regionally labeled with tagged toxin? The motoneurons which innervate voluntary muscle give off many collaterals within the spinal cord, both to synergistic muscle motoneurons and to interneurons. If distal motoneuron, i.e., cholinergic, synapses are labeled with toxin, one would expect synapses of collaterals to be distinguished too. They do, after all, represent synapses of the same nerve cells. The question of diffusion does not seem pertinent, because *in vitro* sections do not have functional blood–brain barriers. Most certainly, this is a problem that should receive close examination.

Several investigations have been designed to maximize the probability of disrupting CNS activity during intoxication. On all occasions, unfractionated toxin was used. Davies *et al.* (1953) made direct injections into the brain. In contrast to results produced by tetanus toxin, botulinum toxin produced no local neurological signs. Injection of the poison into the femoral vein of monkeys evoked an astonishing effect, a completely flattened electroencephalogram (Polly *et al.*, 1965) (*see* Figs. 3 and 4). The results were essentially replicated by Simpson *et al.* (1967), using guinea pigs and cats. EEGs taken on patients with type B botulism were not characteristically abnormal (Koenig *et al.*, 1967).

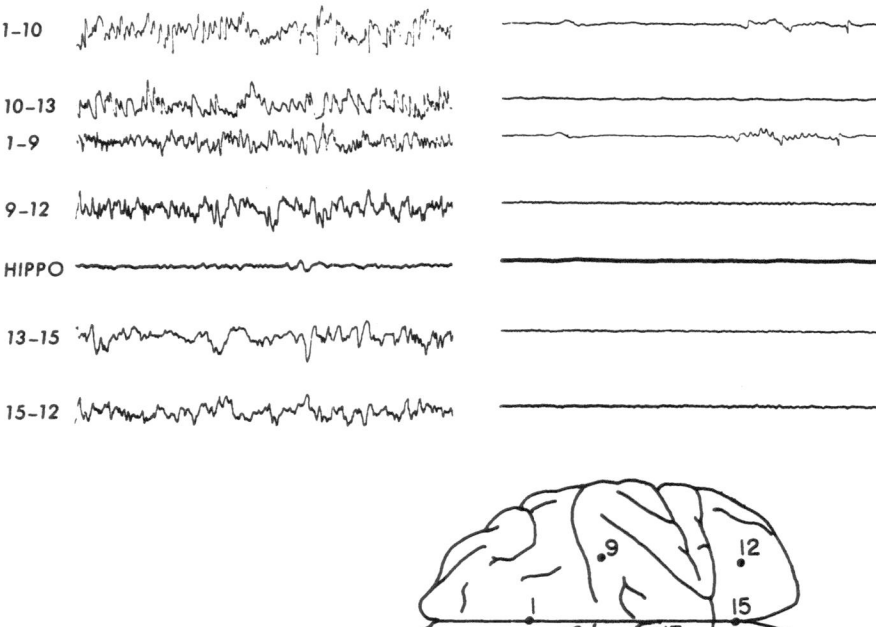

Fig. 3. EEG of monkey that has received multilethal dose of type A botulinum toxin. The recording on the left is a control, and that on the right is 15 min post-toxin injection. Numbering scheme for electrodes is indicated on diagrammatic brain. Shortly after injection, but long before clinical symptoms, botulinum toxin has produced a nearly isoelectric EEG. (Records were obtained through the courtesy of J. A. Vick.)

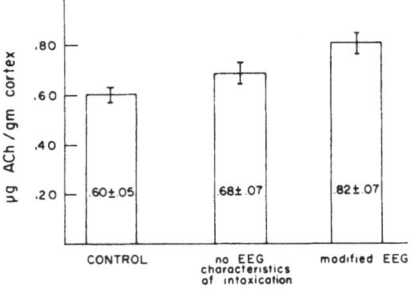

Fig. 4A. Acetylcholine concentration in cortices of botulinal-intoxicated guinea pigs. Levels of ACh are not distinguishably different in controls and poisoned animals without EEG abnormality. However, differences between controls and experimentals are significant after onset of EEG depression. (Reprinted by permission, Simpson et al., 1967.)

Three papers have been suggestive that the cholinergic system within the CNS is affected. Hart et al. (1965) found increases in intoxicated rabbit brain levels of ACh. Simpson (1968a) reported similar changes in rat brain without a concommitant disruption of the EEG. Homogenized and fractionated brain of intoxicated mice showed increased levels of choline and ACh in one fraction, and a diminished number of synaptic vesicles, some of which were distended (Saelens, 1965).

The bulk of study coming from the Soviet Union is compatible with CNS biochemical lesions during botulism. Exemplary studies are those of Mikhailov (1955), Abrosimov (1956), and Ado and Abrosimov (1964). Acute experiments were done largely on cats, although rabbits and rats have been included. These investigations have pointed to a medullary susceptibility during intoxication, and further have raised the possibility that disruption of CNS respiratory centers can contribute to or even cause death.

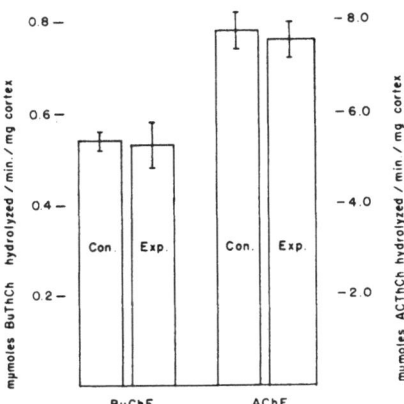

Fig. 4B. Determination of acetylcholinesterase and butyrylcholinesterase activity in the cortices of intoxicated rats. With neither enzyme is there significant alteration in activity. Similar experiments, with similar negative results, have been performed on rat cortex homogenate. (Reprinted by permission, Simpson and Morimoto, 1969.)

From the conglomerate of results, it is not possible to draw any firm conclusions (except that we are in need of definitive research!). Species differences, route of administration, and method of testing—the catchalls used to explain data at odds—are not satisfying explanations. Two alternatives do present themselves. First, it is possible that an agent producing the CNS effects is not simple botulinum toxin, but is a dissociation product of botulinum toxin. It is known that botulinum toxin kept for long periods of time in acetate buffer will dissociate into several products (Riesen, 1965). In this context, it should be mentioned that positive EEG findings were the result of injecting old batches of toxin (Vick, personal communication; Simpson, unpublished results). Second, if CNS effects are not conclusively shown, it could be because either there are no cholinergic synapses in the CNS, or if they do exist their anatomy or physiology is peculiar from PNS cholinergic synapses. Both alternatives are highly assumptive; indeed, differences may yet be resolved on grounds of methodology.

VI. REACTIVE SITES INVOLVED IN NEUROTOXIN ACTIVITY

A. Free Amino Groups

It would be of considerable importance to our understanding of neurotoxin activity, as well as to our awareness of neuromuscular pharmacology, if the reactive groups in neurotoxin could be identified. Attempts at this have been made, but reproducibility has been at a minimum. Equally disconcerting, the majority of studies have been conducted on the hemagglutinin–neurotoxin aggregate, so it is questionable whether these observations are extendable to pure neurotoxin.

Botulinum toxin is a completely proteinaceous material, and its content can be accounted for by nineteen different amino acids (Buehler *et al.*, 1947). No prosthetic groups have been identified, so the biological activity of the toxin must be due to the nature of the amino acids present and their molecular configuration. Schantz and Spero (1957) have examined the effect of ketene ($CH_2{=}CO$) on botulinum toxin type A. Exposure of poison to this very reactive organic compound brought about rapid toxin inactivation. The plot of diminished toxicity versus exposure time to ketene revealed first-order kinetics. Three sites in protein are reactive with ketene: free amino groups, phenolic hydroxyl groups, and sulfhydryl groups. The rate of ketene inactivation did not closely follow the rate of *O*-acetylation, so phenolic hydroxyls are poor candidates. *p*-Chloromercuribenzoic acid interacts with sulphydryl groups; it did not diminish toxicity. Free amino groups appear essential to the biologic activity of botulinum toxin.

In a companion paper, Spero and Schantz (1957) observed the reaction between toxin and nitrous acid in the presence of excess nitrite. The technique was intended to provide additional evidence for the importance of intact free amino groups in botulinum toxin. The kinetics of toxin inactivation were consistent with the data obtained by inactivation of simple amino compounds.

In studies on the pH sensitivity of botulinum toxin, Spero (1958) found that within a narrowly defined range, inactivation was inversely proportional to the ninth power of the hydrogen ion concentration. Auxiliary work on the heat of ionization of nonneutral amino acids suggested that inactivation within this narrow pH range could be due to the specific ionization of the ε-amino group in lysine. Thus dissociation of a single proton from each of nine lysine residues could result in loss of toxicity. One must say that a rather sophisticated analytical probe was being made into what is now known to be a heterogeneous molecule. Indeed, the investigator expressed difficulties incurred in equating observed data with theoretical calculations. In looking back, one is hard-pressed to determine if the conclusions are invalid due to the large, contaminating presence of hemagglutinin, partially valid and applicable to the molecule's integrity of configuration rather than reactive site, or an insightful though yet unreproduced study on the amino group essential to botulinal neuroactivity.

B. Fluorescence and Toxicity

In 1958 and 1959, Boroff and Fitzgerald made the original reports on the fluorescence of botulinum toxin. Treatment with either alkali (pH > 10) or specific antiserum produced a reduction in fluorescence and in toxicity. Both treatments are straightforward, and the results were to be expected. A less easily explained observation was that ferric ion, even at concentrations of 10^{-7} M, could reduce fluorescence and toxicity. On the basis of their findings, the authors suggested a possible relation between the optical properties and the toxic properties of the poison. Specifically, the same region of the molecule might be responsible both for fluorescence and for toxicity. The suggestion was called into question when it was found possible to alter biological activity and fluorescence independently (Schantz et al., 1960). Treatment of botulinum toxin with 6-M urea will nearly abolish toxicity while exerting negligible influence on fluorescence. Conversely, 0.1-M thioglycolate will dramatically reduce fluorescence though slightly diminishing toxicity.

C. Tryptophan

Certainly tryptophan is the most intensively studied amino acid as a possible candidate for location in the reactive locus of botulinum toxin. The experimental motivation grows from the original data on toxin fluorescence, for the maxima of activation and fluorescence are reasonably close to that of tryptophan. It might be asked, why have tyrosine and phenylalanine—both of which are fluorescing amino acids—not been so intensively examined? A possible rationale for excluding tyrosine is that it does not contain free amino groups and it does contain a phenolic hydroxyl, both of which are contrary to expectations of the reactive amino acid. Phenylalanine does not contain any free amino groups when in protein. (Neither does tryptophan, although it does contain an imino group.)

Several treatments which are relatively specific to tryptophan do cause reduction in toxicity. Photo-oxidation in the presence of methylene blue is such a technique, and has been applied (Weil *et al.*, 1957; Boroff and Das-Gupta, 1964). The possibility that methionine, histidine, or cysteine could have been affected was either examined or commented upon (Boroff and DasGupta, 1964). Data did not support the involvement of either methionine or histidine. The authors did not actually investigate cysteine owing to earlier work which tended to eliminate *S*-containing amino acids as essential to neuroparalysis (Schantz and Spero, 1957). A subsequent experiment in which 2-hydroxy-5-nitrobenzylbromide, a reagent nearly specific to tryptophan, was reacted with botulinum toxin produced evidence corroborating the essentiality of intact tryptophan residues (Boroff and DasGupta, 1966). The single disparate comment comes from Gerwing *et al.* (1966), who failed to find any tryptophan in "purified" type B neurotoxin. (The work of Boroff and DasGupta implicating this amino acid was done on type A toxin. However, since all types exert a similar neuroparalytic activity, it is to be expected that reactive regions will prove similar or even identical.) This counterobservation is of questionable importance since neurotoxin prepared by the technique of Gerwing and her coworkers has not proved to be homogeneous (Boroff *et al.*, 1968).

It is the author's bias that attempts to identify a single amino acid as the integral portion of the neurotoxin's reactive locus could be unfruitful. As stated above, the research has been conducted on botulinum toxin and the results extrapolated to neurotoxin. In addition, evidence regarding the importance of an amino acid for biological activity must distinguish whether importance relates to the molecule's configuration or to its reactive site. Even assuming that tryptophan integrity is necessary for the exertion of neuroparalysis, its role may be in maintaining neurotoxin's tertiary configuration. In fact, there is no reason to believe that a single amino acid could account for neurotoxin's mode of action. Single amino acid groups do play large roles in proteins, exerting or halting enzymatic activity, but surely this is not applicable to neurotoxin. More likely, neurotoxin binds to the membrane of the bouton or to the amorphous surface material and thereby blocks channels of ACh passage. Such binding would suggest the involvement of more than a single type amino acid.

Gerwing *et al.* (1966, 1967) are the only ones who have worked analytically with what was claimed to be neurotoxin. A sequence of amino acids was proposed as possibly involved in the poison's reactive locus. But until these workers can rebuff the claim of Boroff *et al.* (1968) that their material is not homogeneous, their data cannot be accepted with confidence.

VII. CONCLUSION

At this point, an understatement may be appropriate. Any significant advance in our understanding of how neurotoxin acts is also a dramatic step in our understanding of neuromuscular pharmacology. Investigators dealing with neurotoxin find themselves in an interesting paradox. They are attempting to decipher pathophysiology nearer the molecular level than knowledge of physiology will support. That is, work is being done to describe how neurotoxin suppresses release or movement of ACh, but neuroscientists know precious little about mechanisms of ACh release or movement.

The paradox is itself a motivation for continuing to study neurotoxin. It is inevitable that study which elaborates the pharmacology of neuromuscular transmission and that study which elucidates the mode of neurotoxin activity will produce companion results.

VIII. REFERENCES

Abrams, A., G. Kegeles, and G. A. Hottle (1946), *J. Biol. Chem.*, **164**:63.
Abrosimov, V. N. (1956), *Arkh. Pat.*, (*Moskva*), **18**:86.
Ado, A. D. and V. N. Abrosimov (1964), *J. Hyg. Epidemiol.*, **8**:433.
Ambache, N. (1949), *J. Physiol.*, **108**:127.
Ambache, N. (1951), *J. Physiol.*, **113**:1.
Ambache, N. and A. W. Lessin (1955), *J. Physiol.*, **127**:449.
Axelsson, J. and S. Thesleff (1959), *J. Physiol.*, **149**:178.
Bishop, G. H. and J. J. Bronfenbrenner (1936), *Amer. J. Physiol.*, **117**:393.
Boroff, D. A. (1955), *J. Bact.*, **70**:363.
Boroff, D. A. (1959), *Internat. Arch. Allergy*, **15**:74.
Boroff, D. A. and B. R. DasGupta (1964), *J. Biol. Chem.*, **239**:3694.
Boroff, D. A. and B. R. DasGupta (1966), *Biochim. Biophys. Acta*, **117**:289.
Boroff, D. A., B. R. DasGupta, and U. Fleck (1963), Chemistry and biological activity of the toxin of *Clostridium botulinum, in* "Proc. 2nd Int. Pharmac. Meet." (H. W. Raudonat, ed.), vol. 9, Macmillan, New York, pp. 93–103.
Boroff, D. A., B. R. DasGupta, and U. Fleck (1968), *J. Bact.*, **95**:1738.
Boroff, D. A. and J. E. Fitzgerald (1958), *Nature*, **181**:751.
Boroff, D. A. and U. Fleck (1967), *J. Pharmacol. Exp. Therap.*, **157**:427.
Boroff, D. A., R. Townsend, U. Fleck, and B. R. DasGupta (1966), *J. Biol. Chem.*, **241**:5165.
Brooks, V. B. (1954), *J. Physiol.*, **123**:501.
Brooks, V. B. (1956), *J. Physiol.*, **134**:264.

Buehler, H. J., E. J. Schantz, and C. Lamanna (1947), *J. Biol. Chem.*, **169**:295.
Bulbring, E. (1946), *Brit. J. Pharmac. Chemother.*, **1**:38.
Burgen, A. S. V., F. Dickens, and L. J. Zatman (1949), *J. Physiol.*, **109**:10.
Cardella, M. A., J. T. Duff, B. H. Wingfield, and C. Gottfried (1960), *J. Bact.*, **79**:372.
Cowdry, E. V. and F. M. Nicholson (1924), *J. Exper. Med.*, **39**:827.
DasGupta, B. R. and D. A. Boroff (1967), *Biochim. Biophys. Acta*, **147**:603.
DasGupta, B. R. and D. A. Boroff (1968), *J. Biol. Chem.*, **243**:1065.
DasGupta, B. R., D. A. Boroff, and E. Rothstein (1966), *Biochem. Biophys. Res. Commun.*, **22**:750.
DasGupta, B. R., D. A. Boroff, and K. Cheong (1968), *Biochem. Biophys. Res. Commun.*, **32**:1057.
Davies, J. R., R. S. Morgan, E. A. Wright, and G. P. Wright (1953), *J. Physiol.*, **120**:618.
Dickson, E. C. and R. Shevky (1923a), *J. Exper. Med.*, **37**:711.
Dickson, E. C. and E. Shevky (1923b), *J. Exper. Med.*, **38**:327.
Drachman, D. B. and B. L. Fanburg (1969), *J. Neurochem.*, **16**:1633.
Duda, J. J. and J. M. Slack (1969), *J. Bact.*, **97**:900.
Duff, J. T., J. Klerer, R. H. Bibler, D. E. Moore, C. Gottfried, and G. G. Wright (1957), *J. Bact.*, **73**:597.
Emmelin, N. (1961), *J. Physiol.*, **156**:121.
Freiman, V. B., A. I. Mikhailov, V. K. Golshmid, K. A. Ahundov, and V. D. Artemenko (1967), Immunochemical study of *Clostrodium botulinum* antigens and sera, *in* "Botulism 1966" (M. Ingram and T. A. Roberts, eds.), Chapman and Hall Ltd., London, pp. 330–335.
Gerwing, J., C. E. Dolman, and H. S. Bains (1965), *J. Bact.*, **89**:1383.
Gerwing, J., C. E. Dolman, D. V. Kason, and J. H. Tremaine (1966), *J. Bact.*, **91**:484.
Gerwing, J., C. E. Dolman, M. E. Reichmann, and H. S. Bains (1964), *J. Bact.*, **88**:216.
Gerwing, J., A. Ko, D. Van Alstyne, and J. H. Tremaine (1966), *Biochim. Biophys. Acta*, **117**:487.
Gerwing, J., B. Mitchell, and D. Van Alstyne (1967), *Biochim. Biophys. Acta*, **140**:363.
Gordon, M., M. A. Fiock, A. Yarinsky, and J. T. Duff (1957), *J. Bact.*, **74**:533.
Guth, L. (1968), *Physiol. Rev.*, **48**:645.
Guyton, A. C. and M. A. MacDonald (1947), *Arch. Neurol. Psychiat.*, **57**:578.
Hart, L. G., R. L. Dixon, J. P. Long, and B. Mackay (1965), *Toxicol. Appl. Pharmacol.*, **7**:84.
Heckly, R. J., G. J. Hildebrand, and C. Lamanna (1960), *J. Exper. Med.*, **111**:745.
Hildebrand, G. J., C. Lamanna, and R. J. Heckly (1961), *Proc. Soc. Exp. Biol. Med.*, **107**:284.
Hilton, S. M. and G. P. Lewis (1955), *J. Physiol.*, **128**:235.
Hubbard, J. I., S. F. Jones, and E. M. Landau (1968), *J. Physiol.*, **194**:355.
Jirmanova, I., M. Sobotkova, S. Thesleff, and J. Zelena (1964), *Physiol. Bohemoslov.*, **13**:467.
Kegeles, G. (1946), *J. Amer. Chem. Soc.*, **68**:1670.
Kitamura, M., S. Sakaguchi, and G. Sakaguchi (1967), *Biochem. Biophys. Res. Commun.*, **29**:892.
Kitamura, M., S. Sakaguchi, and G. Sakaguchi (1968), *Biochem. Biophys. Acta*, **168**:207.
Koenig, M. G., D. J. Drutz, A. I. Mushlin, W. Schaffner, and D. E. Rogers (1967), *Amer. J. Med.*, **42**:208.
Kupfer, C. (1958), *Proc. Soc. Exper. Biol. Med.*, **99**:474.
Lamanna, C. (1948), *Proc. Soc. Exp. Biol. Med.*, **69**:332.
Lamanna, C. (1959), *Science*, **130**:763.
Lamanna, C. and C. J. Carr (1967), *J. Clin. Pharmacol. Therap.*, **8**:286.
Lamanna, C. and H. N. Glassman (1947), *J. Bact.*, **54**:575.
Lamanna, C. and J. P. Lowenthal (1951), *J. Bact.*, **61**:751.
Lamanna, C., O. E. McElroy, and H. W. Eklund (1946), *Science*, **103**:613.
Lowenthal, J. P. and C. Lamanna (1951), *Amer. J. Hyg.*, **54**:432.
Lowenthal, J. P. and C. Lamanna (1953), *Amer. J. Hyg.*, **57**:46.

Marshall, R. and L. Y. Quinn (1967), *J. Bact.*, **94**:812.
Masland, R. L. and G. D. Gammon (1949), *J. Pharmacol. Exp. Therap.*, **97**:499.
Mikhailov, V. V. (1955), *Bull. Exp. Biol. Med.*, **41**:311.
Pak, Z. P. and T. I. Bulatova (1962), *Farmakol. i Toksikol.*, **25**:478.
Polley, E. H., J. A. Vick, H. P. Ciuchta, D. A. Fischetti, F. J. Macchitelli, and N. Montanarelli (1965), *Science*, **147**:1036.
Putnam, F. W., C. Lamanna, and D. G. Sharp (1947), *J. Biol. Chem.*, **165**:735.
Putnam, F. W., C. Lamanna, and D. G. Sharp (1948), *J. Biol. Chem.*, **176**:401.
Resepov, F. F. (1967), A study of *Clotridium botulinum* type F toxin and antitoxin, *in* "Botulism 1966" (M. Ingram and T. A. Roberts, eds.), Chapman and Hall Ltd., London, pp. 323–329.
Riesen, W. H. (1965), Dissociation of type A *Clostridium botulinum* toxin, *in* "Proceedings of a Conference on Botulinum Toxin" (C. C. Hassett, ed.), Edgewood Arsenal Special Publication 100-1, pp. 59–92.
Saelens, J. K., I. Rosenblum, D. M. Serrone, A. A. Stein, and F. Coulston (1965), Choline-C-14 and ACh-C-14 distribution and ultrastructure of brain particles obtained from mice treated with botulinum type A toxin, *in* "Proceedings of a Conference on Botulinum Toxin" (C. C. Hassett, ed.), Edgewood Arsenal Special Publication 100-1, pp. 255–260.
Schantz, E. J. and L. Spero (1957), *J. Amer. Chem. Soc.*, **79**:1623.
Schantz, E. J. D. Stefanye, and L. Spero (1960), *J. Biol. Chem.*, **235**:3489.
Simpson, L. L. (1968a), *J. Neurochem.*, **15** 359.
Simpson, L. L. (1968b), *Toxicon*, **5**:239.
Simpson, L. L. (1971), *Neuropharmacology*, in press.
Simpson, L. L., D. A. Boroff, and U. Fleck (1968), *Exp. Neurol.*, **22**:85.
Simpson, L. L., F. de Balbian Verster, and J. T. Tapp (1967), *Exp. Neurol.*, **19**:199.
Simpson, L. L. and H. Morimoto (1969), *J. Bact.*, **97**:571.
Simpson, L. L. and H. Morimoto (1970), *Neuropharmacology*, **9**:47.
Simpson, L. L. and J. T. Tapp (1967a), *Neuropharmacology*, **6**:485.
Simpson, L. L. and J. T. Tapp (1967b), *Neuropharmacology*, **6**:493.
Spero, L. *Arch.* (1958), *Biochem. Biophys.*, **73**:484.
Spero, L. and E. J. Schantz (1957), *J. Amer. Chem. Soc.*, **79**:1625.
Sterne, M. (1954), *Science*, **119**:440.
Stover, J. H., M. Fingerman, and R. H. Forester (1953), *Proc. Soc. Exp. Biol. Med.*, **84**:146.
Sumyk, G. B. and C. F. Yocum(1968), *J. Bact.*, **95**:1970.
Thesleff, S. (1960), *J. Physiol.*, **151**:598.
Torda, C. and H. G. Wolff (1947), *J. Pharmacol. Exp. Therap.*, **89**:320.
Tyler, H. R. (1963a), *Science*, **139**:847.
Tyler, H. R. (1963b), *Arch. Pathol.*, **76**:55.
Wagman, J. (1954), *Arch. Biochem. Biophys.*, **50**:104.
Wagman, J. (1963), *Arch. Biochem. Biophys.*, **100**:414.
Wagman, J. and J. B. Bateman (1951), *Arch. Biochem. Biophys.*, **31**:424.
Wagman, J. and J. B. Bateman (1953), *Arch. Biochem. Biophys.*, **45**:375.
Weil, L., T. S. Seibles, L. Spero, and E. J. Schantz (1957), *Arch. Biochem. Biophys.*, **68**:308.
Woolley, D. W. (1958), *Proc. Natl. Acad. Sci., USA*, **44**:197.
Wright, G. P. (1955), *Pharmacol. Rev.*, **7**:413.
Zacks, S. I. (1965), Fractionation and fluorescent labeling of botulinum toxin, *in* "Proceedings of a Conference on Botulinum Toxin" (C. C. Hassett, ed.), Edgewood Arsenal Special Publication 100-1, pp. 139–150.
Zacks, S. I., J. F. Metzger, C. W. Smith, and J. M. Blumberg (1962), *J. Neuropathol. Exp. Neurol.*, **21**:610.
Zacks, S. I., M. V. Rhoades, and M. F. Sheff (1968), *Exp. Mol. Pathol.*, **9**:77.

Chapter 15

Botulinum Toxin as a Tool for Research on the Nervous System

Daniel B. Drachman*

Department of Neurology
The Johns Hopkins University
School of Medicine and Hospital
Baltimore, Maryland, U.S.A.

I. INTRODUCTION

In recent years there has been a great increase of interest in the mechanisms by which nerves transfer information to other nerves and to nonneural end organs. New chemical, pharmacological and physiological techniques have been developed to study the variety of neurotransmitter agents and mechanisms which exist in nature. Nevertheless, our knowledge of the sequence of events from synthesis of a transmitter through its ultimate effect at the innervated end-organ is incomplete for any given agent or synapse.

One of the most accessible and extensively studied synapses is the neuromuscular junction (NMJ). It is now widely accepted that transmission across the NMJ is mediated by acetylcholine (ACh) (Eccles, 1964; Katz, 1966). Interest in botulinum toxin as a tool for research in the nervous system is based on its uniquely potent and specific ability to block cholinergic transmission. This property allows the investigator to carry out a "pharmacological dissection" of the NMJ and other cholinergic synapses. By way of background, a brief account of the events which normally occur at the NMJ is given below.

* Supported by NIH Grant HD 04817–01.

II. NEUROMUSCULAR TRANSMISSION

The synthesis of ACh takes place within the cholinergic nerves, presumably at their terminals (Hebb, 1963). Choline is first taken up by a transport system (Marchbanks, 1968), and then combines with the acetate group of acetyl-CoA, in the presence of the enzyme choline acetylase. There has been much debate as to whether ACh is formed in the soluble cytoplasm of the nerve endings or in the synaptic vesicles. This controversy hinges on conflicting experimental evidence on the subcellular localization of choline acetylase. Under certain conditions of ionic concentration and pH, the enzyme is bound to the fraction containing the vesicles, while under other (probably more physiological) circumstances it remains freely soluble in the cytoplasm (Michaelson, 1967). The problem has thus far been investigated in material derived from mammalian brain, and evidence is not yet available for the NMJ.

Storage of ACh takes place in the synaptic vesicles (Whittaker, 1968). These membranous structures are remarkably uniform in size, about 500 Å in diameter, and are found in large numbers at the nerve terminals (de Robertis and Bennett, 1954; Anderssen-Cedergren, 1959). It has been estimated that each vesicle contains approximately 10^3 to 10^4 molecules of ACh (Whittaker, 1965).

Release of ACh from the NMJ occurs both at rest and as a result of conducted impulse activity in the motor nerves. Katz and his coworkers first observed the effects of spontaneously released ACh as small, randomly occurring depolarizations in the region of the motor endplates of isolated muscle fibers (Fatt and Katz, 1950, 1952; Del Castillo and Katz, 1954). In view of the uniformity of size of these miniature endplate potentials (mepps), they postulated that the release of fixed, or quantal, amounts of ACh was responsible for the electrical events. Their findings, which have been amply confirmed, correlate nicely with the ultrastructural evidence, suggesting that each synaptic vesicle contains a fixed, or quantum amount of ACh.

When an electrical impulse is conducted to a motor nerve terminal much larger quantities of ACh are released, giving rise to a greater amplitude endplate potential (epp). The effect of the conducted impulse is to increase the *probability* of release of ACh quanta, but the release mechanism for mepps and epps is thought to be otherwise identical (Del Castillo and Katz, 1954).

The process of ACh release is not yet well understood. It has been suggested, on the basis of indirect evidence, that the ACh-containing vesicles discharge their contents into the synaptic cleft (de Robertis and Bennett, 1954; Del Castillo and Katz, 1955; Hubbard and Kwanbunbumpen, 1968). Calcium ions are necessary for all, or nearly all, ACh release, (Elmqvist and Feldman, 1965; Hubbard *et al.*, 1968) while sodium opposes the calcium effect (Gage and Quastel, 1965). These ionic effects are thought to influence the ACh release mechanism directly, without interfering with conduction of impulses in the nerve terminals (Katz and Miledi, 1965).

The released ACh crosses the synaptic cleft to combine with the specialized receptor site of the postjunctional membrane (PJM). The effect of this interaction is to increase the permeability of the PJM to all ions, notably Na^+ and K^+ (Takeuchi and Takeuchi, 1960). If the amount of ACh released is small, the resulting depolarization is correspondingly small in magnitude and remains confined to the endplate region as a miniature endplate potential. However, if a larger amount of ACh is released, it gives rise to an electrical impulse which is propagated along the muscle membrane, and triggers a sequence of events leading to a contractile response (*see* Nastuk, 1966, for review).

Acetylcholinesterase, which is locally concentrated at the NMJ, inactivates the released ACh extremely rapidly. The speed of this reaction serves to limit the action of ACh spatially and temporally, and to enable the NMJ to react quickly to the next release of ACh (Koelle, 1963).

III. BOTULINUM TOXIN AS A PHARMACOLOGICAL TOOL

Most experiments which have utilized botulinum toxin as a pharmacological tool, have depended heavily upon its accepted action as a presynaptic blocking agent for cholinergic junctions. In order to evaluate such work critically, it will be helpful to consider the attributes of an idealized cholinergic blocking agent, and compare them with the available information about the properties of botulinum toxin.

A. Characteristics of an "Ideal Blocking Agent"

A number of the desirable characteristics of a hypothetical "ideal blocking agent" are outlined below.

Mode of Action
    Blocks cholinergic transmission
    Blocks both spontaneous and impulse-dependent transmission
    Pharmacological locus of action known
    Precise mechanism of action known
Specificity
    Does not directly impair function or structure of nerve or muscle, even after prolonged use
    Blocks *only* cholinergic transmission; no other transmission affected
Generality of Action
    Blocks *all* cholinergic nerve endings

Convenience of Use
    Can be used safely in the laboratory
    May be used to produce local or systemic effect

B. Comparison of Botulinum Toxin with Ideal Model

In general, botulinum toxin conforms remarkably closely to this model, although there are several areas in which more information is still needed.

1. Mode of Action

Present evidence indicates that botulinum toxin acts presynaptically as an extremely powerful blocker of cholinergic transmission. The fact that it eliminates both mepps and epps was first established by Brooks (1956) and has subsequently been confirmed (Thesleff, 1960). This effect is apparently not a consequence of interference with impulse conduction in the motor nerve (Brooks, 1954, 1956), or of inhibition of synthesis or storage of ACh (Burgen *et al.*, 1949; Stevenson and Girvin, 1953; Thesleff, 1960; Simpson, 1968). Evidently, the toxin directly affects the mechanism by which quanta of ACh are liberated from the nerve endings. The attractive possibility that botulinum might interfere with the calcium uptake which is coupled to quantal ACh release seems unlikely in the light of evidence discussed in Chap. 14, and its precise mechanism of action remains a challenging problem.

2. Specificity

Neither the nerve nor the muscle suffers impairment of electrical excitability or conductivity in the presence of complete neuromuscular block produced by botulinum toxin (Bishop and Bronfenbrenner, 1936; Brooks, 1954). The effects of long-term treatment have been only partially worked out, but the available evidence indicates that the only changes in nerve or muscle are secondary "atrophic" consequences of the loss of cholinergic transmission (see below). The microscopic appearance of chronically treated nerves is normal (Jirmanova *et al.*, 1964; Drachman, 1967; Duchen and Strich, 1968), although sprouting of additional fine fibers occurs at the terminals. An electron micrographic study revealed no changes in the fine structure of mammalian or amphibian motor endplates after 3–4 weeks of botulinum treatment (Thesleff, 1960). Guth (1969) has suggested that the electron microscopy should be repeated with the more refined techniques now available, but there is no reason to suspect that any abnormalities would be found.

It is somewhat more difficult to prove that skeletal muscle is not directly damaged by prolonged exposure to botulinum toxin, since it invariably undergoes atrophy under these conditions. However, two lines of evidence support this point. First, the changes in botulinum-treated skeletal muscle are consistent in kind and in degree with the effects of denervation alone (*see* Sec. IV). Second, cardiac muscle remains functionally and morphologically intact even after prolonged treatment with botulinum toxin in the chick embryo (Drachman, 1964). Like skeletal muscle, cardiac muscle is striated, but it differs in not being dependent on its innervation for maintenance of its integrity.

Until recently, there has been no hint of any neurotoxic action of botulinum toxin other than blockade of ACh release. However, Whaler and his co-workers (Rand and Whaler, 1965; Westwood and Whaler, 1968) have recently asserted that botulinum toxin may affect adrenergic transmission either directly or indirectly. This important question is by no means settled, and is discussed in more detail in Sec. V. The possibility that the toxin might block a hypothetical "trophic" substance other than ACh has also been entertained, but lacks any experimental support (*see* Sec. IV). On balance, the evidence still favors the concept that botulinum toxin is extremely selective in its action on cholinergic transmission.

3. Generality of Action

Wherever it has been tried, botulinum toxin has been uniformly effective in blocking all *peripheral* cholinergic synapses including the NMJ, sympathetic ganglia and parasympathetic nerve endings. The situation in the central nervous system, however, has remained unclear. Which, if any, of the central cholinergic synapses can be blocked by systemically or locally administered toxin has not yet been established (*see* Chap. 14, Sec. V).

4. Convenience of Use

From the point of view of convenience as an experimental tool, botulinum toxin requires some special precautions, but has been used safely and successfully by many workers throughout the world. The keystone of protection for laboratory personnel is immunization with the available toxoid preparation (Cardella, 1964). A series of recommendations for laboratory precautions are listed in the Appendix to this chapter.

Because of the rapidity and firmness with which botulinum toxin is bound to muscle, it can be injected locally into a given muscle group where it continues to act for a prolonged period. The dosage must be carefully controlled in order to minimize systemic effects. We have found it desirable to give repeated intramuscular injections at intervals of several days in order to achieve the maximum local effect while keeping the systemic spread to a minimum. Kupfer (1958) injected antitoxin 15 min after the local application of botulinum toxin in order to prevent generalized poisoning. The doses used by various workers have ranged from 0.66×10^{-9} g to 15×10^{-6} g. The purity of the toxin preparation, experimental animal, and site of injection will govern the dosage requirements.

IV. THE "TROPHIC" EFFECTS OF NERVES

A. Scope and Definition of the Problem

In addition to its function as a rapid carrier of impulse-coded information, the nervous system has the remarkable capacity to exert long-term control over the properties of many innervated structures. For example, it makes possible regeneration of the amputated limbs of amphibia; it is necessary for maintaining the structural integrity of certain taste buds in mammals, and of "barbels" in fish; it maintains and regulates the structural and functional characteristics of skeletal muscle (Guth, 1969). Such long-term influences of the nervous system are known as "trophic" effects. Paradoxically, they are most easily recognized by their absence. Denervation of a structure which is dependent on its nerve supply results in "atrophic" changes in its anatomical, physiological, or biochemical properties. We are led to conclude that the intact nerve supply is normally able to prevent these changes by exerting some "trophic influence."

A great many examples of trophic effects have been identified and studied, but the approach of cataloging such evidence has not led to a resolution of the crucial problem of *how* the nerves exert their trophic influences. It should be emphasized that each system in which trophic interactions occur must be considered separately, and different mechanisms undoubtedly exist in the vastly different situations loosely considered together. It is in the field of trophic interactions that botulinum toxin has made its greatest contribution as a research tool.

B. Motor Nerves and Skeletal Muscle

The most widely studied example of trophic interaction occurs in the case of skeletal muscle (Guth, 1968). It is an important problem in its own right, since muscle atrophy occurs commonly in man. However, it also serves as a paradigm of trophic interactions in general.

The immediate effect of denervation of skeletal muscle is motor paralysis. Over the longer term, denervation leads to a series of alterations in the morphology, physiology, and metabolism of muscle, some examples of which are listed in Table I. It is clear that the motor nerves alone supply the trophic influence which is capable of preventing these changes, while the sensory and sympathetic innervations play no significant role (Tower,

Table I.
Examples of Atrophic Effects of Denervation of Muscle

Effect	Observation
Morphological	Fiber atrophy with preservation of striations
	Relative increase in number of nuclei, with rounding, alignment, clumping, pyknosis, and central migration
	Loss of cholinesterase at end plates
	Degeneration of fibers, fatty and fibrous replacement of muscle (late changes)
Physiological	Fibrillations
	Spread of ACh-sensitive zone
	Decreased resting membrane potential
	Slowing of twitch contraction and relaxation
	Acceptance of innervation by foreign nerve
Metabolic	Glycogen decreased
	Phosphorylase activity decreased
	Effects of insulin decreased
	Proteolytic activity increased

1931a,b, 1935). The question of *how* the nerves exert this effect is one of paramount importance.

C. Possible Trophic Mechanisms

In order to approach the problem constructively, it will be useful to list the theoretically possible mechanisms of neuromuscular trophic influence.

Cholinergic Mechanisms

a) Nerve impulses → endplate potentials (epp's) → muscle activity (this sequence may also be termed "usage")

b) Spontaneous quantal release of ACh → miniature endplate potentials (mepp's)

Release of Unknown "Trophic Substances"

Nerve–Muscle Contact

The first possibility, i.e., that active cholinergic synaptic transmission may be involved in the trophic interaction, lends itself to experimental analysis, because ACh is a known substance that can be manipulated in many ways.

The most productive experimental approach to this question has been called the "elimination strategy," and depends to an important extent on the use of botulinum toxin. The logic of this strategy may be outlined as follows:

Select an "endpoint" (i.e., a change that is known to result from denervation of muscle).

Eliminate all cholinergic transmission for an appropriate length of time, without otherwise disturbing the neuromuscular connections. Observe the result of the above procedures and compare it with that of denervation. If the results are identical, then ACh must be essential for transmission of the nerve's trophic influence.

To determine the role of "usage" the muscle should be put to complete rest, while its motor innervation remains otherwise intact. A variety of experimental techniques have been used to produce disuse either by eliminating nerve impulses (Tower 1937; Denny-Brown and Brenner, 1944; Gutmann and Zak, 1961) or by relieving the muscle of its work load (Eccles, 1943; Solandt et al., 1943). Unfortunately, none of these methods create the conditions of complete disuse.

The contribution of spontaneous ACh release can be deduced by comparing the effect of disuse with that of complete ACh blockade; the greater effect of complete blockade is presumably due to its interference with spontaneous release of ACh as well as impulse-directed release. This indirect approach is necessary, because it is not possible to block spontaneous release without affecting impulse transmission.

In principle, the logic of the elimination strategy is simple, but it poses many difficult and interesting problems which remain to be worked out.

Thesleff was the first to utilize botulinum toxin to study this problem. He and his colleagues have demonstrated that prolonged local application of botulinum toxin to skeletal muscle resulted in several physiological effects ("endpoints") like those of prolonged denervation. Within one week, the muscle developed fibrillation potentials (Josefsson and Thesleff, 1961), and spread of the chemosensitive zone (Thesleff, 1960). Both of these findings are characteristic denervation effects. More recent work has shown that botulinum-treated muscle is capable of accepting innervation by an implanted foreign nerve, which is otherwise possible only after denervation (Fex et al., 1966).

The tentative conclusion was that ACh itself may be essential for the trophic influence of the nerve in these situations. Furthermore, because experimental "disuse" does not result in fibrillations, and produces only slight spread of the ACh-receptive zone, it seemed likely that the spontaneous quantal release of ACh might be sufficient to maintain the nerves' trophic effects with regard to these endpoints. Although the success of botulinum toxin in reproducing these physiological effects of denervation was undeniable, the interpretation of the experiments was open to question on several grounds:

a. Does botulinum toxin have any other relevant action in addition to its known blockade of ACh release?

1. Does it cause physical destruction of motor nerves?

2. Does it block some other trophic substance (unknown) *in addition to* ACh?

b. Is botulinum toxin capable of producing atrophy of skeletal muscle in the classical morphogical sense?

The first part of this question has been answered by studies of the histology and ultrastructure of nerves in chronically poisoned animals, as indicated in Sec. III. In order to answer the remaining questions, I have utilized an unusual experimental model, the chick embryo. The advantage of this model is that it permits the use of very large amounts of neuromuscular blocking agents for prolonged periods of time. Because the chick embryo does not require muscular movements for respiration, it readily survives the paralysis produced by systemically administered neuromuscular blocking agents. Injections or infusions of pharmacological agents can be carried out over a broad range of time by a simple method devised specifically for these studies (Drachman and Coulombre, 1962a).

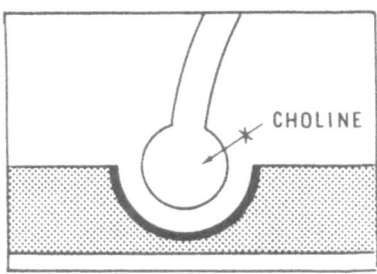

HEMICHOLINIUM

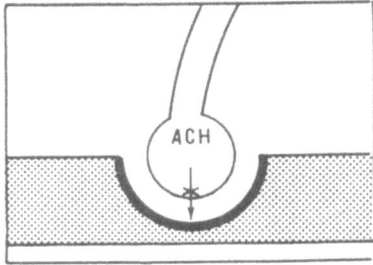

BOTULINUM TOXIN

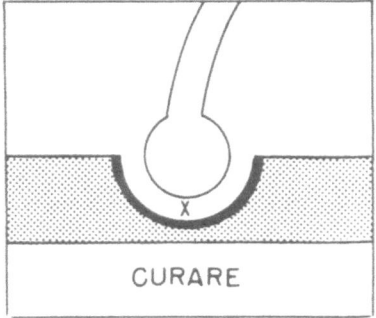

CURARE

Fig. 1. Chief actions of neuromuscular blocking agents. Diagrams represent neuromuscular junctions. X indicates predominant site of blocking action of each agent. Hemicholinium blocks uptake of choline by nerve ending, and interferes with synthesis of ACh. Botulinum toxin blocks release of ACh at nerve terminal. Curare blocks access of ACh to endplate receptor. (From Drachman, 1968.)

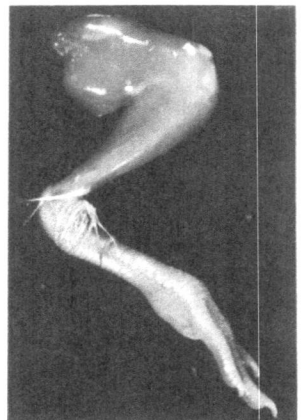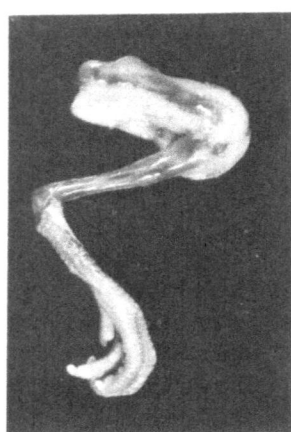

Fig. 2. Botulinum toxin. Limbs of 19-day-old chick embryos, with skin removed. Left: Normal control, with plentiful muscle. Right: Embryo treated with botulinum toxin from 7th to 19th days. Note severe loss of muscle, and replacement by fat (white-appearing material). (From Drachman, 1964, 1968.)

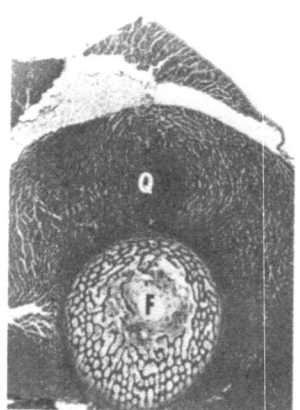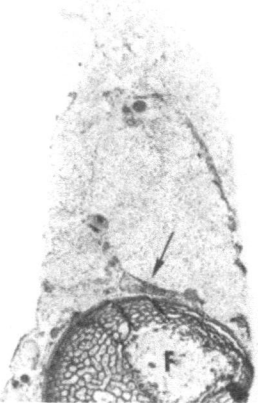

Fig. 3. Botulinum toxin. Transverse sections through anterior thighs of chick embryos at 19 days. Left: Normal control chick embryo. Right: Embryo treated with botulinum toxin. At this low magnification, the dark area represents muscle; the light reticulated area is fat. Note the severe loss of muscle and massive replacement by fat in the botulinum-treated specimen. A small amount of atrophic muscle is indicated by the arrow. Hematoxylin and eosin. ×18 approx. F: Femur; Q: quadriceps muscle. (From Drachman, 1968.)

In a series of experiments, several pharmacological agents that act at different sites in the process of neuromuscular transmission were utilized, and their effects on the microscopic appearance of skeletal muscle were then evaluated (Drachman, 1964, 1967, 1968). In addition to botulinum toxin, the agents used included curare and hemicholinium-3 (HC-3). Curare exerts mainly a post-synaptic action by blocking access of ACh to the receptor at the motor endplate. HC-3 has been shown to prevent the synthesis of ACh at intact nerve endings by blocking the uptake of choline. In high concentrations, it also exerts a curare-like effect. These actions are represented diagramatically in Fig. 1. Neuromuscular blockade brought about by each of these agents produced atrophy, degeneration, and fatty replacement of skeletal muscle, effects identical to those which occur after surgical denervation (Figs. 2 and 3). The intramuscular nerves were not damaged directly. Cardiac muscle functioned normally, and was intact histologically, suggesting that botulinum toxin does not exert a direct toxic effect on striated muscle. Furthermore, disuse did not appear to account for the effects, because tenotomy (a fair approximation of disuse) produced only minimal muscle atrophy, not comparable to the results of cholinergic blockade.

It is most reasonable to conclude that impairment of ACh transmission, the common denominator of action of botulinum toxin, curare, and HC-3, is responsible for the denervation atrophy they produce. By the same token, it would be implausible to assume that these strikingly different pharmacological agents all coincidentally possessed the property of blocking some other "trophic substance" in addition to their known effects on cholinergic transmission. The conclusion from this "multiple pharmacological approach" is simply that cholinergic transmission is essential for maintenance of the nerve's trophic influence on the structure of muscle.

D. Red and White Muscle

In spite of these findings, it still seemed difficult to imagine how ACh might play a role in the regulation of the specialized properties of "red" and "white" muscle. The fact that mammalian skeletal muscles are composed of two main types of fibers which differ in certain physiological and metabolic properties has received a great deal of attention recently. The type of fiber which predominates in "red" muscles, such as the soleus, is marked by slow twitch contraction speed, and by high activity of the enzymes of oxidative and lipid metabolism. By contrast, the fiber type which predominates in "white" muscles, such as the extensor digitorum longus, has a faster twitch speed, and greater activity of the enzymes of anaerobic glycolysis (Denny-Brown, 1921; Romanul, 1964; Dawson and Romanul, 1964; for review, see Guth, 1968). It has recently been established that the specific motor innervation plays an important role in determining these differences in muscle properties. After sectioning and cross-uniting nerves to red and white muscles, both the speeds of contraction (Buller *et al.*, 1960) and the histochemical characteristics (Romanul and Van Der Meulen, 1966) of the muscles become reversed. Denervation results in slowing of both fast and slow muscles (Eccles *et al.*, 1962; Lewis, 1962), and disappearance of the differences in their enzymatic activities (Romanul and Hogan, 1964; Romanul *et al.*, 1964).

In order to explore the question of whether a single transmitter, acetylcholine, could possibly mediate the opposite trophic effects of the nerves to the two types of muscle, we once again made use of the properties of botulinum toxin. Injections of the toxin were made repeatedly into the leg muscles of the rat in order to maintain complete neuromuscular blockade for two to three weeks. At the end of that time the physiological and histochemical properties of the muscles were examined (Drachman and Houk, 1969; Drachman and Romanul, in press). We found that the speed of contraction of the botulinum-treated muscles slowed, as it does after denervation. Similarly, the histochemical changes in red and white muscle were identical to those of denervation. These observations indicate that cholinergic transmission is necessary for the motor nerve to exert its trophic influences on the specialized physiological and enzymatic properties of red and white muscle. On the basis of this evidence alone, one cannot draw the further conclusion that ACh is the *sole* factor responsible for the differentiation of red and white muscle. However, there is a growing body of evidence to suggest that usage (also mediated by ACh) may be an additional factor in determining the speed of twitch contractions (*see* Drachman and Houk, 1969; Salmons and Vrbova, 1969).

E. Other Trophic Neuromuscular Relationships

1. The Role of Motor Innervation in the Trophic Regulation of Muscle Cholinesterase

This is a complex problem which has not yet been fully resolved. Muscle cholinesterase is only partially under the control of the nerve supply, and is partially independent of it. After denervation, cholinesterase activity decreases, but it continues to be maintained by the muscle at a lower level (Stewart and Martin, 1966; Rose and Glow, 1967; Guth 1969a).

In order to determine the role of cholinergic transmission in the regulation of cholinesterase, several investigators have made use of botulinum toxin. It should be pointed out that botulinum toxin has no direct effect on cholinesterase (Sumyk and Yocum, 1968; Simpson and Morimoto, 1969). Stromblad (1960) measured the cholinesterase activity of whole muscle after prolonged botulinum treatment and denervation. In both situations, the cholinesterase activity was markedly reduced, although the effect of denervation was more pronounced than that of botulinum toxin. However, the muscle weight was so severely reduced in the botulinum-treated rats that the cholinesterase *concentration* per gram of muscle appeared essentially normal. Sonneson and Thesleff (1968) studied the recovery of cholinesterase activity (presumably due to resynthesis of the enzyme) after the use of the irreversible cholinesterase inhibitor (DFP). They found that cholinesterase activity returned somewhat more slowly in denervated and botulinum-treated muscles than in control muscles.

Guth and his associates (1964) have introduced a method for separately measuring endplate and nonjunctional, or "background" muscle cholinesterase, which may help to clarify the problem of trophic control of the enzyme activity. For example, they found that disuse decreases only the background cholinesterase, while denervation produces a loss of both endplate and background cholinesterase (Guth, 1969b). This method has not yet been applied to experiments using botulinum toxin.

2. Effects of Botulinum Toxin on Motor Nerves

In previous sections evidence has been cited which indicates that botulinum toxin does not directly injure nerves or nerve endings. However, certain changes have been noted which may represent *secondary* responses on the part of the motor nerves. These observations raise questions about possible trophic influences in reverse, which the periphery may exert upon the nerve supply.

In 1968 Duchen and Strich reported that motor nerve endings develop a remarkable pattern of outgrowth after botulinum toxin treatment. Experimentally, they injected botulinum toxin locally into mouse leg muscle and observed the histological appearance of the nerve endings for periods up to several months. Sprouting began at about the same time as muscle atrophy, earlier in the red soleus muscle than in the predominantly white gastrocnemius. The new growth originated from the terminal arborizations of the motor nerve fibers at the endplates, spreading out to form complex branched arrangements. The new nerve sprouts were apparently unable to establish functional connections for many weeks, as judged by the continuing paralysis and atrophy. However, recovery eventually took place, beginning sooner and progressing more rapidly in the soleus than in the gastrocnemius muscle.

This work is of interest because it represents a new approach to the very important problem of reinnervation of denervated muscle. It has long been known that when a motor nerve is cut, the nearby motor nerves undergo sprouting of axons, in apparent attempt to re-supply the denervated muscle (Edds, 1953). The stimulus for this new growth has been sought, thus far in vain. The botulinum toxin experiments show that nerve damage is not necessary for the process to occur. The fact that muscle atrophy begins at about the same time as sprouting suggests that some feature of the atrophy process evokes the response of new nerve growth. Whatever this factor may be, it is tempting to speculate that impairment of cholinergic transmission serves as the trigger, according to the following scheme:

botulinum toxin blocks ACh → muscle atrophy → nerve sprouting

This system would seem to be a particularly favorable one for the study of the nature of nerve regeneration and sprouting.

Watson (1969) investigated the nucleic acids of motor neurons after intramuscular botulinum injection or surgical section of the axon. He found an increase in the nucleic acid content of the nucleoli and cell bodies of motor neurons, similar in time course for both treatments. He suggested that the nucleic acid change was related to the nerve sprouting as described above.

Drachman (1967) studied the spinal cords of chick embryos treated for various periods of time with botulinum toxin (*see* above). In one group treated for seven days, the anterior horn cells were normal in number and appearance although muscular atrophy was present. This observation, confirmed the point that muscular atrophy can occur while the motor neurons are structurally intact. However, in another group of chick embryos treated for 12 days, there was a definite reduction in the number of motor neurons. Many of the remaining cells showed the pathological picture of central chromatolysis, with cellular rounding, peripheral location of nuclei, and prominence of nucleoli. This finding is consistent with the phenomenon of retrograde degeneration of motor neurons which occurs in the embryo or young neonate after loss of the "peripheral field of innervation." The muscle atrophy in this group was so profound as to lead in turn to secondary degeneration of the motor neurons. Similar observations have been made in the chick embryo after limb-bud amputation (Bueker, 1943) and in the new born mouse as a result of removal of individual muscles (Romanes, 1946).

F. Conclusions

In the work summarized above, botulinum toxin served as an important tool in the study of certain "trophic" neuromuscular relationships. Interpretation of the experimental findings depends critically on the specificity of action of botulinum toxin. If, as seems likely, botulinum toxin blocks ACh completely, but has no other significant action at the neuromuscular junction, then one may conclude that ACh is essential for transmission of the nerve's trophic influences to muscle. However, it remains to be determined whether ACh alone can replace all the trophic functions of motor nerves, or whether other cofactors, as yet unidentified, may be involved as well. Because there is no critical evidence against ACh as the trophic transmitter in these situations, and because there is no sound evidence favoring the transmission of some other trophic substance, the simplest and most economical explanation of the facts is that ACh itself may serve as the transmitter of trophic influences from nerve to muscle. As yet, the actual mechanism of acetylcholine's actions as a trophic transmitter has not been established. However, it seems unlikely that it serves as an essential nutrient factor for muscle (*see* Drachman, 1968, for discussion), or that it triggers the release of some other trophic cofactor. I prefer the alternative that trophic influences are integrally related to the known physiological actions of ACh at the end plate.

V. BOTULINUM TOXIN AND THE AUTONOMIC NERVOUS SYSTEM

A. Parasympathetic Nervous System

The early work of Dickson and Shevky (1923) first established that the actions of the parasympathetic nervous system could be blocked by botulinum toxin. In rabbits and cats treated with toxin they noted a progressive block of the vagus nerve, manifested by a decrease in its effect on cardiac slowing and intestinal motility. There was a block of the effect of stimulation of the chorda tympani on the flow of saliva, a failure of bladder contraction and erection of the penis on stimulation of the pelvic nervi erigentes, and abolition of pupillary contraction on stimulation of the oculomotor nerve. Ambache (1949, 1951) analyzed the parasympathetic blockade further by the ingenious use of local injections into the short ciliary nerve–pupilloconstrictor system of the cat. He was able to produce selective blockade of either the pre- or the postganglionic fibers, and concluded that both sets of fibers were cholinergic. He also established the important point that the sudomotor nerves are paralyzed by botulinum toxin. These nerves are cholinergic, although they belong anatomically to the sympathetic nervous system.

Hilton and Lewis (1955) utilized the cholinergic blocking properties of botulinum toxin to study the neural control of vasodilatation in the submandibular salivary gland. They found that stimulation of the chorda tympani no longer produced vasodilatation or salivary secretion after toxin treatment. They concluded that a single set of cholinergic fibers in the chorda tympani is normally responsible for both actions. It had previously been supposed that the vasodilator fibers were noncholinergic, on the basis of the observation that atropine at certain dose levels selectively blocked salivary secretion without affecting vasodilatation. Hilton and Lewis also made the interesting observation that the preganglionic fibers were blocked several hours earlier than the postganglionic ones.

Emmelin (1961) studied the effects of prolonged botulinum toxin treatment on the chemosensitivity of the salivary gland. He devised an ingenious technique for administering the toxin via the salivary duct. Finding that the normal salivary flow would wash the injected agent out before it had a chance to become fixed to the gland, he administered a parasympatholytic agent systemically at the same time as he introduced the intraductal botulinum toxin. This blocked the secretion of saliva long enough to allow the toxin to take effect. Within one week, the sensitivity of the gland to sympathomimetic and parasympathomimetic drugs increased, as measured by the volume of saliva secreted. The sensitivity reached its maximum at three weeks, and declined gradually thereafter. This result is consistent with the known effect of section of the chorda tympani, a purely cholinergic parasympathetic nerve. It is curious that supersensitivity develops to both cholinergic and adrenergic drugs after abolition of control by a cholinergic nerve. In a sense, this is another example of "trophic" control mediated by the transmitter, ACh.

In order to determine whether the motor nerves to the bladder are cholinergic, Carpenter (1967) measured the mechanical responses and liberation of ACh from rat bladder after acute botulinal poisoning. He found a marked, but not quite complete, loss of contraction, and concomitant drop in ACh release on stimulation of the motor nerves. Carpenter noted that parasympathetically innervated viscera were more vulnerable to type D toxin than to type A.

Ambache and Lessin (1955) have made use of botulinum toxin to distinguish the site of action of a variety of pharmacological agents. Using the isolated guinea pig or rabbit ileum, they compared the effects of various pharmacological agents on botulinum-treated and control preparations. Drugs like nicotine which normally act via the nerves have no effect after the nerves are blocked by botulinum toxin. On the other hand, the effects of drugs which act directly on smooth muscle, such as muscarine, are unaltered by the botulinum treatment.

B. Sympathetic Nervous System

It has been widely accepted for the past 20 years that the sympathetic nervous system is virtually immune to the effects of botulinum toxin. Ambache (1949, 1951) reported that sympathetic nerve stimulation still elicited a maximal pupillary response in cats which had received 200–300 times the dose of botulinum toxin necessary to paralyze the cholinergic pupilloconstrictor fibers. Similarly, the retractor of the nictitating membrane remained responsive to sympathetic stimulation after very large doses of toxin, although the magnitude of the response was somewhat reduced. Ambache emphasized the resistance of the sympathetic fibers to botulinum toxin although he was unable to exclude the possibility that "a fraction of the reduction . . . might be due to a lesion of adrenergic fibers." Kupfer (1958) studied the long-term effects of botulinum toxin on rabbits and found that the cholinergic blockade persisted for as long as six months, but the response to sympathetic stimulation was normal. In the salivary gland preparation of Hilton and Lewis (1955) sympathetic stimulation "gave its typical secretory and complex vascular response," although somewhat reduced, at a time when cholinergic blockade was complete. Most recently, Vincenzi (1967) used the rabbit's sinoatrial node to reexamine the problem. He found once again that the cholinergic response was completely blocked, while there was sparing of the adrenergic fibers.

In general, these observations support the classical concept of susceptibility of cholinergic fibers and insensitivity of adrenergic fibers to the effects of botulinum toxin. Against this background it was particularly startling when Rand and Whaler (1965) declared that sympathetic transmission is indeed impaired by botulinum toxin, and supported their contention by several different lines of evidence.

In their original study, Rand and Whaler tested the responses to sympathetic stimulation of the guinea pig vas deferens, the rabbit ileum, and the cat piloerector muscle, after treatment with botulinum toxin. In each case they used large doses of toxin (10,000 to 30,000 LD_{50}/ml in $vitro$, and 200,000 LD_{50}/hair tuft in the cat's tail), and waited for many hours for the effects to develop. They were candid in reporting a number of inconsistent results, in which the responses of control preparations faded or the responses of botulinum-treated preparations remained normal. Despite these inconsistencies, most of their preparations showed markedly reduced responsiveness to sympathetic stimulation after botulinum toxin treatment. Interpretation of these findings is very difficult, but it is particularly hazardous in the case of the guinea pig vas deferens. In this preparation, the ganglion cells are spread out along the nerve, mainly within a few millimeters of the muscle tissue, making it difficult to be certain whether a stimulus is exciting a pre- or postganglionic fiber. Westwood and Whaler (1968) attempted to circumvent this problem by using a series of pharmacological agents and different stimulus parameters, but their methods were of questionable specificity, and their results once again variable.

All of these experiments are open to the criticism that an $indirect$ effect of transmitter release (i.e., the contractile response) was measured, but the same criticism applies to virtually all work in which botulinum toxin has been used. In spite of the technical difficulties, the major experimental observations that some effects of sympathetic nerve stimulation are reduced by large amounts of botulinum toxin may be tentatively accepted. However, we would reserve judgement as to whether norepinephrine release is actually affected, pending a detailed analysis of the events at the sympathetic nerve ending.

If botulinum toxin should, in fact, be proven to block the release of norepinephrine at adrenergic nerve endings, it would have certain fundamental implications for our understanding of neurotransmission. First, it may provide support for the "Burn–Rand" hypothesis (1965) of adrenergic transmission. According to this concept, the nerve impulse releases a minute amount of ACh which in turn triggers the liberation of norepinephrine. Botulinum toxin may conceivably impair adrenergic transmission by blocking the intermediate cholinergic step. Alternatively, it may indicate that the action of botulinum toxin is less specific than has been supposed. Botulinum toxin may block the release of transmitters other than ACh via interference with some common mechanism. Needless to say, this would undermine the interpretation of experiments based on the specificity of action of botulinum toxin. In this regard, we are on much safer ground in using a "multiple pharmacological approach" as described in Sec. IV B.

VI. BOTULINUM TOXIN AS A MARKER OF CHOLINERGIC SYNAPSES: A POSSIBLE FUTURE USE

It would be extremely useful to have a reliable method for the anatomical identification of cholinergic synapses. In the past, the histochemical demonstration of AChE has been used as one indicator of cholinergic transmission. However, this enzyme occurs rather widely in nature and cannot be regarded as specific. An ideal marker substance would attach exclusively to cholinergic synapses wherever they occur. The bond should be lasting, and the substance easily identified. Because of its remarkable affinity for the neuromuscular junction, botulinum toxin might be thought of as a possible marker substance. Zacks and his associates (1962, 1968) have been able to attach ferritin or fluorescent labels to the toxin molecule, and have studied its localization by ultraviolet light and electron microscopy. They have found the tagged botulinum toxin in the synaptic clefts of skeletal muscle, but have noted no binding to brain or other organs. This finding would be consistent with the reported lack of central action of the toxin, and would, of course, limit its usefulness as a marker. It is possible that the brief times of exposure which Zacks used (up to 30 min) were insufficient to allow the toxin to attach to less avid sites. Nevertheless, tagged botulinum toxin may still prove useful for studies of the peripheral nervous system.

VII. THE ROLE OF MOVEMENT IN THE DEVELOPMENT OF JOINTS: A MODEL SYSTEM

Most of the experimental applications of botulinum toxin make use of its property as a blocker of cholinergic transmission. The muscular paralysis which this inevitably causes is at best an incidental side effect, and more often presents a difficult problem in maintaining respiration of the experimental animal. However, the paralyzing effect has proven particularly useful for our recent studies of embryonic joint development.

The problem was one which had been studied in the 1920s: What role does movement play in the development of limbs and joints? The early experiments utilizing culture or grafting techniques emphasized that recognizable bones and joints could develop in embryonic limb fragments isolated from extrinisic influences (Murray, 1926; Fell and Canti, 1934; Hamburger and Waugh, 1940). However, morphogenesis of the isolated joints was neither complete nor perfect, and gross distortions of the skeletal structures often occurred under these conditions. It seemed reasonable that some of these abnormalities might be due to immobility of the limbs; the joint is a structure so specifically adapted for motion that it might logically require movement to perfect its development. Transplantation and culture techniques are too crude to resolve this point, since they inevitably alter the environment of the developing limb. In order to sort out the contribution of movement to joint development, it is necessary to use an experimental method capable of paralyzing the embryo's muscular contractions without producing other conditions adverse to growth and development. We therefore utilized the technique by which neuromuscular blocking agents, such as botulinum toxin, could be injected or infused directly into the extra-embryonic blood vessels of the developing chick embryo (Drachman and Coulombre, 1962a). By this means, we were able to produce muscular paralysis for periods up to 12 days while allowing the embryos to develop in the eggs under otherwise normal circumstances.

The results of muscular paralysis fell into certain consistent patterns, depending on the experimental treatments:

A. Soft-Tissue Ankylosis

In this group, the embryos were paralyzed for a relatively brief period of time with one of the reversible blocking agents, such as curare, and were then allowed to develop further until the normal hatching time (21 days).

These specimens showed soft-tissue ankylosis of multiple joints, with all the peri- and intra-articular structures serving to maintain the fixed postures. The postures of the deformed limbs simply reflected the normal embryonic positions of the chick. The severity of joint ankylosis was roughly proportional to the duration of the previous paralysis (Drachman and Coulombre, 1962b).

B. Abnormalities of Joint Cavities and Other Articular Structures

In this group, treatment was begun at a stage before joint cavity formation, and the embryos were *kept paralyzed* until they were sacrificed at later stages of development. Articular cavities failed to develop in the paralyzed joints, although the preparatory changes in the cellular architecture proceeded otherwise normally. "Fusion" occurred across the presumptive joints, first by loose fibrovascular tissue and later by compact fibrous connective tissue, cartilage, or bone. The shape of the articular surfaces lacked fine sculptural details. Certain accessory articular structures which are important to the mechanical function of the joints failed to develop. These included some sesamoids and all adventitious cartilages and intra-articular ligaments. Certain skeletal prominences which normally give attachment to muscles were absent or distorted in the paralyzed embryos (Drachman and Sokoloff, 1966; Drachman and Murray, in press).

The principles derived from these studies appear to have wide application. The soft tissue ankylosis produced by transient immobilization faithfully reproduces certain deformities which occur in man. The pathogenetic mechanism suggested by this model is now generally thought to apply to clubfoot or arthrogryposis multiplex congenita, in the human. The important, but restricted, role of movement in the primary development of joints is now thoroughly established.

ACKNOWLEDGMENTS

The author is indebted to Dr. E. Schantz, Fort Detrick, Maryland, for his generous gifts of botulinum toxin used in many of the experiments quoted here.

VIII. REFERENCES

Ambache, N. (1949), *J. Physiol.*, **108**:127.
Ambache, N. (1951), *J. Physiol.*, **113**:1.
Ambache, N. and A. W. Lessin (1955), *J. Physiol.*, **127**:449.
Andersson-Cedergren, E. (1959), *J. Ultrast. Res. Suppl.*, **1**:5.
Bishop, G. H. and J. J. Bronfenbrenner (1936), *Amer. J. Physiol.*, **117**:393.
Brooks, V. B. (1956), *J. Physiol.*, **134**:264.

Bueker, E. D. (1943), *J. Exp. Zool.*, **93**:99.

Buller, A. J., J. C. Eccles, and R. M. Eccles (1960), *J. Physiol.*, **150**:417.

Burgen, A. S. V., F. Dickens, and L. J. Zatman (1949), *J. Physiol. (London)*, **109**:10.

Burn, H. and M. J. Rand (1965), *Ann. Rev. Pharmac.*, **5**:163.

Cardella, M. A. (1964), Botulinum toxoids, *in* "Botulism, Proceedings of a Symposium," U.S. Public Health Service, Cincinnati.

Carpenter, F. G. (1967), *J. Physiol.*, **188**:1.

Dawson, D. and F. C. A. Romanul (1964), *Arch. Neurol.*, **13**:263.

Del Castillo, J. and B. Katz (1954), *J. Physiol. (London)*, **124**:560.

Del Castillo, J. and B. Katz (1955), *J. Physiol.*, **128**:396.

Denny-Brown, D. (1929), *Proc. Roy. Soc. B*, **104**:371.

Denny-Brown, D. and C. Bolnner (1944), *Arch. Neurol. Psychiat.*, **51**:1.

de Robertis, E. and H. S. Bennett (1954), *Fed. Proc.*, **13**:35.

Dickson, E. C. and R. Shevky (1923), *J. Exp. Med.*, **37**:711.

Drachman, D. B. (1964), *Science*, **145**:719.

Drachman, D. B. (1967), *Arch. Neurol.*, **17**:206.

Drachman, D. B. (1968), The role of acetylcholine as a trophic neuromuscular transmitter, *in* "Ciba Foundation Symposium on Growth of the Nervous System" (G. E. W. Wolstenholme and M. O'Connor, eds.), J. & A. Churchill Ltd., London, p. 251.

Drachman, D. B. and A. J. Coulombre (1962a), *Science*, **138**:144.

Drachman, D. B. and A. J. Coulombre (1962b), *Lancet*, II:523.

Drachman, D. B. and J. Houk (1969), *Amer. J. Physiol.*, **216**:1453.

Drachman, D. B. and P. D. F. Murray (1969), *J. Embryol. Exp. Morphol.*, **22** No. 3:349.

Drachman, D. B. and F. C. A. Romanul, *Arch. Neurol.*, in press.

Drachman, D. B. and L. Sokiloff (1966), *Developmental Biol.*, **14**:401.

Duchen, L. W. and S. J. Strich (1968), *Quart. J. Physiol.*, **53**:84.

Eccles, J. C. (1964), "The Physiology of Synapses," Springer-Verlag, Berlin.

Eccles, J. C., R. M. Eccles, and W. Kozak (1962), *J. Physiol.*, **163**:324.

Edds, M. V. (1953), *Rev. Biol.*, **28**:260.

Elmqvist, D. and D. S. Feldman (1965), *J. Physiol.*, **181**:487.

Emmelin, N. (1961), *J. Physiol.*, **156**:121.

Fatt, P. and B. Katz (1950), *Nature (London)*, **166**:597.

Fatt, P. and B. Katz (1952), *J. Physiol. (London)*, **117**:109.

Fell, H. and R. B. Canti (1934), *Proc. Royal Soc. Bull.*, **116**:316.

Fex, S., B. Sonesson, S. Thesleff, and J. Zelena (1966), *J. Physiol.*, **184**:872.

Gage, P. W. and D. M. J. Quastel (1966), *J. Physiol.*, **185**:95.

Guth, L. (1968), *Ann. Rev. Physiol.*, **48**:645.

Guth, L. (1969a), *Neurosci. Res. Prog. Bull.*, **7**:1.

Guth, L. (1969b), *Exp. Neurol.*, **24**:508.

Guth, L., R. W. Albers, and W. C. Brown (1964), *Exp. Neurol.*, **10**:236.

Gutmann, E. and R. Zak (1961), *Physiol. Bohemoslov.* **10**:493.

Hamburger, V. and M. Waugh (1940), *Physiol. Zoo.*, **13**:367.

Hebb, C. (1963), Formation, storage and liberation of acetylcholine, *in* "Handbuch der Experimentellen Pharmakologie" (G.B.Koelle, ed.), Chap. 3, Springer-Verlag, Berlin.

Hilton, S. M. and G. P. Lewis (1955), *J. Physiol.*, **128**:235.

Hogan, E. L., D. M. Dawson, and F. C. A. Romanul (1965), *Arch. Neurol.*, **13**:274.

Hubbard, J. I. and S. Kwanbunbumpen (1968), *J. Physiol.*, **194**:407.

Hubbard, J. I., S. F. Jones, and E. M. Landau (1968), *J. Physiol.*, **194**:355.

Jirmanova, I., M. Sobotkova, S. Thesleff, and J. Zelena (1964), *Physiol. Bohemoslov.*, **13**:467.

Josefsson, J. O. and S. Thesleff (1961), *Acta Physiol. Scand.*, **51**:163.

Katz, B. (1966), "Nerve, Muscle and Synapse," McGraw-Hill, New York.

Katz, B. and R. Miledi (1965), *Proc. Royal Soc.*, **161**:496.

Koelle, G. B. (1963), Cytologic distribution and physiologic functions of cholinesterases, *in* "Handbuch der Experimentellen Pharmakologie," Chap.6, Springer-Verlag, Berlin.

Kupfer, C. (1958), *Proc. Soc. Exp. Biol. Med.*, **99**:474.
Lewis, D. M. (1962), *J. Physiol.*, **161**:24P.
Marchbanks, R. M. (1968), *Biochem. J.*, **110**:533.
Michaelson, I. A. (1967), *Ann. N.Y. Acad. Sci.*, **144**:387.
Murray, P. D. F. (1926), *Proc. Linnaean Soc.*, **51**:187.
Nastuk, W. (1966), *Ann. N.Y. Acad. Sci.*, **135**:110.
Rand, M. J. and B. C. Whalter (1965), *Nature*, **206**:588.
Romanes, G. J. (1946), *J. Anat.*, **80**:117.
Romanul, F. C. A. (1964), *Arch. Neurol.*, **11**:355.
Romanul, F. C. A. and E. L. Hogan (1964), *Arch. Neurol.*, **13**:263.
Romanul, F. C. A. and J. P. Van Der Meulen (1966), *Nature*, **212**(5068):1369.
Rose, S. and P. H. Glow (1967), *Exp. Neurol.*, **18**:267.
Salmons, S. and G. Vrbova (1969), *J. Physiol.*, **201**:535.
Simpson, L. L. (1968), *J. Neurochem.*, **15**:359.
Simpson, L. L. and H. Morimoto (1969), *J. Bact.*, **97**:571.
Solandt, D. Y., R. C. Parridge, and J. Hunter (1943), *J. Neurophysiol.*, **6**:17.
Sonesson, B. and A. Thesleff (1968), *Life Sciences*, **7**:411.
Stevenson, J. W. and G. T. Girvin (1953), *Atti VI Congr. Int. Microbiol.*, **4**:133.
Stewart, D. M. and A. W. Martin (1966), *Exp. Neurol.*, **16**:299.
Stromblad, B. C. R. (1960), *Experientia*, **26**:458.
Takeuchi, A. and N. Takeuchi (1960), *J. Physiol. (London)*, **144**:52.
Thesleff, S. (1960), *J. Physiol. (London)*, **151**:598.
Tower, S. (1931a), *Bull. Johns Hopkins Hosp.*, **48**:115.
Tower, S. (1931b), *Brain*, **54**:99.
Tower, S. (1935), *Amer. J. Anat.*, **56**:1.
Tower, S. (1937), *J. Comp. Neurol.*, **17**:241.
Vincenzi, F. F. (1967), *Nature*, **213**:394.
Watson, W. E. (1969), *J. Physiol.*, **202**:611.
Westwood, D. A. and B. C. Whaler (1968), *Brit. J. Pharmac. Chemother.*, **33**:21.
Whittaker, V. P. (1965), The application of subcellular fractionation techniques to the study of brain function, Chap. 2, *in* "Progress in Biophysics and Molecular Biology," vol. 15, Pergamon Press, New York.
Whittaker, V. P. (1968), *Neurosciences Research Program Bulletin*, MIT, **6**:27.
Zacks, S. I., M. V. Rhoades, and M. E. Sheff (1968), *Exp. and Mol. Pathol.*, **9**:77.
Zacks, S. I., J. F. Metzger, C. W. Smith, and J. M. Blumberg (1962), *J. Neuropath. Exp. Neurol.*, **21**:610.

IX. APPENDIX

Laboratory Handling of Botulinum Toxin

1. All individuals working with botulinum toxin should be immunized with polyvalent toxoid (available from National Communicable Disease Center, Atlanta, Georgia 30333).
2. Eating, drinking, and smoking are not permitted in the laboratory.
3. Mouth pipetting is not permitted. A suitable mechanical device is used instead.
4. When using botulinum toxin, laboratory shoes and a surgical gown (fastened in back) are worn. A scrub suit and disposable rubber gloves are worn when concentrated toxin is used. Gowns are autoclaved after use.

5. Careful hand washing with a detergent and water is carried out after using botulinum toxin (surgical scrub technique).

6. Glassware may be decontaminated by autoclaving, or immersion in 10% formalin for 10 min. Immersion in NaOH or sodium hypochlorite has also been recommended.

7. Biological specimens treated with botulinum toxin are fixed in formalin to inactivate the toxin. They may be disposed of by incineration.

8. Antitoxin should be available in the laboratory, in case of accidental contact by nonimmunized individuals. (Lederle Laboratories, Pearl River, New York, 10965 supplies types A and B; Connaught Medical Research Laboratories, Willowdale, Ontario, Canada, types A, B, and E.)

9. Avoid using chipped or sharp glassware, so as to prevent accidental cuts.

It should be emphasized that immunization of all laboratory workers is the keystone of protection. These precautions are derived from a questionnaire sent by the author to other workers in the field, and have been practiced consistently in his laboratory.

Index